Data Analytics in Healthcare Research
Tools and Strategies

Volume Editors

David T. Marc, MBS, CHDA
Ryan H. Sandefer, MA, CPHIT

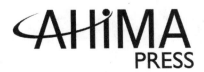

ISBN: 978-1-58426-443-9
AHIMA Product No.: AB107114

AHIMA Staff:
Caitlin Wilson, Assistant Editor
Jason O. Malley, Vice President, Business and Innovation
Ashley R. Latta, Production Development Editor
Pamela Woolf, Director of Publications

For more information, including updates, about AHIMA Press publications, visit
http://www.ahima.org/publications/updates.aspx

American Health Information Management Association
233 North Michigan Avenue, 21st Floor
Chicago, Illinois 60601-5809
ahima.org

Brief Table of Contents

PART II

Online Resources

CSV Excel Worksheets

Data Dictionary

Entity-relationship Diagram

Frequently Asked Questions

SQL Queries

R Scripts

Detailed Table of Contents

_____

Online Resources

CSV Excel Worksheets

Data Dictionary

Entity-relationship Diagram

Frequently Asked Questions

SQL Queries

R Scripts

About the Editors and Authors

Volume Editors

David Marc, MBS, CHDA is an assistant professor and the graduate program director for health informatics at the College of St. Scholastica in Duluth, MN. Mr. Marc is an accomplished speaker and researcher with a breadth of experience around health data analytics. Previously, Mr. Marc was employed at a biotech company where he developed predictive data models for the diagnosis of neurological and immunological diseases. Mr. Marc has a master's degree in biological sciences from the University of Minnesota.

Ryan Sandefer, MA, CPHIT is an assistant professor and chair of the health informatics and information management department at the College of St. Scholastica in Duluth, MN. Mr. Sandefer is on the Editorial Advisory Board and Review Panel for Perspectives in Health Information Management. He is an elected Board member and the Chair of the American Health Information Management Association (AHIMA) Council for Excellence in Education, is the past-Chair of the CEE's Research and Periodicals Workgroup, and currently sits on the AHIMA Foundation's Graduate Resource Alliance. Mr. Sandefer earned his master's degree in political science at the University of Wyoming.

Chapter Authors

Danika E. Brinda, PhD, RHIA, CHPS is an assistant professor and HIT consultant in the HIIM department at the College of St. Scholastica. She has served as adjunct faculty with Rasmussen College, was regional manager for HIM at Allina Hospitals and Clinics, and was manager of revenue cycle improvement at Allina Hospitals and Clinics. She earned her master's degree in HIM at the College of St. Scholastica and her PhD in information technology at Capella University.

Dilhari R. DeAlmeida, PhD, RHIA, is an assistant professor in the department of health information management at the University of Pittsburgh. She received her bachelor of science degree in cell and molecular biology from University of Toronto, Canada. Prior to joining the HIM department, she has over 12 years of experience working in government, academic, and the private sector in the field of molecular biology. She received her master of science (HIS/RHIA option) and doctorate degrees from the University of Pittsburgh. Her dissertation research involved evaluating the ICD-10-CM coding system for documentation specificity and reimbursement, and she is an AHIMA-approved ICD-10-CM/PCS trainer. In addition to teaching both the undergraduate and graduate HIM courses, her current research focuses on research use case development and data analytics in healthcare, including building clinical alerts for early detection of acute kidney injury within an electronic health record system.

Susan H. Fenton, PhD, RHIA, FAHIMA is the associate dean of academic affairs at the University of Texas Health Science Center at Houston (UTHealth) School of Biomedical Informatics. Dr. Fenton teaches health informatics standards and health informatics safety and security, among other topics. She has served as principal investigator (PI) for various grants, including a recently concluded $5.4 million university-based training grant from the Office of the National Coordinator and a $900,000, two-year health IT workforce research and training grant from the Texas Governor's Office. Dr. Fenton has conducted several ICD-10-CM/PCS-related studies including an examination of the adequacy of clinical documentation, the impact upon coder productivity, and the calculation of comparability ratios for quality measure reporting. She is currently co-PI of a pilot study examining the use of industrial engineering techniques in addressing the causes of catheter-associated urinary tract infections. The textbook, *Introduction to Healthcare Informatics*, which Dr. Fenton coauthored with Sue Biedermann, was published by AHIMA Press in July of 2013. Previously, she served as Director of Research at AHIMA and was Director of Health Information Management for the Veterans Health Administration Headquarters. Among other honors, Dr. Fenton has received the 2012 AHIMA Triumph Award for Research. She holds a PhD in Health Services Research from the Texas A&M School of Rural Public Health, an MBA from the University of Houston, and a BS in Health Information Management from UTMB, Galveston.

Linda Kloss, MA, RHIA, FAHIMA is founder and president of Kloss Strategic Advisors, Ltd., providing thought leadership and advisory services to health information business leaders, provider organizations, and healthcare associations on health information asset management, health data analysis, governance, and change leadership. In 2011, Ms. Kloss was appointed to a four-year term on the National Committee on Vital and Health Statistics (NCVHS) and co-chairs its Privacy, Confidentiality, and Security Subcommittee. NCVHS advises the Secretary of Health and Human Services on national health information policy. Previously, Ms. Kloss served as CEO of AHIMA from 1995 to 2010, leading a period of unprecedented growth and expanded influence for this well respected professional association of over 64,000 health information management professionals worldwide. In 2007, *Modern Healthcare* named her as one of the top 25 women in healthcare and to the list of the top 100 people in healthcare from 2002 to 2007. She earned a masters degree in organization development with a concentration on nonprofit change leadership from DePaul University and a baccalaureate degree in health information management from the College of St. Scholastica.

Sally K. Koski, PhD, RN is an associate professor in the graduate nursing program at the College of St. Scholastica. She teaches courses related to research, systems leadership, and informatics. Her research interests include rural health, online learning, and consumer engagement in healthcare. Dr. Koski has numerous presentations and publications focusing on rural health, e-health, and transdisciplinary academic-community/industry partnerships in healthcare. Dr. Koski currently serves as a subject matter expert on the Minnesota e-Health Roadmap project, a grant reviewer for several state grant programs, and a manuscript reviewer for three nursing journals.

Pam Oachs, MA, RHIA, is an assistant professor in the College of St. Scholastica's healthcare informatics and information management department. She teaches courses related to health information technology, system development and implementation, workflow redesign, healthcare management, and applied research. She has most recently participated in a collaborative student/faculty grant promoting the use of a personal health record in vulnerable populations. She has more than 15 years of healthcare experience. Her career has included a variety of positions, both managerial and professional, in the areas of utilization management, quality improvement, medical staff credentialing, Joint Commission coordination, information technology, project management, and patient access. She has authored several articles and chapters including the prior three editions of this textbook. She has been involved in system implementations, both small and large, in a variety of healthcare settings. She has served on the Board of Directors of the Minnesota Health Information Management Association and the Northeastern Minnesota Health Information Management Association.

Shauna Overgaard, MHI, is an adjunct professor in the College of St. Scholastica's healthcare informatics and information management department, where she teaches a course in healthcare data analytics. She is a PhD student of biomedical health informatics and biostatistics at the University of Minnesota and an adjunct professor at the College of St. Scholastica. Her clinical research has largely focused on the analysis of MRI, DTI, and fMRI neuroimaging data as well as proteomic and genomic phenotypic data for psychiatric and neurological disorders. Shauna spent several years working in a clinical research setting, designing, implementing, and supervising research studies; building database systems for automated clinical data entry and extraction; and analyzing and interpreting clinical outcomes data. While working on her master's degree, she was awarded a UPHI fellowship and specialized in healthcare information exchange. She is an IPHIE Fellow, a Merrill H. Knotts Fellow, and is AMIA student working group co-member-at-large (doctoral/PhD). Shauna is currently working at the Mayo Clinic in Rochester MN, completing her dissertation pertaining to the development of bioinformatic tools in neuroimaging and genomic modeling for the early identification and diagnosis of Alzheimer's disease.

Brooke N. Palkie, EdD, RHIA is an associate professor in the College of St. Scholastica's health informatics and information management department. She teaches courses related to clinical quality; compliance; and clinical classifications, vocabularies, terminologies and data standards. She has recently led a collaborative and interdisciplinary grant assisting an independent behavioral health organization transition to DSM-5 and ICD-10 for documentation, billing, and reporting purposes. With 14 years of healthcare experience—including management and professional positions in health information management, quality, corporate compliance, and consulting—she is a frequent presenter at both state and national meetings and conferences, and has authored several articles, white papers, and textbook chapters. She has also served in several capacities at the state and regional levels of the Minnesota Health Information Management Association.

David S. Pieczkiewicz, PhD, is the director of graduate studies and clinical assistant professor at the University of Minnesota's Institute for Health Informatics. He received a BA with honors in anthropology from Case Western Reserve University, an MA in biological anthropology from the University of Kansas, and a PhD in Health Informatics from the University of Minnesota. After receiving his doctorate in 2007, he served as a National Library of Medicine-funded postdoctoral fellow at the Marshfield Clinic Research Foundation in Wisconsin, until rejoining the University of Minnesota in 2010 as a faculty member. David is an active instructor in the informatics program, teaching courses in basic informatics, databases, computer programming, analytics, and data visualization. In 2015, he was the recipient of the Outstanding Advising and Mentoring Award from the university's graduate and professional student assembly. His academic and research interests include data and information visualization, data science, human-computer interaction and usability, and epidemiology.

Patricia Senk, PhD, RN is an assistant professor in the department of graduate nursing at the College of St. Scholastica. She teaches courses related to health information technology, quality improvement, program evaluation, outcomes research, epidemiology, and biostatistics. She is also the program director for the nursing informatics certificate program. She has worked in healthcare for over 30 years in direct patient care, quality improvement, and nursing research, which has focused on healthcare informatics and the representation of nursing knowledge in an electronic medical record.

Piper Svensson-Ranallo, PhD is the founder of Six Aims for Behavioral Health, a nonprofit organization whose mission is to accelerate development of the evidence base for mental health. The organization focuses on the effective use of information technologies and the use of best informatics practices to achieve this goal. Dr. Ranallo completed her undergraduate training at UCLA where she studied psychology and neuroscience. She completed her doctoral training at the University of Minnesota, researching gaps in the health information infrastructure relative to mental health; her dissertation research focused on gaps in standards and information models for representing mental health assessment data. She has published papers related to the use of health information technology in behavioral health and is currently developing information models to support the collection of high-quality data in this domain. Dr. Ranallo is committed to demarginalizing mental health in the field of informatics and to improving the quality of life for those suffering with mental health conditions.

Amy L. Watters, EdD, RHIA, FAHIMA is an assistant professor and director of the HIM graduate program at the College of St. Scholastica. She has more than 15 years of HIM experience in a variety of positions, including release of information, HIM and admitting management in acute care settings, product management at a software and consulting firm, and HIPAA security experience at a multispecialty physician group. She has participated in AHIMA work groups and is a member of the Foundation Scholarship Committee. She has served on the board of the Minnesota Health Information Management Association, as president of the Northeastern Minnesota Health Information Management Association, and currently serves on the board of the MN chapter of HIMSS. In 2011, she was awarded fellowship in AHIMA in recognition of her contributions to the field of HIM.

Valerie J. M. Watzlaf, PhD, RHIA, FAHIMA is an associate professor in the HIM department in the School of Health and Rehabilitation Sciences (SHRS) at the University of Pittsburgh. She also holds an appointment in the Graduate School of Public Health. In these capacities, Dr. Watzlaf teaches and performs research in health information management, epidemiology, quality improvement, statistics, and long-term care. She has worked and consulted for several healthcare organizations in health information management, long-term care, and epidemiology. Dr. Watzlaf has served on numerous AHIMA Task Forces, Committees, and Councils; was the chairperson of AHIMA's Coding, Policy, and Strategy Committee; and most recently served as a board member on AHIMA's Foundation of Research and Education (FORE). She is also on the Editorial Advisory Board for the Journal of AHIMA and for Perspectives in HIM, a national peer-reviewed online journal within AHIMA. She received the AHIMA Research Award in October 2001 and became a Fellow of AHIMA in April 2003. Dr. Watzlaf received her bachelor of science degree in health records administration, master of public health, and doctorate degree in epidemiology from the University of Pittsburgh.

Preface

Data Analytics—The New Healthcare Frontier

The ability to collect, manage, analyze, and report data is becoming increasingly important for all professionals, and this is particularly important in healthcare where massive amounts of data are being collected regarding patient demographics, diagnoses, procedures, preferences, and so on. Healthcare is facing major issues related to rising costs and decreasing quality. As the healthcare industry continues to transition from cost-based reimbursement to value-based payments, organizations will increasingly look to their data as an asset. The culture of quality and accountability will require stakeholders to leverage their data to better predict clinical outcomes, track patient populations more effectively, coordinate care more seamlessly, adopt clinical best practices more widely, and generally improve the patient experience of care. It truly is a new frontier of healthcare, and data and analytics are front and center.

The purpose of this textbook is to introduce healthcare data analytics through a hands-on approach with working with data across the analytics continuum. This book gives readers a unique opportunity to extract data from a very large SQL database, clean the data using Microsoft Excel, and import the data into the RStudio data analytics software for statistical analysis and data visualization. Each chapter is related to a specific research question (from nursing home quality to hospital readmissions). The data needed to answer each research question are included in the MySQL database accompanying this textbook. Readers have the opportunity to replicate each study—from data extraction to statistical analysis to interpretation of findings.

Part I of the book introduces readers to background concepts related to data analytics. Chapter 1 provides an overview of open source software and open source data, and an introduction to data analytics techniques and statistical procedures. It also describes the steps required to download and use the software and data related to this textbook. Chapter 2 provides readers with an introduction to the basics of data and information governance and the criticality of data analytics for governance programs. Chapter 3 describes the importance of privacy and security protocols when conducting data analytics for research in healthcare. Chapter 4 includes a discussion of database concepts and principles, and provides an in-depth discussion of how to use the database accompanying this textbook effectively. Similarly, chapter 5 provides an in-depth introduction to the RStudio Statistical Software, the software used for all analyses conducted in this textbook.

The Part II of the book (chapters 6 through 16) provides step-by-step cases of research studies using open source data and open source software. Each chapter provides background for why the research is needed, formally states the research question and statistical hypotheses, describes the steps required to extract the data from the MySQL database and import the data into the RStudio analytics application, and explains how to interpret the findings and present the results. These chapters allow readers to engage with data analytics using a hands-on, research-driven approach. Throughout the book, readers will be exposed to both simple and complex database programming syntax. Readers will also be exposed to basic descriptive statistics, inferential statistics such as two-way ANOVAs, regression models, data mining techniques, and advanced data visualizations techniques.

It is our fundamental belief that learning is improved through experience. This text is intended to help bridge data analytics theory and practice by integrating the data, the software, and steps into one research study.

Ryan Sandefer and David Marc

Acknowledgments

We would like to acknowledge the time and effort that so many individuals have put into this book, including the authors and their families for the support. Our families for their understanding for the nights spent burning the midnight oil. And our peers for the critical reviews and feedback on manuscript drafts. Finally, we want to thank all of the educators for pushing data analytics competencies into curriculum.

AHIMA Press would like to thank Murad Moqbel, PhD, MBA for his technical review and feedback on this text.

Downloadable Resources

To utilize this textbook, you will need to download MySQL Workbench, R, and RStudio. In this section you will find download instructions for Windows as well as Mac OS X. After you have downloaded the following software, follow the instructions to connect to the database for both Windows and Mac OS X.

Setting Up MySQL Workbench on Windows

Step 1

To download the most recent version of MySQL Workbench, visit http://dev.mysql.com/downloads/ and click **DOWNLOAD**, which is listed under MySQL Workbench (see figure 0.1).

Figure 0.1.   Downloading MySQL for Windows: Step 1

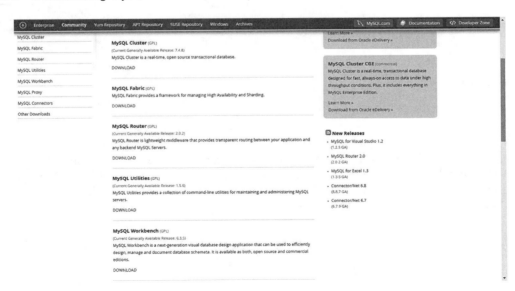

Step 2

Next, download the MySQL Installer for your Windows operating system (do not select the ZIP Archive). Under Other Downloads, choose one of the following:

- If your Windows operating system is 32-bit, download the **Windows (x86, 32-bit), MSI Installer**.
- If your Windows operating system is 64-bit, download the **Windows (x86, 64-bit), MSI Installer** (see figure 0.2).

If you are unsure what bit version your operating system is and you are using Windows 7 or above, go to the following webpage: https://support.microsoft.com/en-us/kb/827218. The bit version of your Window's operating system will be listed under Automatic Version Detection Results.

Figure 0.2.   Downloading MySQL for Windows: Step 2

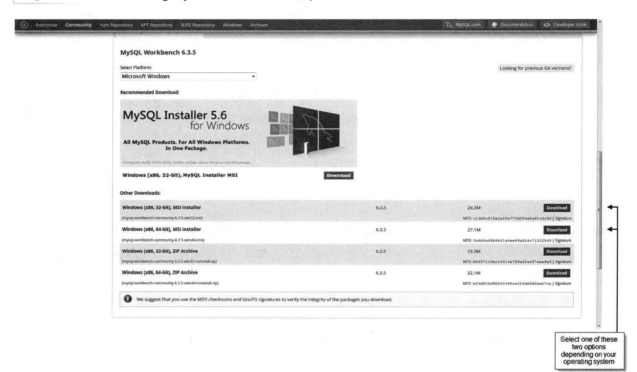

Callouts added to screen shot by AHIMA.

Step 3

It is not necessary to login or sign up for an Oracle Web account. Simply bypass this step by clicking **No thanks, just start my download** (see figure 0.3). The software will begin to download to the folder that you have defaulted for downloads, such as the Downloads folder or Desktop. If the file does not automatically appear, you may need to navigate to the downloaded file to execute. Click Run when prompted.

Figure 0.3.   Downloading MySQL for Windows: Step 3

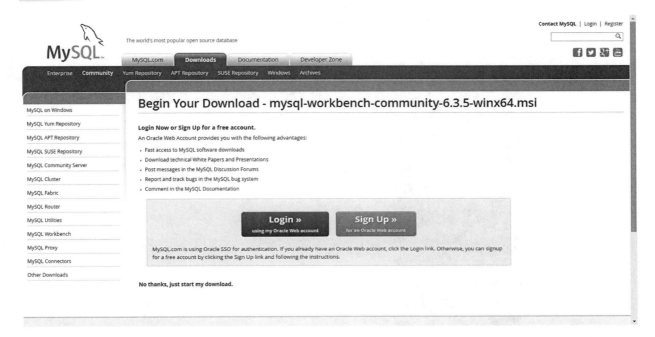

Prerequisite Software

MySQL Workbench requires some prerequisite software to run on Microsoft Windows operating systems. You may see a dialog box instructing you to download these prerequisite software packages. Click OK (see figure 0.4). If your machine includes the prerequisite software, you will not see this message. If you do receive this message, you can find links to download the prerequisite software listed under MySQL Workbench Prerequisites: from this link: http://dev.mysql.com/downloads/workbench/.

Figure 0.4.   Downloading MySQL for Windows: prerequisite software

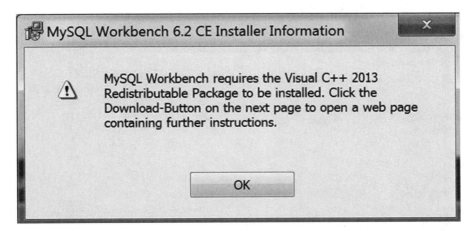

Another dialog box may appear that explains that the installation ended prematurely. Click Download Prerequisites to continue with the setup. You will be directed to a page that will ask you to download the prerequisites. Follow each link and follow the associated instructions. Once you have downloaded the required libraries, navigate back to the download webpage shown in figure 0.2 and restart your download by clicking the appropriate MSI installer.

Step 4

When the setup wizard appears. Click Next (see figure 0.5).

Figure 0.5.   Downloading MySQL for Windows: Step 4

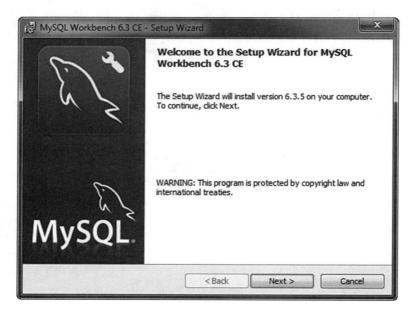

Step 5

The default destination folder can remain the same. Click Next (see figure 0.6).

Figure 0.6.   Downloading MySQL for Windows: Step 5

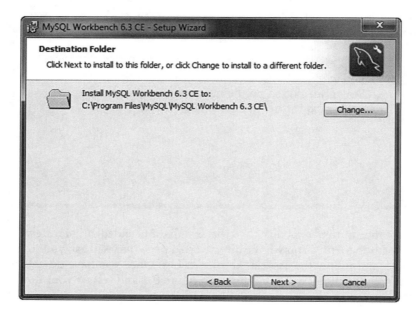

Step 6

The next window of the dialog box will ask you to choose a setup type. Make sure the Complete option is selected (default), and then click Next (see figure 0.7).

Figure 0.7.   Downloading MySQL for Windows: Step 6

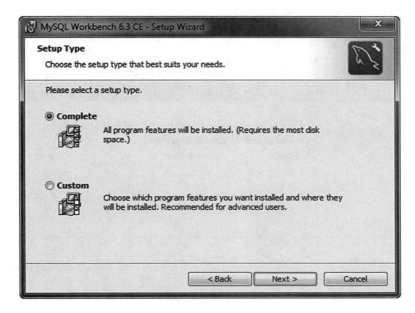

Step 7

The final dialog box will ask you if you want to review or change any installation settings. Click Install (see figure 0.8).

Figure 0.8.   Downloading MySQL for Windows: Step 7

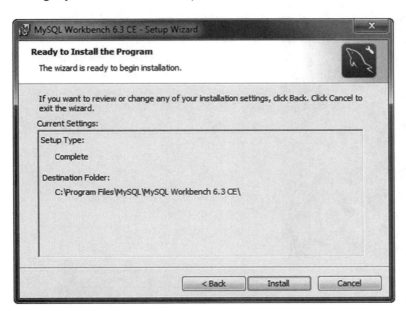

Step 8

Windows may open two dialog boxes asking if you want to allow the program to install software on the computer and to make changes to the computer. Click Yes on both dialog boxes (see figure 0.9), the software will download to your computer.

Figure 0.9.   Downloading MySQL for Windows: Step 8

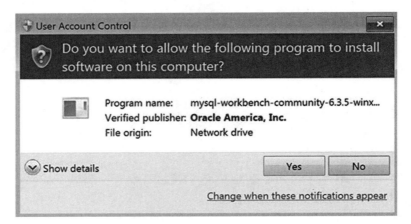

Once the wizard has completed, select Finish to complete download of MySQL Workbench (see figure 0.10).

Figure 0.10.   Downloading MySQL for Windows: Step 8

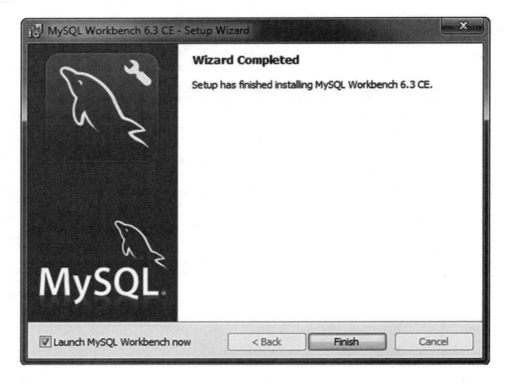

Setting Up R Studio on Windows

Step 1

RStudio requires the most up-to-date version of R. To download R, go to http://www.r-project.org and click **download R**, which is listed in the first paragraph of text (see figure 0.11).

Figure 0.11.   Downloading R for Windows: Step 1

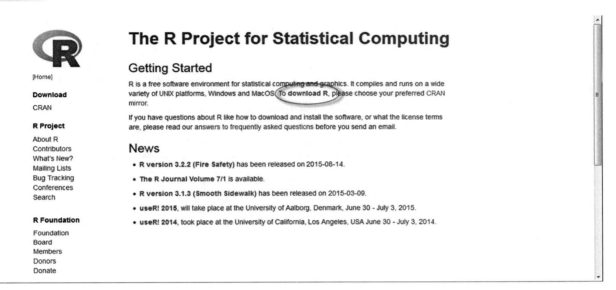

Source: Used with permission from R.

Step 2

On the CRAN Mirrors page, click the 0-Cloud option for downloading R (see figure 0.12). You may select either link under 0-Cloud.

Figure 0.12.   Downloading R for Windows: Step 2

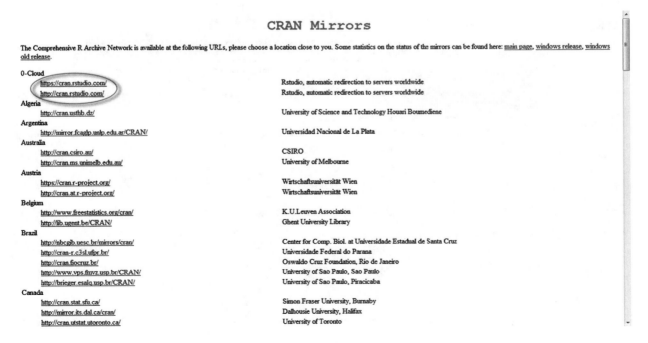

Source: Used with permission from R.

Step 3

On the download page, click Download R for Windows (see figure 0.13).

Figure 0.13.   Downloading R for Windows: Step 3

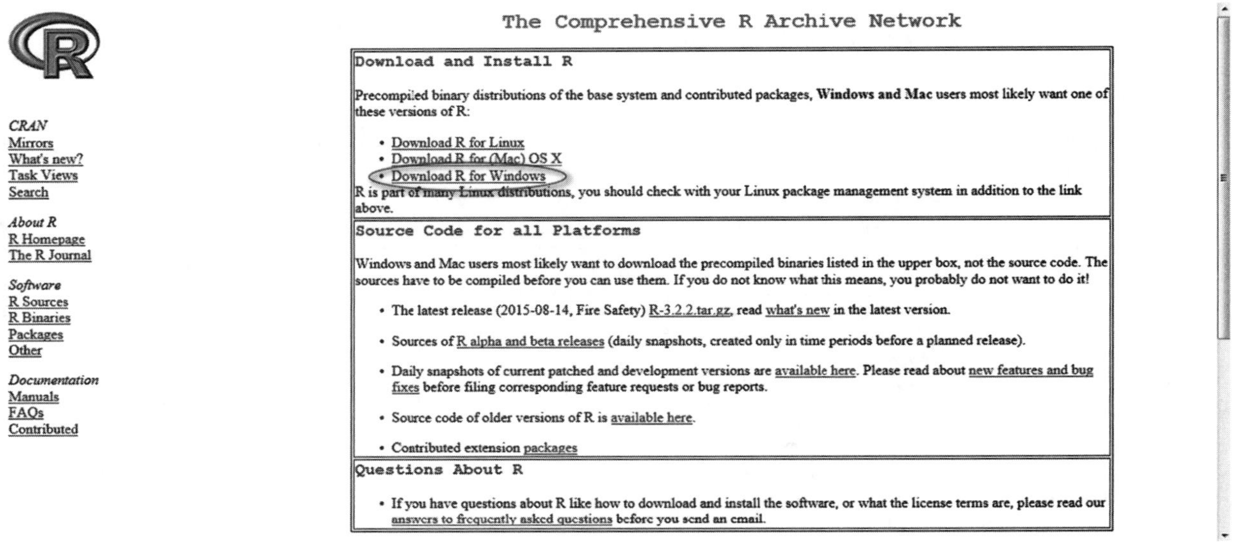

Source: Used with permission from R.

Step 4

On the R for Windows page, click **Install R for the first time** (see figure 0.14).

Figure 0.14.   Downloading R for Windows: Step 4

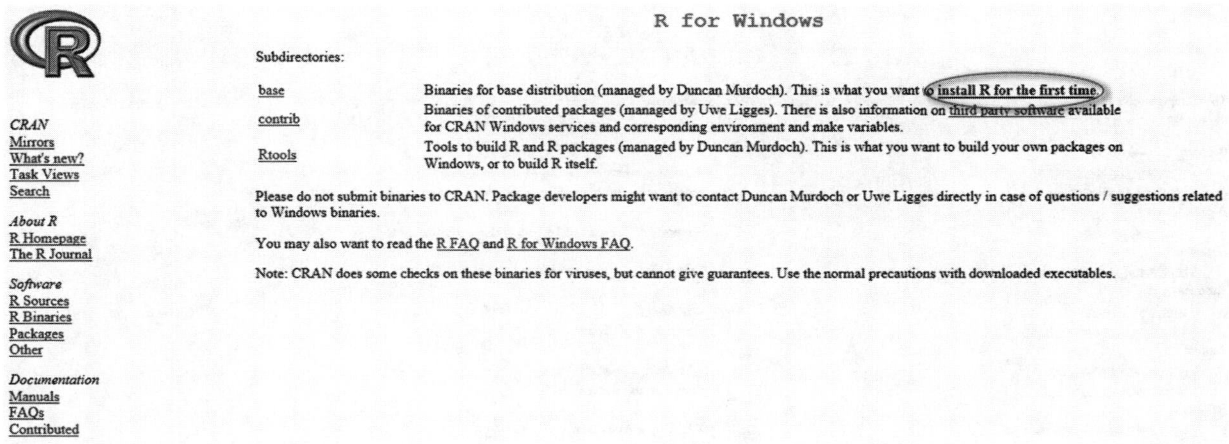

Source: Used with permission from R.

Step 5

The next step is to click **Download R 3.2.2 for Windows** (or the most current version), and then click Run when prompted (see figure 0.15).

Figure 0.15. Downloading R for Windows: Step 5

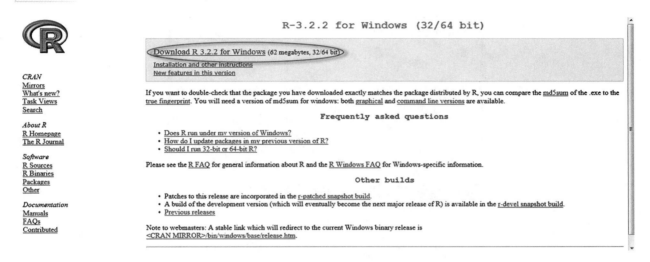

Source: Used with permission from R.

Step 6

A dialog box may appear asking if you want the program to make changes to your computer. You may receive a security warning; if so, click Yes or Run to run the program.

You will then go through a set-up process. Select all of the default settings. Follow the installation wizard instructions shown in the following series of figures (see figure 0.16).

Figure 0.16. Downloading R for Windows: Step 6

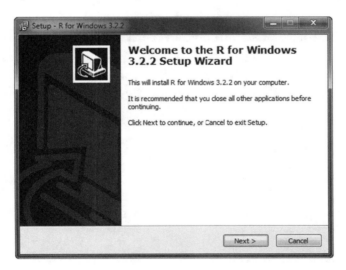

(Continued)

Figure 0.16. Downloading R for Windows: Step 6 *(Continued)*

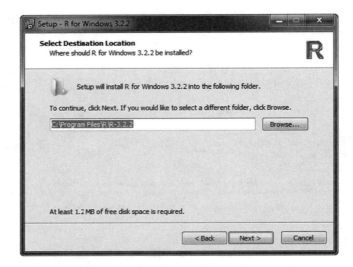

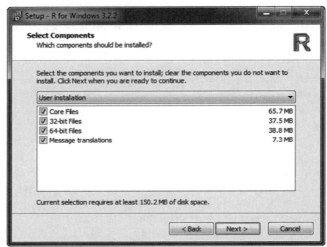

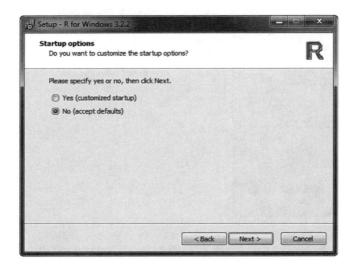

(Continued)

Figure 0.16.   Downloading R for Windows: Step 6 *(Continued)*

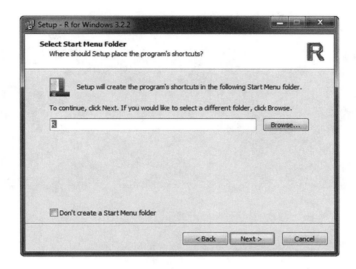

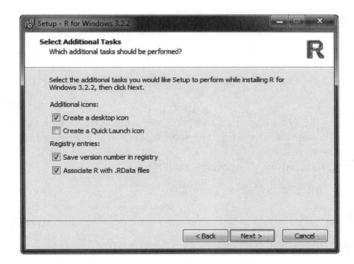

Source: Used with permission from R.

When your have completed your installation, click Finish. You will see two R icons on your desktop.

Step 7—Downloading R Studio

The next step in the process is to download R Studio—it is a separate application than the base R platform which you just downloaded. To download the most recent version of R Studio, go to http://www.rstudio.com and click the Download RStudio button on the homepage (see figure 0.17).

Figure 0.17.   Downloading RStudio for Windows: Step 7

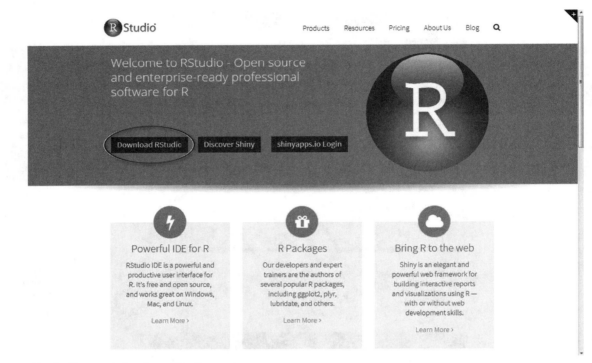

Source: Used with permission from RStudio.

Step 8

The page that opens will provide you choices for which version of RStudio to download. Scroll down and select the Desktop option. (You may select either the icon or Desktop.) (See figure 0.18.)

Figure 0.18.   Downloading RStudio for Windows: Step 8

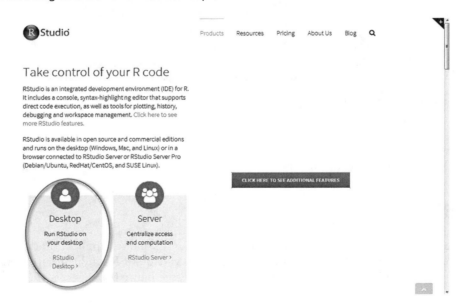

Source: Used with permission from RStudio.

Step 9

Click the DOWNLOAD RSTUDIO DESKTOP button (see figure 0.19).

Figure 0.19.   Downloading RStudio for Windows: Step 9

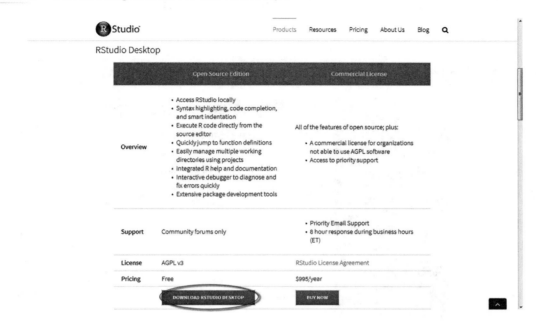

Source: Used with permission from RStudio.

Step 10

Now select the download for your operating system. Click **RStudio 0.99.489 Windows Vista/7/8/10 Installer** (see figure 0.20), and then click Run.

Figure 0.20.   Downloading RStudio for Windows: Step 10

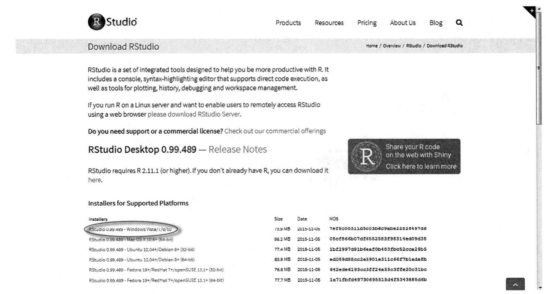

Source: Used with permission from RStudio.

Step 11

The RStudio wizard should appear. However, a dialog box may open and ask you if you want to allow the program to make changes to your computer. If it opens, click Yes or Run. After clicking Yes, a RStudio setup will open.

Follow the instructions from the wizard to install RStudio. Select all of the default settings by continuing to select Next or Install on each screen through the wizard (see figure 0.21).

Figure 0.21.   Downloading RStudio for Windows: Step 11

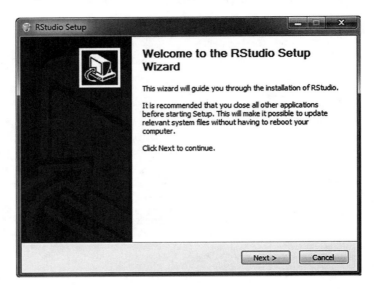

Source: Used with permission from RStudio.

Step 12

After you have successfully installed RStudio using the wizard, open the RStudio Application from the Start menu: Start | All Programs | RStudio | RStudio (see figure 0.22).

Figure 0.22.   Downloading RStudio for Windows: Step 12

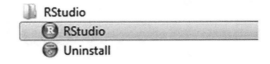

Step 13

Once you have opened RStudio, the software application should look similar to figure 0.23. Continue to page xliv for instructions to connect to the database. For detailed instructions and a summary of the components of the RStudio interface, see chapter 5.

Figure 0.23.   Downloading RStudio for Windows: Step 13

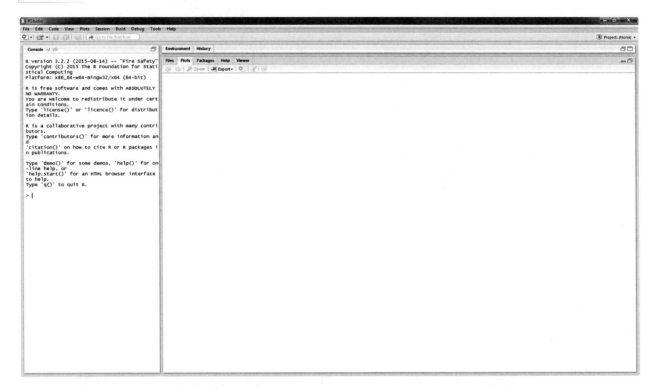

Source: Used with permission from RStudio.

Setting Up MySQL on Mac OS X

Step 1

To download the most recent version of MySQL Workbench on your Mac, visit http://dev.mysql.com/downloads/ and click **DOWNLOAD**, which is listed under MySQL Workbench (see figure 0.24).

Figure 0.24.   Downloading MySQL for Mac OS X: Step 1

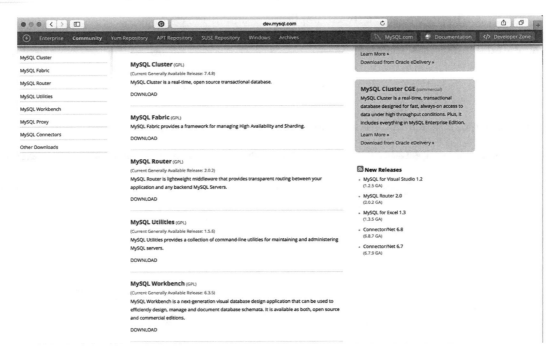

Step 2

Ensure that MySQL 6.3.5 (or most recent version) is listed under the Generally Available (GA) Releases tab and also ensure that Mac OS X is the selected platform in the drop-down window. Click the Download button (see figure 0.25).

Figure 0.25.   Downloading MySQL for Mac OS X: Step 2

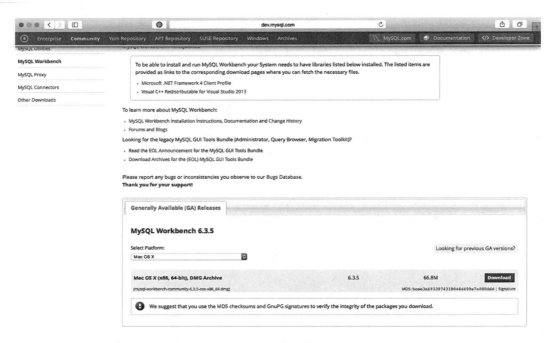

Step 3

It is not necessary to login or sign up for an Oracle Web account. Bypass this step by clicking **No thanks, just start my download**. (See figure 0.26.)

Figure 0.26.   Downloading MySQL for Mac OS X: Step 3

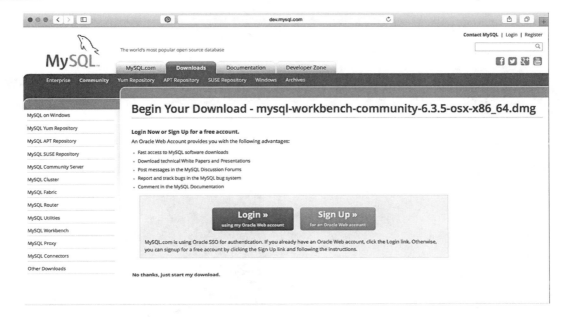

Step 4

The software will begin to download to the folder that you have defaulted for downloads, such as the Downloads folder or Desktop. Using the Finder, navigate to the downloaded file that will be titled **mysql-workbench-community-6.3.5-osx-x86_64.dmg**. Double-click the file begin the installation. A window will open that requires you to drag the MySQL Workbench icon into the Applications folder—complete that step to start the installation process (see figure 0.27).

Figure 0.27.   Downloading MySQL for Mac OS X: Step 4

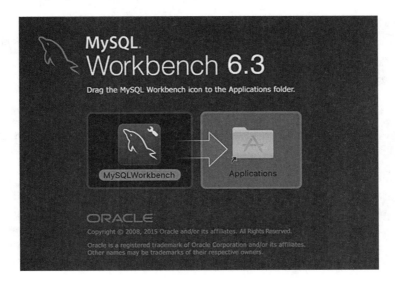

Step 5

After you have successfully dragged the MySQL Workbench icon into the Applications folder, the software will be installed and you can find the MySQL Workbench icon listed in your Applications folder and on your Dock (see figure 0.28). Double-click the MySQL Workbench icon to open the application. A dialog box will appear asking if you want to open the application. Click Open.

Figure 0.28.   Downloading MySQL for Mac OS X: Step 5

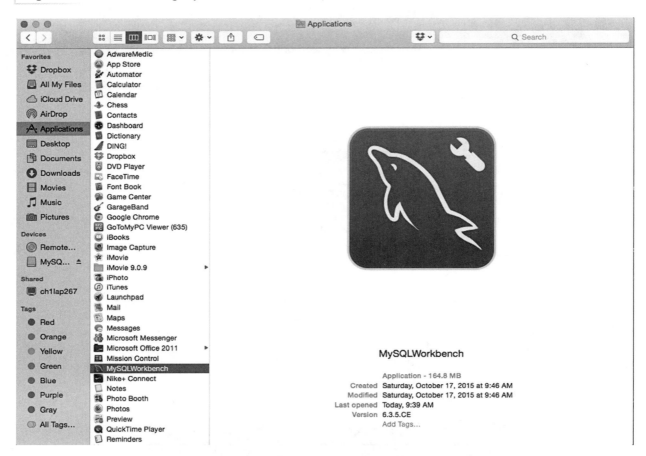

Step 6

You have successfully downloaded and installed MySQL Workbench on your computer. Once you have opened MySQL Workbench, you should see an application interface that looks similar to figure 0.29.

Figure 0.29.   Downloading MySQL for Mac OS X: Step 6

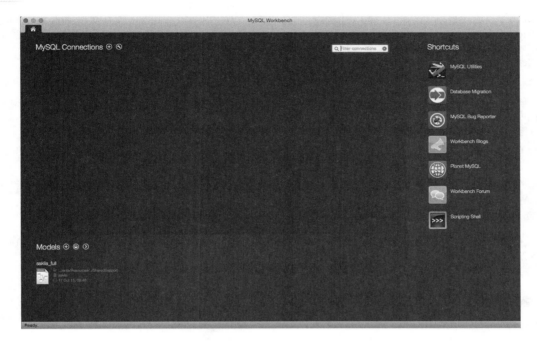

Setting Up R Studio on Mac OS X

Step 1

RStudio requires the most up-to-date version of R. To download R, go to http://www.r-project.org and click **download R** (see figure 0.30).

Figure 0.30.   Downloading R for Mac OS X: Step 1

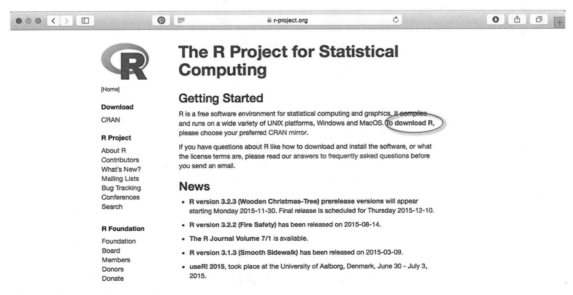

Source: Used with permission from R.

Step 2

On the CRAN Mirrors page, click the 0-Cloud option for downloading R (see figure 0.31). You may select either option.

Figure 0.31.   Downloading R for Mac OS X: Step 2

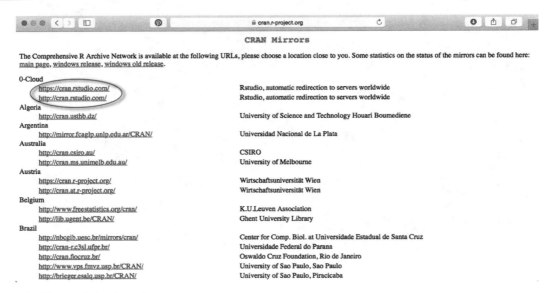

Source: Used with permission from R.

Step 3

On the download page, click **Download R for Max OS X** (see figure 0.32).

Figure 0.32.   Downloading R for Mac OS X: Step 3

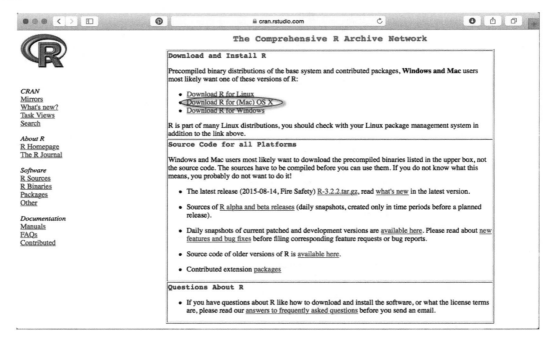

Source: Used with permission from R.

Step 4

You will be required to select the appropriate download file based upon your current operating system. Select either Snow Leopard, Mavericks, or the appropriate version for your current operating system. If you do not know your operating system, you can find it by going to the Apple icon in the upper left-hand corner and selecting About This Mac. If you are currently running Mavericks or above, please be sure to select the Mavericks option as it automatically installs required X Quartz software (see figure 0.33). If you are using an earlier version of Mac OS X, follow the instructions on the R website to download the appropriate software.

Figure 0.33.   Downloading R for Mac OS X: Step 4

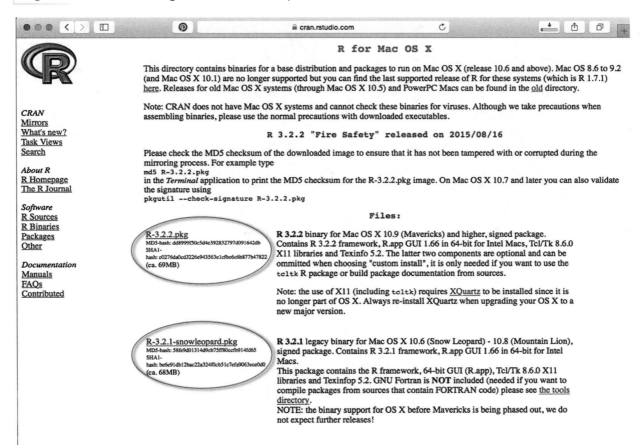

Source: Used with permission from R.

After clicking the appropriate download file, the file with automatically download to your default download folder and will be titled **R-3.2.2.pkg** or **R-3.2.1-snowleopard.pkg**. Open the file and follow the installation instructions, selecting the default options.

Step 5

The next step in the process is to download R Studio—it is a separate application than the base R platform which you just downloaded. To download the most recent version of R Studio, go to http://www.rstudio.com and click the Download RStudio button on the homepage (see figure 0.34).

Figure 0.34.   Downloading RStudio for Windows: Step 5

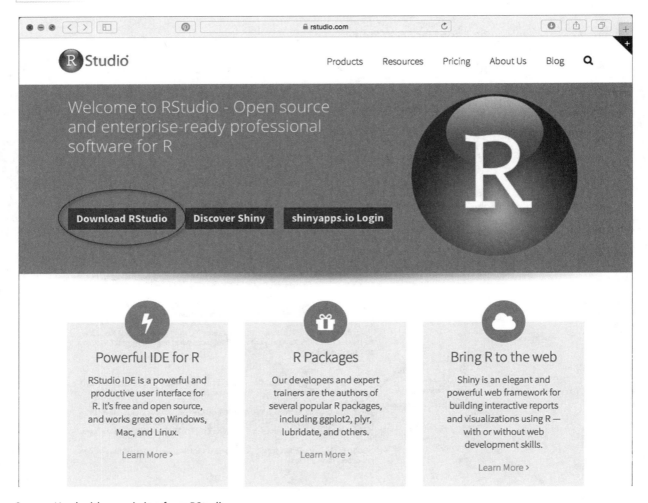

Source: Used with permission from RStudio.

Step 6

The page that opens will provide you choices for which version of RStudio to download. Scroll down and select the **Desktop** option. (You may select either the icon or Desktop.) (see figure 0.35).

Figure 0.35.   Downloading RStudio for Windows: Step 6

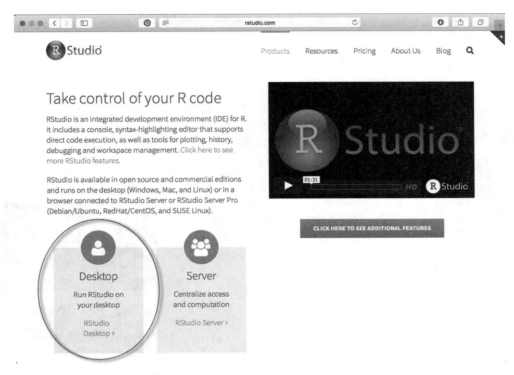

Source: Used with permission from RStudio.

Step 7

Click the **DOWNLOAD RSTUDIO DESKTOP** button (see figure 0.36).

Figure 0.36.   Downloading RStudio for Windows: Step 7

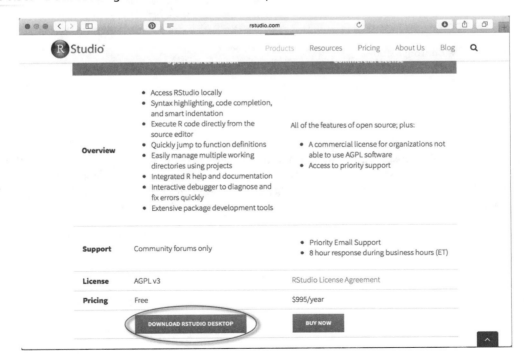

Source: Used with permission from RStudio.

Step 8

Select the download for your operating system. Select **Mac OS X 10.6+ (64-bit)** (see figure 0.37).

Figure 0.37.   Downloading RStudio for Mac OS X: Step 8

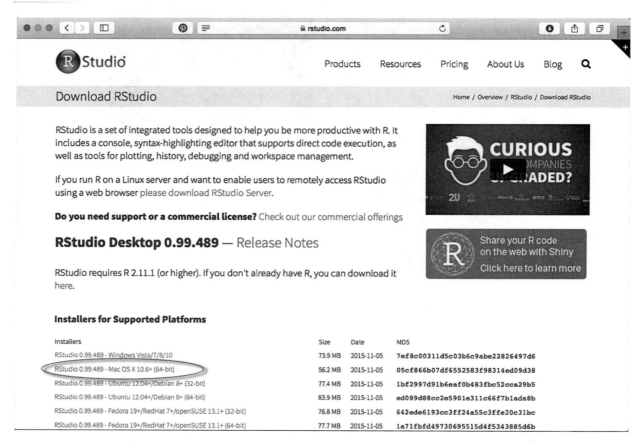

Source: Used with permission from RStudio.

Step 9

After clicking the Mac OS X installer, the file with automatically download to your default download folder and will be titled **RStudio-0.99.484.dmg,** or a more up-to-date version. Open the file and follow the installation instructions. **Please note:** When you open the RStudio-0.99.484.dmg file, it is *critical* to drag the RStudio icon into the Applications folder to successfully install the software (see figure 0.38).

Figure 0.38.   Downloading RStudio for Mac OS X: Step 9

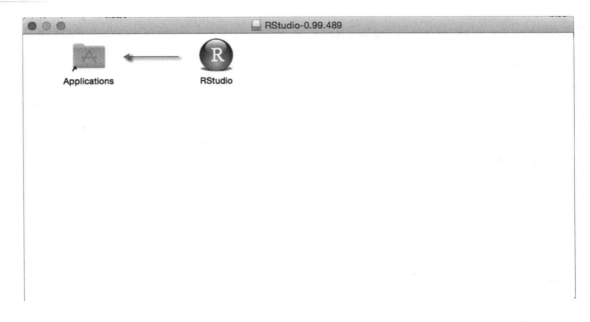

Step 10

After you have installed the software, open RStudio, which can be found in the Applications folder or on the Dock (see figure 0.39).

Figure 0.39.   Downloading RStudio for Mac OS X: Step 10

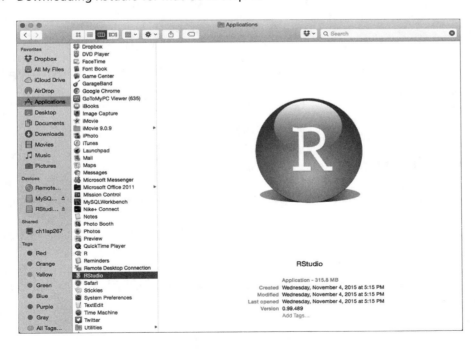

Step 11

The RStudio application window should look like figure 0.40. For detailed instructions and a summary of the components of the RStudio interface, see chapter 5.

Figure 0.40.   Downloading RStudio for Mac OS X: Step 11

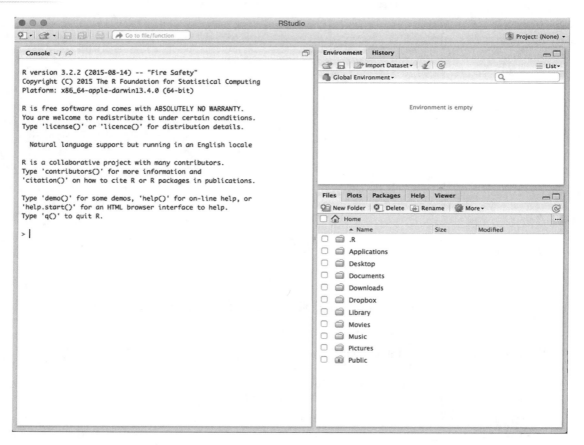

Source: Used with permission from RStudio.

Connecting to the Database

The following are connection instructions to connect to the database. The following instructions will work on both Windows and Mac OS X.

Step 1

Open MySQL Workbench by going to Start | All Programs | MySQL | MySQL Workbench or Finder | Applications | MySQL Workbench.

Step 2

Create a new connection by clicking the + icon next to the text MySQL Connections. See figure 0.41.

Figure 0.41.   MySQL Connections

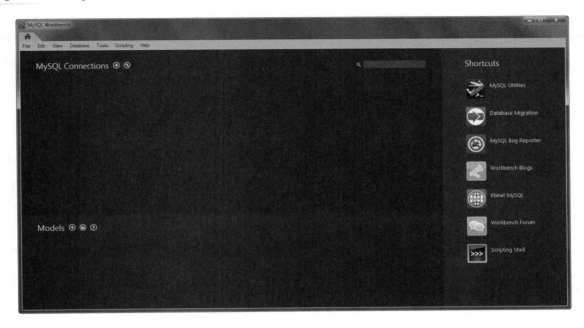

Step 3

In the Setup New Connection window, enter the following information in the following textboxes (see figure 0.42):

Connection Name: **TextbookData**
Hostname: **mysql.ab107114-ahima.org**
Username: **ahima_ab107114**
Default Schema: **ab107114**

Figure 0.42.   Setup New Connection

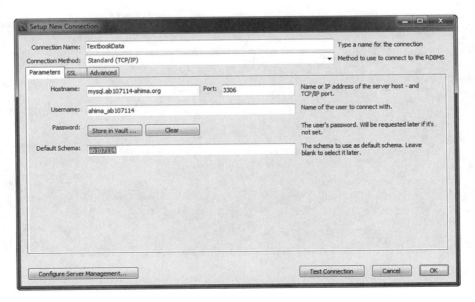

Step 4

Click the Store in Vault... or Store in Keychain... button. In the Store Password For Connection window that appears, enter the following information in the Password textbox: **DataAnalytics**, and click OK (see figure 0.43).

Figure 0.43.   Store password for connection

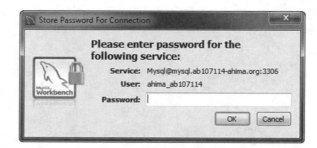

Step 5

In the Setup New Connection window, click OK.

Step 6

A box will now appear with the name TextbookData (figure 0.44). This box represents the connection to the database. Double-click the TextbookData box to access the database.

Figure 0.44.   TextbookData database

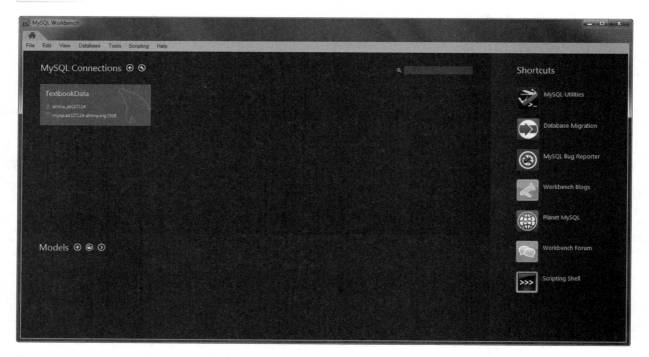

You are now connected to the database.

Part I

Chapter 1

Data and Information Governance

Linda Kloss, MA, RHIA, FAHIMA and Pamela Oachs, MA, RHIA, CHDA, FAHIMA

Learning Objectives

- Differentiate between data governance and information governance
- Articulate how data governance is integrated in the analytics life cycle
- Illustrate each of the building blocks of enterprise information management
- Develop a model for adoption of an information governance strategy
- Define the foundational principles for information governance
- Illustrate a model for data quality management
- Describe the inseparable relationship between data governance and data analytics

Key Terms

Accountable care organizations (ACOs)
Data analytics life cycle
Data governance
Data normalization
Enterprise information management (EIM)
Information governance
Information management (IM) life cycle

The complexity of healthcare delivery, the focus on value-based healthcare, the growth of patient involvement, and the ever-changing legal and regulatory environment have created a huge demand for quality data and information. Healthcare data are proliferating at an extraordinary pace due to rapid advancement, acceptance, and implementation of technology. There is a growing need in the healthcare industry to strengthen health information management (IM) and governance. The persistent breaches of personal health information; the increased prevalence of medical identity theft and healthcare fraud; data integrity and quality issues; inconsistency in how data are gathered, managed, and utilized; and complex error remediation are all challenges enhanced by new technology and changing work processes (Kloss 2015). Effective governance of data and information is imperative to the trusted and meaningful use of health information systems for effective decision making.

Health Data and Information Governance

Healthcare is undergoing changes in payment and care delivery models embedded in an incentivized environment encouraging adoption of technology; new requirements, such as those identified through the EHR Incentive Program or the Hospital Value-Based Purchasing Program, make the accuracy, timeliness, accessibility, and integrity of data and information critical. Clinical data capture, documentation, and content management require principles, guidelines, and standards to ensure consistency and accuracy for meaningful use of this information.

Data and information governance aim to ensure greater accountability for data and information quality and more consistent definitions and policies for IM. Governance can proactively identify issues, reactively resolve issues, and help enforce standards. An effective governance program includes methodologies to identify data quality issues effectively, ensure that workflows are well documented and established, ensure data owners are held responsible for data quality, and establish roles and responsibilities to ensure consistent data standards (Walton 2013, 1).

Definitions of Data and Information Governance

Data governance and information governance are often used interchangeably; however, they address different levels of governance. **Data governance** has an operational focus on policies, processes, and practices that address accuracy, validity, completeness, timeliness, and integrity of the data. The focus of data governance is on data at the business unit, functional area, or departmental level. Each department has representatives identified as data stewards. Data stewards are those employees who are most knowledgeable about the data generated and used in their department and best able to ensure the quality of the data in which they work (Dimick 2013). Data governance begins with ensuring that master data, such as identifiers, demographics, codes, classifications, and other data that are used across systems and are critical for effective analytics, are as accurate and complete as possible. This is done through the development of data dictionaries, database architecture, policy, and process. Analytics is prompting a greater focus on data governance in healthcare.

Information governance focuses on strategic goals and is a broader concept specifying an accountability framework and decision rights to ensure effective and efficient use of information across the enterprise to achieve its goals (Dimick 2013). Information governance is value driven, interdisciplinary, multifocal, and holistic through work across the organization reducing functional silos (Kloss 2013). A strong information governance program assesses risks, identifies and understands gaps, and allows advanced planning for developing policies, procedures, and tools that enable proactive management of data and information enterprise-wide (Warner 2013, 1). The American Health Information Management Association (AHIMA) defines information governance as "an organization-wide framework for managing information throughout its life cycle and supporting the organization's strategy, operations, regulatory, legal, risk, and environmental requirements" (Empel 2014, 30).

AHIMA has developed an information governance framework specific to the healthcare industry that establishes eight principles as a foundation for information governance programs. This framework is called Information Governance Principles for Healthcare (IGPHC) (Empel 2014). The principles are

1. Accountability: Senior leadership must be responsible for oversight.
2. Transparency: Information governance processes and activities must be open and consistent with business needs.
3. Integrity: Data and information must be authentic, reliable, and complete.
4. Protection: Information must be safe from breach, corruption, and loss.
5. Compliance: The information governance program must comply with applicable laws, regulations, standards, and organizational policies.
6. Availability: Data retrieval must be timely, accurate, and efficient.
7. Retention: Information must be maintained for an appropriate time considering legal, regulatory, fiscal, operational, and historical requirements.
8. Disposition: Information no longer required to be maintained by applicable laws or organizational policy should be properly disposed of (Eastwood 2014; Empel 2014).

Data and information governance are both critically important in order to manage information across the enterprise. In healthcare, data and information governance provide a mechanism for ethical decision making about the capture and use of health information and allow for the availability of trusted information that can be used for the public good (Kloss 2013). Data governance focuses on the oversight of the quality of data and establishes policies related to how they are defined, captured, structured, stored, and retrieved. Information governance focuses on the control and use of information created from data and establishes polices related to how information is used, shared, and analyzed by the organization (Johns 2015).

Governance in the Analytics Life Cycle

The **information management (IM) life cycle,** shown in figure 1.1, illustrates how information moves from origination to archival and/or deletion. The steps are comprised of the following stages:

- Design: What is the data definition? Do the data already exist? How are the data currently stored?
- Acquire: What methods will be used to collect the data? Are the data already being collected?
- Process: Where and in what format will the data be stored? What protections are in place to ensure quality data? How will the data be retrieved?
- Use: Who will have access? How will information be distributed?
- Dispose: Do the data and information need to archived? Can they be destroyed? (Kloss 2015)

The IM life cycle begins with an assessment of the need for the information requested. Determining the requirements for the information, if and how it is currently stored, and the need for new data collection is critical for maintaining integrity and avoiding redundancy. This is the design stage. Acquisition of the data to avoid duplication of work and consistency is the next step in the life cycle. Processes for storage, proper retrieval, changes and corrections of content, and protection of the information is the critical next step. Access and use of the information needs to be properly delineated as data are accessed and used for decision making. Finally, the last step of the IM life cycle is the disposal of the information through archiving or destruction. When information is no longer relevant and there are no regulatory requirements to keep it, it should be disposed of in order to minimize cost and risk (Kloss 2015). The decision to dispose of any healthcare-related information must be a conscientious and informed decision.

The **data analytics life cycle** identifies the phases of a data mining project in which data are obtained and analyzed to determine trends or patterns (LaTour et al. 2013). The IM life cycle identifies the phases involved in gathering information for decision making and eventual archival or destruction (Kloss 2015). Both require a strong initial phase of business and data understanding so that preliminary design will achieve the identified objectives effectively without redundancy, rework, or inconsistent information. Data preparation and data modeling in the data analytics life cycle allow the opportunity to ensure data integrity prior to analysis, evaluation, and use in decision making.

An example of a data analytics life cycle is the Cross-Industry Standard Process for Data Mining (CRISP-DM) model. This model guides data mining projects using the following phases:

- Business understanding: Gather background information and define the business objectives. What is the problem that needs to be solved?
- Data understanding: What data already exist and do they meet the needs? What is the format of the data? What is the quality of the data? Are they complete, accurate, and consistent?
- Data preparation: Ensure the data are free from errors. Are errors, inconsistencies, and missing fields removed?
- Data modeling: What data are required in the model to meet the objective? What are the relationships between the data? How will the model be tested?
- Evaluation: Did the results meet the business objective? Were there any flaws in the results? Is there a more streamlined method to approach the problem?
- Deployment: Present the results and findings of the data analysis. How can the results be used to solve the identified problem and make improvements? How can improvements be maintained? (IBM Corporation 1994, 2011)

Figure 1.2 illustrates the CRISP-DM process model.

The components of the IM life cycle and those of the data analytics life cycle are closely aligned. Starting a project with a disciplined evaluation of the information needs, obtaining an understanding of the business requirements, and following that information through the life cycle is an example of strong governance. Figure 1.3 illustrates the compatibility of these models.

Understanding the business requirements and project objectives in the data analytics life cycle is analogous to the design phase of the IM life cycle where the goal is to gain an understanding of the need for and

Figure 1.1.   Information management life cycle

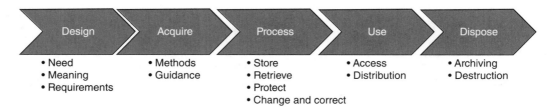

Source: Kloss 2015, 20.

Figure 1.2.   CRISP-DM model for data analytics

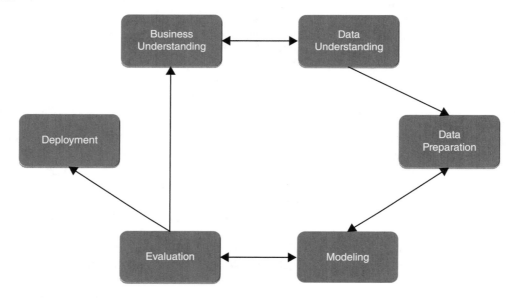

Source: IBM Corporation 1994, 2011.

meaning of the project. Next, the initial data gathering occurs. In the acquisition phase of the IM life cycle and data understanding phase of the data analytics life cycle, problems with the data are identified and insights into what the data mean and what may be missing occur. Guidance and methods for acquiring the data are shared to ensure the right data are collected. The process phase of the IM life cycle encompasses the data analytics components of data preparation, data modeling, and evaluation. This is the largest area of the data analytics project. Data are normalized and cleansed for use in the chosen data analysis technique. The data model is thoroughly evaluated to ensure it meets the business objectives. In comparison, the process phase ensures data are stored, protected, accurate, and available for retrieval. The phases of use and deployment ensure the information is organized and presented in a way that is valuable for the needs of the user. This phase may be generating a report or establishing a data analytics process for continual evaluation. Disposal at the appropriate time is a part of the IM life cycle—from creation to destruction (Kloss 2015; IBM Corporation 1994, 2011).

The data analytics and the IM life cycles work very similarly throughout an analysis project. From beginning to end, policies and decisions need to be made regarding data capture, data standards, data modeling, data and information analysis, and information usage all the way through to archival and destruction. Information governance provides the structure and framework for the phases of these life cycles.

Figure 1.3. Comparison of IM life cycle to data management life cycle

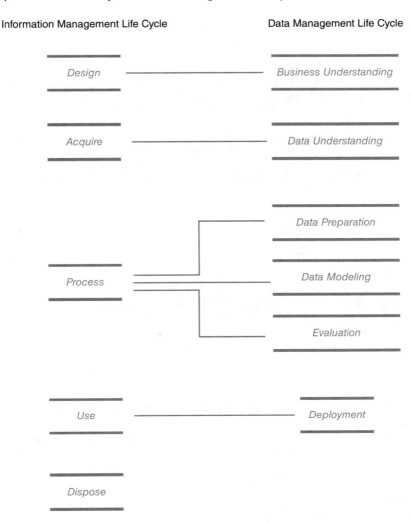

Information Management Life Cycle

Data Management Life Cycle

Design — Business Understanding

Acquire — Data Understanding

Data Preparation

Process — Data Modeling

Evaluation

Use — Deployment

Dispose

Enterprise Information Management

Enterprise information management (EIM) is a set of managerial functions encompassing the life cycle of data and information. It goes beyond the activities involved in each of the life cycle phases by establishing policies, processes, procedures, and training to ensure quality work within each phase. It includes managing functions that support the use of information for decision making, it describes the process for capturing and determining meaning from clinical data, it refers to the integrity of information across the life cycle, it ensures compliance, and it advances the value of information assets. To make informed decisions throughout the enterprise, clinical and business leaders need access to accurate information. EIM organizes the work of governance by bringing issues, recommendations, draft policies, and status reports forward for consideration so that governance can be performed efficiently (Kloss 2015).

A data governance model that illustrates EIM functional areas such as data life cycle management, data architecture, metadata management, business intelligence, data quality management, and terminology management is shown in figure 1.4 (Kloss and Johns 2014). This model incorporates additional components of people, processes, content, and technology.

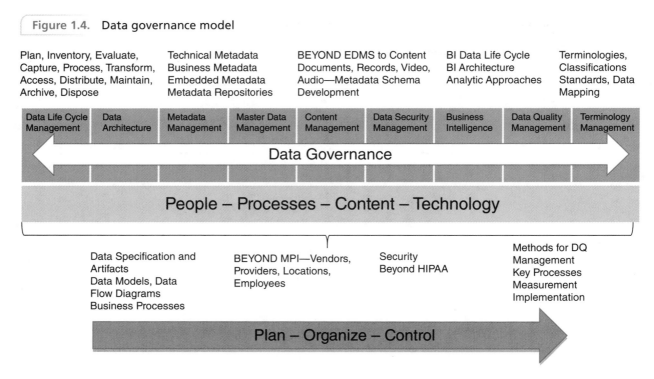

Figure 1.4. Data governance model

Source: Kloss and Johns 2014.

Each functional area, despite the model used, should have a purpose and scope identified; goals and measures of success established; a data governance structure, processes, and communication plan finalized; funding identified and approved; decision rights identified; and accountability assigned (Kloss and Johns 2014).

EIM focuses on managing information as an enterprise-wide asset (Johns 2015) and consists of five building blocks (LaTour et al. 2013):

1. Integrity and Quality
2. Privacy, Confidentiality, and Security
3. Information Design and Capture
4. Content and Records Management
5. Information Access and Use

Information governance encompasses the building blocks that define the governance scope. Figure 1.5 illustrates a model for each of the EIM building blocks for information governance (Kloss 2015, 49). The model shows the integrity and quality block and the privacy, security, and confidentiality block as the foundational elements to the other three building blocks that reflect the IM life cycle from capture to life cycle management and use.

The following sections will look at each of these building blocks in more detail in relation to data analytics.

Information Design and Capture

The use of information governance methodology at the point of data capture can help to improve the efficiency and quality of data as they are collected so that they are complete and accurate for later information use, interoperability, and further reuse. Redundancy can be reduced through standardization of the design for data and information capture. Free text, structured and unstructured data formats, metadata, usage (transactions and analytics), technology used, and software updates and upgrades all need to be considered in the information design and capture phase (Kloss 2015).

Figure 1.5. EIM building blocks for information governance

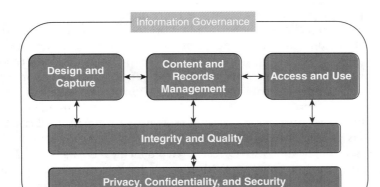

Source: Kloss 2015, 49.

Growing consumer interest in healthcare and use of patient-generated health data (PGHD) challenges this component of EIM. Historically, patients have reported their health information to providers, which is documented in the patient record; however, the method of capture is becoming more variable in recent years with the advancement in technology. PGHD may now come from health information documented via patient portal, biometric information transmitted from home monitoring equipment, or activity updates from personal fitness trackers or mobile apps (Deering 2013). An information governance framework, including organizational policies and procedures to define optimal use of PGHD, is critical to ensure reliable capture, distribution, and use of PGHD (AHIMA 2015).

Determining what information is required and how it will be captured requires a multidisciplinary approach. The users have the best knowledge of the information needed and can offer the information necessary to best design methods of data capture. Experts with knowledge of the capabilities of the applications, data management tools and standards, secondary uses of information, and applicable obligations are also necessary. EIM begins with intentional design and data capture to support predictive analytics, clinical analytics, and advanced research (Kloss 2015).

Content and Records Management

As health records become increasingly electronic, effective governance to manage content and records across the enterprise, regardless of type or media, is critical. The governance and enterprise management of electronically stored information (ESI) consisting of databases, e-mail, web pages, and cloud servers is a growing challenge. As ESI increases, enterprise content management systems are needed to organize electronic documents so they are accessible across systems. Being able to access current data dictionaries, understanding ESI, as well as understanding retention policies is important for those seeking data (Kloss 2015).

Identifying and approving the content for designated record sets (including the official electronic health record [EHR] and approving policies for authentication of entries in the EHR), covering record amendments and corrections, access and disclosure for paper and e-discovery, and legal hold issues are all a part of the content and records management building block. Also included in the content and records management component is a comprehensive retention schedule for all types and formats of information (Kloss 2015).

PGHD are important not only in the information design and capture EIM building block but also in the content and records management building block. Policies are needed regarding whether PGHD will be used for treatment purposes and decision making and, therefore, part of the legal health record. When PGHD is received, providers will need to know how to handle receipt of the information and be aware of liability issues. Content considered a part of the legal health record is subject to all applicable regulations related to privacy, security, use, maintenance, disclosure, and retention (AHIMA 2015).

Information Access and Use

Analytics requires policies, procedures, and processes to acquire information and prepare it for use through cleansing and normalization. Information must be trusted before it is used for decision making. Information governance strategies need to include an understanding of the uses and the user's needs. Clinical analytics for population health and quality improvement studies, consumer engagement, and information exchange are all current drivers for information governance to ensure access to useful and trusted information (Kloss 2015).

Healthcare delivery is an information intensive industry. The more complex the data and the more data sharing that occurs, the more there is a need for a framework for understanding the data (Wright n.d.). Data analytics and information governance need a strong synergy. An example of this need is illustrated in **accountable care organizations (ACOs)**, which consist of groups of providers that voluntarily practice coordinated care to reduce unnecessary duplication of services and avoid medical errors (CMS 2015). ACOs need to be able to exchange data on their patient population. Meeting quality measures related to care coordination, patient safety, prevention, and patient or caregiver experience is critical. If ACOs are not able to share and analyze data using the same terminologies and standards, their success will be at risk. Important in this effort is **data normalization**, which includes adopting standardized code sets and terminologies. Normalization ensures that data from across care settings are not redundant, are logically stored, and can be aggregated for analysis of performance and patient outcomes (Levy 2013).

Clear policy on information access and use comes from the Mayo Clinic. The Mayo Clinic and most large medical centers and healthcare systems face the challenge of collecting, organizing, retrieving, and analyzing vast quantities of data for research, quality improvement, outcomes analyses, business analyses, and best practice development. This information exists in multiple disparate databases, registries, and departmental systems. Systematic normalization of this data including consistent information models and shared vocabulary must be recognized as a critical need for enterprise systems. Mayo recognized this need and began development of a data warehouse that they called the Mayo Enterprise Data Trust (EDT). "EDT is a collection of data from internal and external transactional systems and data repositories, optimized for business intelligence and ad hoc delivery" (Chute et al. 2010, 2). Data related to practice, research, education, and administration are integrated from all Mayo sites allowing for consistent information access and use (Chute et al. 2010).

Information Integrity and Quality

Information integrity and quality are critical to effective use and valid decision making. A distrust of data creates barriers to meaningful use. Core attributes for information integrity and quality include the requirement that data are accurate, complete, timely, and valid (Kloss 2015). The information should represent what it is intended to represent.

Data quality is a foundational building block of EIM. AHIMA's data quality management model, shown in figure 1.6, describes a set of data quality characteristics that can be used to determine the level of quality when considering data for analysis. Those characteristics are data accuracy, accessibility, comprehensiveness, consistency or reliability, currency, definition, granularity, precision, relevancy, and timeliness (Bronnert et al. 2012).

In healthcare, the primary data set used to initiate patient care is the enterprise master patient index (EMPI). The EMPI is the database used across a healthcare organization that holds unique and current patient identifiers making it critical that this database be a focus for accurate, consistent, and reliable data. Similar to the EMPI, health information exchanges (HIEs) need to ensure accurate records. Historical information is maintained and patient matching algorithms match new patient demographic information against existing information. Likely demographic matches are identified and subsequently reviewed by the HIE staff. Corrections are made as necessary when duplicate health records are identified and then the duplicate patients are merged or linked. Many HIEs also receive Health Level Seven International (HL7) merge messages from each exchange participant. These messages are routed into a work queue and patients are electronically and manually merged, linked, or updated. The processes to correct demographic data depend on the individual HIEs and their agreements with the participating hospitals or providers. At a minimum, the HIE's policy should clearly state who can initiate a correction, what notifications are required (by whom and to whom), and within what time frame of the correction. Clear and concise policies and procedures are required at both the organizational and HIE levels to ensure corrections are handled in an appropriate manner (AHIMA 2012).

Figure 1.6.   AHIMA data quality management model

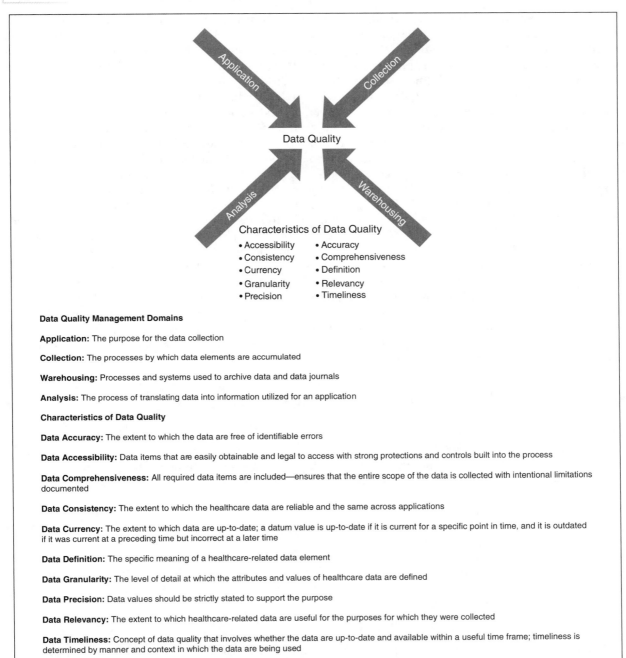

Data Quality Management Domains

Application: The purpose for the data collection

Collection: The processes by which data elements are accumulated

Warehousing: Processes and systems used to archive data and data journals

Analysis: The process of translating data into information utilized for an application

Characteristics of Data Quality

Data Accuracy: The extent to which the data are free of identifiable errors

Data Accessibility: Data items that are easily obtainable and legal to access with strong protections and controls built into the process

Data Comprehensiveness: All required data items are included—ensures that the entire scope of the data is collected with intentional limitations documented

Data Consistency: The extent to which the healthcare data are reliable and the same across applications

Data Currency: The extent to which data are up-to-date; a datum value is up-to-date if it is current for a specific point in time, and it is outdated if it was current at a preceding time but incorrect at a later time

Data Definition: The specific meaning of a healthcare-related data element

Data Granularity: The level of detail at which the attributes and values of healthcare data are defined

Data Precision: Data values should be strictly stated to support the purpose

Data Relevancy: The extent to which healthcare-related data are useful for the purposes for which they were collected

Data Timeliness: Concept of data quality that involves whether the data are up-to-date and available within a useful time frame; timeliness is determined by manner and context in which the data are being used

Source: Bronnert et al. 2012.

Decisions regarding what data to collect, data definitions, and how the data are captured can be valuable toward error prevention. Errors can be prevented at the source through established policies, procedures, standards and training, or they can be identified and resolved later. Systems and processes should be designed to prevent errors in the first place (Kloss 2015). This is the overall intent of information governance.

Privacy, Confidentiality, and Security

When working with healthcare data, personally identifiable and other confidential information should be available only to authorized individuals for authorized use, to ensure any security risks are proactively managed and to comply with all industry regulations. While data analysis and reporting should be supported, policies and procedures must be in place to ensure privacy, confidentiality, and respectful use of patient information. Privacy, confidentiality, and security of healthcare data are also a foundational building block to EIM.

Protected health information (PHI) defined under the Health Insurance Portability and Accountability Act (HIPAA) Privacy Rule is information related to past, present, or future physical or mental health conditions; the provision of healthcare to an individual; or the past, present, or future payment for the provision of healthcare to an individual along with information that identifies the individual (HHS OCR 2012). For use in research and analysis, this PHI must be deidentified. "The process of de-identification, by which identifiers are removed from the health information, mitigates privacy risks to individuals and then supports the secondary use of data for comparative effectiveness studies, policy assessment, life sciences research, and other endeavors" (HHS OCR 2012, 5). There are two acceptable methods for deidentification under HIPAA: (1) expert determination method—use of statistical methods proven to render information not individually identifiable; and (2) safe harbor method—deletion of 18 specified identifiers (HHS OCR 2012; UC Regents 2015). See chapter 2 for more information about the HIPAA Privacy Rule.

This EIM building block includes access controls; risk assessment and mitigation planning; compliance audits; and privacy, confidentiality, and security policies. Policies and practices need to be reviewed, and training needs to be offered routinely. Risks to data privacy and security include those related to people, policy, technology, and information as noted in information governance models. Major risks include those related to access and disclosure, information integrity, fraud, technology, and organizational and human negligence (Kloss 2015). This is a highly regulated and sensitive area to which researchers and analysts need to pay close attention when designing a study.

Models for Information Governance Strategy Adoption

Information governance must have strong administrative support to be successful. When building a case for an information governance plan, it is critical to understand the current environment and where there may be areas of opportunity that can advance the organization's strategic priorities. Information governance and data analytics work together strategically to offer and use trusted data in efforts to

- reduce operating costs,
- demonstrate benchmark levels of quality and safety,
- improve care management,
- establish performance-based contracting,
- ensure accurate and timely reimbursement,
- avoid data breaches,
- promote evidence-based medicine, and
- facilitate business decisions related to mergers or new services (Kloss 2015).

Sutter Health is a large integrated nonprofit health system that recognized the need for a defined governance structure focused on critical data-dependent business needs related to strategic organization goals and objectives. They established consistent policies through a policy framework for EIM, standard operating procedures, and a clear monitoring system to ensure accuracy and availability of data while ensuring data security. Sutter Health realized that to adequately define the scope of the information governance program, cultural assumptions need to be challenged; and they needed to look beyond the EHR and consider all data sources. Defining the organization's information assets is an important step. A data governance council was developed to help translate business objectives into data management strategy and enforce compliance with established policies (Reno and Kersten 2013).

The Mayo Clinic is another large integrated nonprofit health system that has developed an EIM initiative that includes enterprise data governance, enterprise data modeling, enterprise vocabulary, and enterprise managed metadata management. Each component of Mayo's EIM initiative works together to ensure trustworthy data for the enterprise to use in reporting and analytics activities. Mayo's enterprise data governance (EDG) oversees all of the organization's data as an enterprise asset through a data governance committee. EDG establishes and enforces policies, procedures, and standards to optimize Mayo's enterprise data assets and is responsible for activities that improve modeling, standardization, and quality of enterprise data and metadata. EDG is responsible for the definition of vocabularies and reference information used in Mayo's data (Chute et al. 2010). The success of Mayo's EIM initiative is largely due to the well-established governance structure that has been built and supported.

Information governance is critical to the meaningful use of trusted data within an organization. Recommendations for establishing an information governance program include the following:

- Create a vision to drive change; raise awareness of the value of the organization's information assets.
- Convene a steering committee, assign key roles, and engage executive leadership.
- Consider all functions of the information life cycle in defining your governance program's scope.
- Conduct an assessment to determine the current state: Are policies in place? Are standards defined?
- Develop a time frame using a multiphased approach.
- Take an incremental approach; identify areas that will achieve the greatest impact (Reno and Kersten 2013).

Figure 1.7 illustrates a model for adoption that may encourage and engage senior leaders. It includes a means to engage executive sponsors through a case for change, design the governance program including a vision and charter, begin formal governance through working groups and metrics, and design critical mechanisms such as orientation and training to ensure success.

Information is a valuable asset, and it should be managed and governed as such. Information governance sets policies and practices to increase the value of information assets while supporting effective use and protection. High-value information is treated as an asset, is governed and managed across the enterprise, and is managed across its life cycle from creation to destruction (Kloss 2015).

Figure 1.7. Information governance adoption model

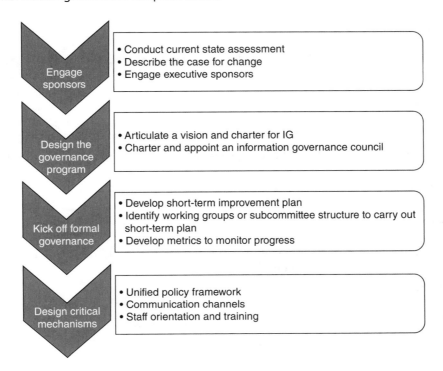

Source: Kloss 2015, 35.

Data Analytics and Governance—Inseparable

Data analytics and governance through EIM is critical to effective data use. Each of the following EIM building blocks is closely aligned with effective data analytics:

- Design and capture: Analytics can be an impetus for improving data dictionaries across systems and collecting data with closer attention to their eventual use.
- Content and record management: Analytics creates new data set, database, and report library management needs, all of which need policies and procedures grounded in sound practice with governance oversight.
- Access and use: Analytics will drive key organizational priorities regarding how trusted data and information are used both centrally and locally at multifacility organizations.
- Integrity and quality: As data are cleansed for analytics, data quality problems will be identified and can be used to identify improvements in data capture moving forward.
- Privacy, confidentiality, and security: Rules are required regarding who is authorized to access what levels of analytic data. These may be role-based authorizations and may require some level of analytic training.

As analytics becomes an integral part of healthcare and critical decision making, ensuring data integrity, data quality, data understanding, and authorized use is necessary. Information governance offers the structure including policies, procedures, best practices, and standards to ensure the availability of trusted data to analyze in a meaningful way to answer questions, advance research, and make decisions.

Review Exercises

Instructions: Choose the best answer.

1. Which of the following is not one of AHIMA's foundational principles for information governance?
   a. Protection
   b. Acquisition
   c. Transparency
   d. Accountability

2. The information management life cycle includes all the phases except:
   a. Acquire
   b. Dispose
   c. Analyze
   d. Use

3. Those most knowledgeable about the data generated and used in their department are:
   a. Data stewards
   b. Data analysts
   c. CIOs
   d. Programmers

4. What process ensures that data from across care settings are standardized and not redundant, are logically stored, and can be aggregated for analysis?
   a. Analysis
   b. Reporting
   c. Governance
   d. Normalization

Instructions: Answer the following on a separate piece of paper.

5. Describe how analytics relates to the five building blocks of enterprise information management.

References

American Health Information Management Association. 2015 (February). Practice brief: Including patient-generated health data in electronic health records. *Journal of AHIMA* 86(2):54–57.

American Health Information Management Association. 2012. Ensuring Data Integrity in Health Information Exchange. AHIMA Thought Leadership Series. http://library.ahima.org/xpedio/groups/public/documents/ahima/bok1_049675.pdf

Bronnert, J., J.S. Clark, B.S. Cassidy, S. Fenton, L. Hyde, C. Kallem, and V. Watzlaf. 2012. Data quality management model (updated). *Journal of AHIMA* 83(7):62–67.

Centers for Medicare and Medicaid Services. 2015 (January 6). Accountable Care Organizations (ACO). https://www.cms.gov/Medicare/Medicare-Fee-for-Service-Payment/ACO/index.html

Chute, C.G., S.A. Beck, T.B. Fisk, and D.N. Mohr. 2010 (March–April). The enterprise data trust at Mayo Clinic: A semantically integrated warehouse of biomedical data. *Journal of the American Medical Informatics Association* 17(2):131–135. http://www.ncbi.nlm.nih.gov/pmc/articles/PMC3000789/

Deering, M.J. 2013 (December 20). Issue Brief: Patient-Generated Health Data and Health IT. http://www.healthit.gov/sites/default/files/pghd_brief_final122013.pdf

Department of Health and Human Services, Office of Civil Rights. 2012 (November 26). Guidance Regarding Methods for De-identification of Protected Health Information in Accordance with the Health Insurance Portability and Accountability Act (HIPAA) Privacy Rule. http://www.hhs.gov/ocr/privacy/hipaa/understanding/coveredentities/De-identification/hhs_deid_guidance.pdf

Dimick, C. 2013 (November–December). Governance apples and oranges: Differences exist between information governance, data governance, and IT governance. *Journal of AHIMA* 84(11):60–62.

Eastwood, B. 2014 (November 13). Inside AHIMA's Framework for Healthcare Information Governance. http://www.cio.com/article/2847153/healthcare/inside-ahimas-framework-for-healthcare-information-governance.html

Empel, S. 2014 (October). The way forward: AHIMA develops information governance principles to lead healthcare toward a better data management. *Journal of AHIMA* 85(10):30.

IBM Corporation. 1994, 2011. IBM SPSS Modeler CRISP-DM Guide. ftp://public.dhe.ibm.com/software/analytics/spss/documentation/modeler/14.2/en/CRISP_DM.pdf

Johns, M.L. 2015. *Enterprise Healthcare Information Management and Data Governance*. Chicago, IL: AHIMA Press.

Kloss, L.L. 2015. *Implementing Health Information Governance: Lessons from the Field*. Chicago, IL: AHIMA.

Kloss, L.L. 2013 (September). Leading innovation in enterprise information governance. *Journal of AHIMA* 84(9):34–38.

Kloss, L. and M. Johns. 2014 (July 28). Data Governance: What's Under the Covers? AHIMA Assembly on Education. Chicago, IL.

LaTour, K.M., S. Eichenwald Maki, and P.K. Oachs. 2013. *Health Information Management: Concepts, Principles and Practice*. Chicago, IL: AHIMA.

Levy, B. 2013 (January 24). The Significance of Normalizing Your Data to the Future of Healthcare [blog]. http://blog.healthlanguage.com/blog/bid/208917/The-Significance-of-Normalizing-Your-Data-to-the-Future-of-Healthcare

Reno, D. and S.K. Kersten. 2013 (May). Getting serious about information governance. *Journal of AHIMA* 84(5):48–49.

UC Regents. 2015. Compliance Program. http://www.ucdmc.ucdavis.edu/compliance/guidance/privacy/deident.html

Walton, J. 2013 (July 2). Data Governance Best Practices for Healthcare, Health IT. http://ehrintelligence.com/2013/07/02/data-governance-best-practices-for-healthcare-health-it/

Warner, D. 2013 (December 4). IG 101: What Is Information Governance? http://journal.ahima.org/2013/12/04/ig-101-what-is-information-governance/

Wright, G. n.d. Data Modeling in the Healthcare Industry [white paper]. http://www.teradata.com/resources/white-papers/Data-Modeling-in-the-Healthcare-Industry-eb5301/

Chapter 2

Data Analytics and Privacy and Security

Danika E. Brinda, PhD, RHIA, CHPS and Amy L. Watters, EdD, RHIA, FAHIMA

Learning Objectives

- Explain the impact of the HIPAA privacy and security regulation on the analysis of health information for research
- Discuss the privacy regulations that impact human subjects' research and how they relate to one another
- Describe the deidentification requirement and methods and how they relate to research
- Define a limited data set and determine when a data use agreement is required
- Examine the breach notification regulation and its impact on research
- Discuss patients' privacy rights in relation to research

Key Terms

Accounting of disclosure
Administrative safeguards
Authorization
Breach notification
Business associates
Clinical trial
Common Rule
Covered entities
Data use agreement
Deidentification
Expert determination method
Health Insurance Portability and Accountability Act of 1996 (HIPAA)
HITECH-HIPAA Omnibus Privacy Act
Human subject protection regulations
Informed consent
Institutional Review Boards (IRB)
Limited data set
Organizational safeguards
Physical safeguards
Privacy Rule
Protected health information (PHI)
Reidentification
Research
Safe harbor method
Security Rule
Technical safeguards

Electronic health records have increased the need and desire for analyzing patient data to improve healthcare delivery and decision making while lowering healthcare costs. These improvements are critical to the health and well-being of patients, healthcare organizations, and society at large. Although the collection and availability of data has grown tremendously with the evolution of technology, this has also intensified concerns regarding confidentiality. In order to maintain the privacy and security of patient data, researchers must be knowledgeable of the applicable standards, rules, and regulations, and organizations must have policies and procedures in place to ensure the protection of that data.

Overview of HIPAA Privacy and Security Rules

Striking a balance between maintaining data privacy and allowing access to enough detailed information for effective research to occur is a considerable challenge for researchers and healthcare organizations. The **Health Insurance Portability and Accountability Act of 1996 (HIPAA)** exists to provide regulations to guide organizations as they strive to find that balance. HIPAA was enacted to ensure health insurance portability, establish standards for electronic claims and national identifiers, protect against fraud and abuse, and assure the privacy and security of **protected health information (PHI)**, which is individually identifiable health information held or transmitted by a covered entity or business associate (HIPAA 1996). Title II of HIPAA, known as the administrative simplification provisions, contains the Privacy and Security Rules, which provide regulations on the use of PHI for research purposes. HIPAA provides only the minimum requirements regarding privacy and security. States are free to adopt more stringent regulations thereby requiring knowledge of both federal and state requirements that are necessary for compliance.

The Standards for Privacy of Individually Identifiable Health Information, commonly known as the **Privacy Rule** (45 CFR Part 160, Subparts A & E of Part 164), was established to assure the protection of health information. Specifically, the goal of the Privacy Rule is "to assure that individuals' health information is properly protected while allowing the flow of health information needed to provide and promote high quality healthcare and to protect the public's health and well being" (HIPAA 1996). The Privacy Rule was established with three goals in mind, all of which align with the goals of healthcare research:

1. to protect and enhance the rights of healthcare consumers by providing them access to their health information and control of the inappropriate use of that information;
2. to improve the quality of healthcare in the United States by restoring trust in the healthcare system; and
3. to improve the efficiency and effectiveness of healthcare delivery by creating a national framework for privacy protection that builds on the efforts of states, health systems and organizations, and individuals (HIPAA 1996).

The purpose of the Security Standards for the Protection of Electronic Protected Health Information, or the **Security Rule** (45 CFR Part 160 & Subparts A & C of Part 164), is to operationalize the protections identified in the Privacy Rule by addressing the technical and nontechnical safeguards that organizations called **covered entities** put in place to secure individuals' electronic PHI (e-PHI) (HHS n.d.). A covered entity is defined as a health plan, healthcare clearinghouse, or healthcare provider that transmits health information electronically in connection with a transaction covered by the HIPAA Transaction Rule. By definition, researchers are not considered covered entities; however, the Privacy and Security Rules could apply to researchers who work at a covered entity or hybrid institution, or who provide care to subjects as part of their research (Gunn et al. 2004).

The Security Rule specifies "a series of administrative, technical, and physical security procedures for covered entities to use to assure the confidentiality, integrity, and availability of e-PHI" (HIPAA 1996). It identifies **administrative safeguards** to manage the activities needed to establish security measures; **physical safeguards** to identify measures to protect information systems, buildings, and equipment from natural and environmental hazards; **technical safeguards** to protect access and control of e-PHI; and **organizational safeguards** so that arrangements are made to protect e-PHI between organizations (Key Health Alliance n.d.). All of the safeguards are intended to protect the privacy of health information as covered entities continue to adopt new and evolving technologies to improve patient care. The Privacy Rule and the Security Rule only apply to covered entities.

Although organizations were required to be in compliance with the Privacy and Security Rules in 2003 and 2005, respectively, they were impacted in 2009 when the Health Information Technology for Economic and Clinical Health (HITECH) Act was enacted to promote the adoption and meaningful use of health information technology as part of the American Recovery and Reinvestment Act (ARRA). The HITECH Act established more detailed provisions and strengthened the requirements included in the HIPAA Privacy and Security Rules by establishing mandatory breach reporting requirements and several tiers of penalties for breaches, establishing new enforcement responsibilities and new privacy requirements such as new accounting requirements for the electronic health record, and extending requirements to the business associates of covered entities (Key Health Alliance n.d.). In response, the US Department of Health and Human Services (HHS) Office for Civil Rights (OCR) published the final omnibus rules in 2013 to address many of the HITECH requirements. The rule is officially titled "Modifications to the HIPAA Privacy, Security, Enforcement, and Breach Notification Rule Under the Health Information Technology for Economic and Clinical Health Act, and the Genetic Information Nondiscrimination Act; Other Modifications to the HIPAA Rule," but is often referred to as the HITECH-HIPAA Omnibus Privacy Act.

The **HITECH-HIPAA Omnibus Privacy Act**

- strengthens the privacy and security of patient health information,
- modifies the breach notification rule,
- strengthens privacy protections for genetic information by prohibiting health plans from using or disclosing such information for underwriting,
- makes business associates of HIPAA covered entities liable for compliance,
- strengthens limitations on the use and disclosure of PHI for marketing and fundraising, and
- allows patients increased restriction rights (Key Health Alliance n.d.).

Additionally, the HIPAA Omnibus Rule changed the regulations to allow for authorization of future research studies with an appropriate and adequate description of how the PHI will be used in the future research through compound authorizations. Compound authorizations combine the use and disclosure of PHI with other legal permissions, which is prohibited by the current HIPAA Privacy Rule. However, this provision was amended by the Omnibus Rule, which permits combining an authorization for the use and disclosure of PHI for a research study with authorization for other permissions for the same study, including informed consent to participate in the study. The Omnibus Rule allows for both conditioned (requiring a signed authorization for research-related treatment) and unconditioned (research-related treatment is not conditioned on a signed authorization) authorizations for research to exist on the same form as long as the authorization form clearly differentiates between the two and allows the individual to opt out of the unconditioned research activities. In addition, the authorization must give participants an opt-in option; combined authorizations that only allow the individual to opt out of the unconditioned research are not permitted. This provision applies to all types of research studies except for authorization to use and disclose psychotherapy notes, which may not be combined with any other authorization (AHIMA 2013).

The OCR indicates that more provisions will be established in the future. The omnibus rule does not address all of the HITECH privacy requirements. For example, the requirement for accounting of disclosures, which would require facilities to track every access of health information, is not included. It is anticipated that the OCR will release provisions related to this and other requirements at a later date.

Regulations in Research

The Privacy Rule defines the conditions under which PHI may be used or disclosed by covered entities for research. The Privacy Rule also requires that individuals be informed of uses and disclosures of their health information for research purposes. The Privacy Rule was designed to build upon two already existing US Department of Health and Human Services (HHS) federal protection standards related to research: the Federal Policy for the Protection of Human Subjects, also known as the Federal Policy or the Common Rule (45 CFR Part 46, Subpart A) and the Food and Drug Administration's (FDA) human subject protection regulations (21 CFR Parts 50 and 56). Most research involving human subjects operates under these regulations, which have provisions that are similar, yet separate from the Privacy Rule's research requirements. These human subject protection regulations, which apply to most federally funded and to some privately funded research, include protections to ensure subjects' privacy and the confidentiality of their information (HHS 2013).

The Office for Human Research Protections (OHRP) oversees the **Common Rule**, which governs research that is conducted on human beings if funded by 1 of 18 federal agencies. The Common Rule has three requirements intended to protect research subjects:

1. Proposed research is reviewed by an **Institutional Review Board (IRB)**, a formally designated group that reviews and monitors research involving human subjects (FDA 2014).
2. The **informed consent** of research subjects, assuring that subjects are aware that they are participating in research, and are well informed about the study, its risks, and its benefits.
3. Institutional assurance of compliance with the regulatory requirements (Williams 2005).

The Common Rule has not been adopted by all agencies that fund research; however, in order to receive funding or conduct research at one of the agencies that has adopted it, researchers must abide by the appropriate regulations. Federal law does not require that research conducted without federal money should follow the Common Rule regulations, though some private companies voluntarily choose to do so.

The US Food and Drug Administration (FDA) **human subject protection regulations** governs clinical investigations of products such as drugs and medical devices, and also has federal regulations for the protection of human subjects. Many of the FDA's federal regulations are similar to those found in the Common Rule. Like the Common Rule, the FDA requires informed consent, IRB review, and assurance of compliance. Unlike the Common Rule, the FDA regulations target clinical trials related to evaluating products for marketing, regardless of the funding source, rather than basic research, in addition to other subtle differences (Williams 2005).

The Privacy Rule allows covered entities to use and disclose PHI for treatment, payment, and healthcare operations (TPO). Often third parties are involved in such processes, referred to as **business associates.** A business associate is a person or entity that performs functions that involve the use or disclosure of PHI on behalf of, or provides services to, a covered entity (HHS 2003). In order to disclose PHI to business associates, the Privacy Rule requires covered entities to develop business associate agreements to document the procedures used to safeguard patient data. Researchers are not considered business associates, nor are business associate agreements required for disclosures of PHI to researchers as long as the researcher has met the other requirements of the Privacy Rule (Gunn et al. 2004).

When human subjects' research involves the use or disclosure of PHI by a covered entity, the Privacy Rule must be adhered to. **Research** is defined in the Privacy Rule as "a systematic investigation, including research development, testing, and evaluation, designed to develop or contribute to generalizable knowledge" (45 CFR 164.501) (HHS 2013). Covered entities and business associates may use and disclose PHI for research with authorization from the patient. The Privacy Rule requires that covered entities obtain a signed and dated **authorization** form from the patient before using or disclosing the patient's PHI. The authorization must contain core elements and required statements as outlined by HIPAA (see table 2.1). Authorization should not be confused with informed consent. Laws and regulations requiring researchers to obtain a subject's consent to participate in a study still apply. Depending on the type of study, researchers may need to obtain both informed consent for study participation as well as authorization to use and disclose PHI. Some organizations choose to include both on one form.

The Privacy Rule indicates that there are instances where PHI may be used or disclosed without authorization by the research participant. A covered entity may always use or disclose PHI for research purposes if it has been deidentified in accordance with 45 CFR 164.502(d), Uses and Disclosures of Protected Health Information: General Rules, and 164.514(a)-(c), Other Requirements Relating to Uses and Disclosures of Protected Health Information, of the Rule (HIPAA 1996). PHI may also be used or disclosed by a covered entity without authorization under the following circumstances:

1. An Institutional Review Board (IRB) or Privacy Board provides consent.
2. The PHI is being used or disclosed solely to prepare a research protocol or for other purposes preparatory to research.
3. The PHI is used or disclosed solely for research on the PHI of decedents.
4. A data use agreement between the covered entity and the researcher is in place allowing the covered entity to disclose a limited data set to the researcher for research, public health, or healthcare operations (HHS 2013).

Table 2.1.   Required elements of HIPAA's valid authorization

#	Section 1: Requirements for Authorization to Disclose Patient Health Information or Records (45 CFR §164.508(c) - HIPAA)
1	Authorization is written in plain language.
2	Authorization identifies the name of the patient whose PHI is being disclosed.
3	Authorization identifies the type of information to be disclosed.
4	Authorization identifies the names or classes of persons or types of healthcare providers authorized to make the disclosure.
5	Authorization identifies the names or classes of persons or types of healthcare providers authorized to whom the organization may make the disclosure.
6	Authorization identifies the purpose of the disclosure.
7	Authorization contains the signature of the patient or patient's authorized legal representative.
8	If signed by an authorized legal representative, the authorization identifies the relationship of that person to the patient.
9	Authorization includes the date on which the authorization is signed.
10	Authorization identifies the time period for which the authorization is effective and expiration date or event.
11	Authorization contains a statement informing the individual regarding the right to revoke the authorization in writing and a description of how to do so.
12	Authorization contains a statement informing the individual about the organization's ability or inability to condition treatment, payment, enrollment, or eligibility for benefits.
13	Authorization contains a statement informing the individual about the potential for information to be redisclosed and no longer protected by the federal Privacy Rule.
14	Authorization contains a statement that if an organization is seeking the authorization, a copy must be provided to the individual signing the authorization.
15	Authorization contains a statement that the individual may inspect or copy the health information disclosed.
16	Authorization includes a statement regarding assessment of reasonable fees for copy services.

Source: AHIMA 2012.

There is also a transition provision under the Privacy Rule, which allows a covered entity to use and disclose PHI that was created or received for research either before or after the compliance date of April 14, 2003 provided that the covered entity received authorization or legal permission, informed consent of the individual, or a waiver of informed consent by an IRB prior to the compliance date (HHS 2013).

Deidentification

The amount of data that are available electronically have increased, seemingly making it easier for organizations to use the data for research; however, under the HIPAA Privacy Rule the information cannot be used for research unless authorized by the patient first. There are scenarios where PHI may be used without a consent, though, and the HIPAA Privacy Rule defines when information can be used without the consent of the patient (AHIMA 2013). HIPAA allows for specific identifiers to be removed from patient data to allow facilities to conduct research without a patient consent through deidentification. The process of deidentification allows researchers to access and use PHI for conducting research while remaining in compliance with privacy regulations.

HIPAA's Deidentification Requirement

The **deidentification** requirement is defined in the HIPAA Privacy Rule (CFR 164.514) as "health information that does not identify an individual and with respect to which there is no reasonable basis to believe that

Figure 2.1.   Department of Health and Human Services deidentification methods

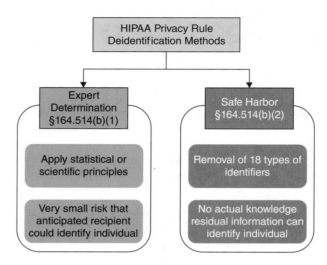

Source: HHS 2012, 7.

the information can be used to identify an individual is not individually identifiable health information" (HHS 2012). By adequately deidentifying the data, the protected health information is unable to be linked back to a specified individual.

The deidentification standard established an implementation specification allowing the covered entity to determine that the protected health information could not identify a specific individual. The regulation defines two specific methodologies for this determination to occur: **expert determination method** and **safe harbor method** (HHS 2012). The expert determination method of deidentification is done by applying a statistical and scientific method to determine the risk of protected health information being identified based on the specific identifiers that are within the protected health information (Warner 2013; HHS 2012). The safe harbor method of deidentification requires the removal of 18 specific identifiers from the protected health information (HHS 2012). Only by the correct application of these two specified methodologies will the information be considered deidentified. Once the information meets the criteria of deidentification, the information is no longer protected under the HIPAA Privacy Rule because the data are no longer considered protected health information. Figure 2.1 depicts the two methodologies for determining that data are deidentified.

Expert Determination Method

The first method of deidentification is expert determination, which requires a person with appropriate statistical and scientific principles knowledge and expertise to deem that the information has a low probability of reidentification. The expert determination process is conducted by applying statistical and scientific methods to determine the low risk of the information being identified based on the identifiers that were removed from the protected health information (Warner 2013; HHS 2012). The expert determination methodology is challenging as the regulations do not specify the requirement or statistical level at which the deidentified information is considered to have a small risk of being reidentified.

To proceed with the expert determination process, the first step for a covered entity is to find an individual who is determined to be an expert in statistical, mathematic, and scientific principles. The HIPAA Privacy Rule does not define a specific degree or designation that would qualify a person to be an expert with deidentification. A covered entity should look for an individual who can prove knowledge and expertise in statistical methods, mathematical methods, and scientific methods. Additionally, past experience with and knowledge of health information deidentification methodologies should be an experience requirement (Warner 2013; HHS 2012). As part of the requirements for deidentification under the expert determination method, the covered entity needs to have a process in place to keep documentation that supports the methods used, the results, and analysis that support the justification that the information is deidentified (HHS 2012).

The HIPAA deidentification regulation does not specify the methodology the expert has to use to determine what the risk is to the data for reidentification purposes. The process for expert determination of deidentification has four recommended steps as outlined by the Department of Health and Human Services:

- Step 1: The facility should choose the expert for the deidentification analysis
- Step 2: Determine the statistical and scientific method to be used to determine the risk of reidentification
- Step 3: The expert applies the method to the deidentified data
- Step 4: Analyze and assess the risk to the deidentified data (LaTour et al. 2013)

If the risk of reidentification is too large, the data would be analyzed and additional identifiers would be removed and the process would start over again. If the deidentified data were determined to have a very small risk, or low probability, of reidentification, the expert would document the statistical and scientific method used for analysis and the results to support the determination (HHS 2012). The expert deidentification process is illustrated in figure 2.2.

The HIPAA requirements do not specify a foundation for applying the statistical or scientific methods; however, in the original HIPAA Privacy Rule the deidentification standard referenced the principles defined

Figure 2.2.   Process for expert determination of deidentification

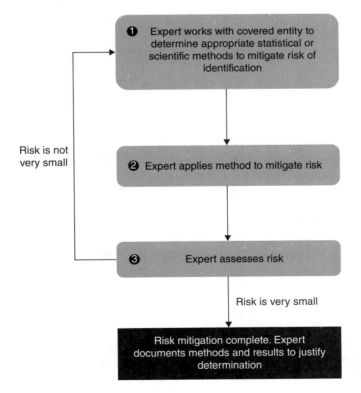

Source: HHS 2012, 13.

by the Federal Committee on Statistical Methodology (HHS 2012). There are four specified principles under this methodology:

- Replicability: Prioritization of the healthcare data into levels or risks by how often the information will consistently occur throughout the data set on a specified individual.
- Data source availability: Determination of information and data sources that are outside of the deidentified data set that include specific patient identifiers and replicability of data. Additionally, who has access and is permitted to view these other data sources becomes a factor in this analysis.
- Distinguishability: Determination of the degree to which the individual data can be easily distinguished with the deidentified data set.
- Assess risk: The higher the replicability, data source availability, and distinguishability, the greater the chance and risk for reidentification of the data (HHS 2012).

While not defined in the HIPAA privacy regulations, this is a process and methodology that an expert can use in the process of evaluating the risk to reidentify the data.

Safe Harbor Deidentification Method

The safe harbor method of deidentification takes a much different approach than the expert determination method. Rather than focusing on the statistical risk of information being reidentified, the safe harbor method requires the removal of 18 data elements out of the protected health information. It doesn't require any statistical analysis or review after the removal of the individually identifiable health information. The following are the 18 data elements that must be removed:

- Patient names
- All geographic subdivisions smaller than the state of residence (street address, city, county, precinct, zip code)
- All elements pertaining to dates except for the year (birth date, admission date, discharge date, death date, and all ages over 89, including year of birth)
- Telephone numbers
- Fax numbers
- E-mail addresses
- Social Security numbers
- Health plan beneficiary numbers
- Account numbers
- Certificate or license numbers
- Vehicle identification numbers and serial numbers (VIN, license plate number)
- Device identifiers and serial numbers
- Web universal resource locators (URLs)
- Internet protocol (IP) addresses
- Biometric identifiers, including finger and voice prints
- Full-face photographs and any comparable images
- Any other unique identifying number, characteristic, or code (HHS 2012; AHIMA 2001)

All 18 elements must be removed in order for the data to meet the safe harbor deidentification method (HHS 2012). After all elements are removed from the data set, the covered entity must attest that there is no actual knowledge that the information alone or in combination with other information could potentially identify an individual (AHIMA 2001).

One of the data elements also has further information and description that require a covered entity to protect and remove the information. For example, under the removal of the geographical information, the first three digits of the zip code can be used and the information will still be deemed deidentified; however, if the combined total of the population of all the geographical locations that start with the first three digits is 20,000 people or fewer, the first three digits of the zip code cannot be used in the data (HHS 2012). In 2000, the United States Census Bureau deemed that there are 17 zip codes that must be omitted from the data as they meet the criteria based on less than 20,000 individuals for the first three digits used. Those zip codes are included in table 2.2.

Table 2.2.   Seventeen restricted zip codes (first three digits) from 2000 census

036	692	878
059	790	879
063	821	884
102	823	890
203	830	893
556	831	

Source: HHS 2012, 24.

Table 2.3.   Samples for safe harbor's unique identifying number, characteristic, or code requirement*

Identifying Number Examples	Identifying Code Examples	Identifying Characteristic Examples
Clinical trial number	Barcode for patient supplies used in patient care	Patient occupation
Research participant ID	Barcode on patient's wristband	Family relationships
Assignment of numbers	Unique medication codes	Publicized clinical event information

*Please note this is not an exhaustive list.

A challenging component of the safe harbor deidentification method is the last specified element, which is "any other unique identifying number, characteristic, or code." Without any additional detail or information, a covered entity must determine if information and details within the data could be traced back to an individual person on number element (AHIMA 2001). There are three main categories that fall under this element's definition: identifying number, identifying code, or identifying characteristic (HHS 2012). There is not an official list of what may be included in each of these categories. Rather, the covered entity is required to evaluate and determine if a data element could potentially identify a patient. Table 2.3 provides some examples of what may fall into this category.

Besides removing the 18 key characteristics, a covered entity should read through all the information in the patient record to determine if any other data points would fall into the category of unique identifying number, characteristic, or code. The goal of the safe harbor deidentification method is to assure that no information could be reidentified.

Reidentification

The second specification under the deidentification standard states that a covered entity may implement a methodology to allow for **reidentification** of the deidentified information. This can be done by assigning specific codes to the data or other means of record identification (HHS 2012). The HIPAA requirement does not specify a particular format or methodology for specific coding or record keeping for purposes of reidentification. The only requirement is that the specific code or identification method cannot be derived from any information relating to the patient. The code or identification cannot create any means of identification of the individual. An example would be to assign a specific code to each of the deidentified information that is linked to the specific patient, but kept separate from the data being deidentified.

In addition, the covered entity needs to ensure that they protect the security of the record identification used for reidentification. The covered entity should implement proper safeguards and control mechanisms to guarantee that the codes used for reidentification are not used or disclosed in any way. The coded information should only be available and used for the purpose of reidentification by the covered entity (HHS 2012). Covered entities need to ensure that they are aware and properly protecting the information that could identify the information in a deidentified data set. Using the previous example, the coded data set for the deidentified information should be kept in a separate location and should not be released to anyone using the deidentified data for research purposes. The coded data set should be kept in a specific area with limited access, potentially to only one or two individuals.

HIPAA's Limited Data Set

Another method for use of patient information without authorization under the HIPAA Privacy Rule is defined by the **limited data set** regulation. HIPAA regulation CFR 164.514(e) states that the covered entity is allowed to use or disclose protected health information for research purposes without an authorization from the patient if:

1. the information provided is considered a limited data set
2. a data use agreement is established prior to the use or disclosure of the information (HHS-NIH 2014)

Under the HIPAA Privacy Rule, a limited data set is defined as a data set that excludes 16 of the direct patient identifiers from the data. Similar to the list of identifiers removed for the purposes of deidentification, the limited data set excludes the same identifiers, except the data can include statement, zip code, elements of data, and other identifying numbers, characteristics, or codes that are not direct identifiers (HHS-NIH 2014). The intent of a limited data set is to allow for use or disclosure of protected health information for the purpose of research, public health activities, and healthcare operations (HHS-NIH 2014). The identifiers that must be removed from the data to qualify as a limited data set are defined as follows:

1. Names
2. Any geographical location that could identify an individual household (street address, PO box)
3. Telephone number
4. Fax numbers
5. E-mail addresses
6. Social Security numbers
7. Medical record numbers
8. Health plan beneficiary identifiers
9. Account numbers
10. Certificate or license numbers
11. Vehicle identifiers and serial numbers
12. Medical device identifiers and serial numbers
13. Web universal resource locators (URL)
14. Internet protocol (IP) address
15. Biometric identifiers, including finger and voice prints
16. Full face photographic images (HHS-NIH 2014)

Data Use Agreement

While an authorization from the patient is not required for use of a limited data set, covered entities are required to establish a **data use agreement** when they disclose a limited data set to a third party. A data use agreement is defined as "an agreement into which the covered entity enters with the intended recipient of a limited data set that establishes the ways in which the information in the limited data set may be used and how it will be protected" (HHS-NIH 2014). While the data use agreement is not the same as a business associate agreement, the purpose and intent of the documents parallel each other. The purpose of the data use agreement is to set forth an agreement with the third party on the purposes or use of the information and how the information is protected (Amatayakul 2002). A data use agreement must include the following elements:

* Establish that the information that was used or disclosed was declared a limited data set prior to use or disclosure
* Establish who is officially permitted to use or receive the limited data set

- Establish the purpose of the limited data set use
- Establish that the recipients will not use or disclose the limited data set outside the scope of the agreement
- Establish that the recipient will apply the appropriate safeguards to protect the information
- Establish that the recipient will inform the covered entity of potential use or disclosure outside of the agreement that they become aware of
- Establish that any subcontractor or agent of the recipient who gets access to the limited data set agrees to the same restrictions and agreements
- Establish that the recipient will not re-identify the individuals or contact the individuals
- Establish the terms of the data use agreement (AHIMA/HIMSS 2011)

The data use agreement must clearly state and outline each of the requirements in order to provide adequate safeguards and guarantees that the information will be kept safe and only used for the intended purpose. It is important to assure that the data use agreement is put into place and executed prior to the exchange of the limited data set. The data use agreement should be signed by the appropriate individual(s), such as administration or the privacy officer, at the covered entity as well as at the recipient of the limited data set.

Breach Notification and Research

While many regulations exist to protect the privacy and security of PHI during research, healthcare organizations need to be aware that unauthorized uses and disclosures of any PHI during a research process may be considered a data breach under the updated regulations. In 2009, the American Recovery and Reinvestment Act (ARRA) was signed into law causing many changes to the HIPAA Privacy and Security regulations. In the Health Information Technology for Economic and Clinical Health Act (HITECH) section of the ARRA, one of the largest regulation provisions to privacy and security was the new requirement related to **breach notification**. The breach notification regulation created a new process for covered entities and business associates to investigate and evaluate if a breach occurred for an unauthorized use or disclosure of protected health information. The regulation also created a short timeline for investigation, conclusion, and notification of the potential breach (Kempfert and Reed 2011; Dimick 2010, Boerner 2009). In the 2009 regulation, a breach was defined as "an impermissible or unauthorized acquisition, access, use, or disclosure of PHI…that poses a significant risk of financial, reputation, or other harm to the individual" (Kempfert and Reed 2011, 266). In January 2013, the HIPAA Omnibus Rule was published, which changed breach notification processes for organization.

In the final HITECH-HIPAA Omnibus Act of 2013, the breach notification regulation changed, causing organizations to reevaluate their breach notification policies. Under the final regulation, a breach is defined as

> an impermissible use or disclosure under the Privacy Rule that compromises the security or privacy of the protected health information. An impermissible use or disclosure of protected health information is presumed to be a breach unless the covered entity or business associate, as applicable, demonstrates that there is a low probability that the protected health information has been compromised based on a risk assessment. (Kastel 2013)

One of the biggest changes between the 2009 interim breach notification rule and the 2013 final rule was the removal of the risk of harm analysis of the breach. The risk of harm analysis requirement was replaced with a more objective risk assessment of the breach, which at a minimum must address:

1. The nature and extent of the PHI involved in the data breach, including the types of identifiers and likelihood of the reidentification
2. The unauthorized person (people) who used the PHI or to whom it was disclosed
3. Whether the PHI was viewed, acquired, or redisclosed
4. The extent to which the risk to the PHI has been mitigated (Kastel 2013)

A covered entity and business associate should assure that an internal investigation process is established that evaluates each of these four objectives at a minimum. Based on the information needed to submit a data breach notice to the Department of Health and Human Services, additional data elements need to be included to submit the data besides the information from the risk assessment. These data elements include:

- Breach start date
- Breach end date
- Discovery start date
- Discovery end date
- Approximate number of people impacted
- Type of breach (hacking or IT incident, improper disposal, loss, theft, unauthorized access/disclosure)
- Location of breach (desktop computer, electronic medical record, e-mail, laptop, network server, other portable electronic device, paper or films, other—must enter a location)
- Type of protected health information involved (clinical, demographic, financial, other—must enter details)
- Brief description of the breach
- Safeguards in place prior to breach (none, Privacy Rule safeguards, Security Rule administrative safeguards, Security Rule technical safeguards, Security Rule physical safeguards)
- Individual notice provided start date
- Individual notice provided end date
- If substitute notice was required
- If media was notified
- Actions taken in response to breach (HHS 2015)

An organization and business associate should establish a process to collect the same data elements each time a data breach investigation is completed.

The breach notification requirement forced covered entities and business associates to establish policies and procedures to investigate an unauthorized use or disclosure of health information to determine if a breach occurred, conclude the investigation, and to notify affected individuals and the secretary of the Department of Health and Human Services within 60 days of date of discovery of the breach (Kempfert and Reed 2011; Boerner 2009). If the number of individuals impacted by the breach exceeds 500, a healthcare organization must notify and report the incident to the local media as well as the individuals impacted by the breach and the secretary of the Department of Health and Human Services (Boerner 2009, Dimick 2010). With the new timeline and reporting requirements, healthcare organizations must assure they have proper reporting process and incident management processes in place.

Additionally, the HIPAA Omnibus Rule defines three exceptions to the breach notification rule requirement.

1. The PHI was not intentional, and the individual or individuals that received the information have the requirement to keep the information confidential.
2. The access to the PHI was unintentional by a workforce member, and the person or persons receiving the information have a right to keep the information confidential.
3. The healthcare organization believes in good faith that the protected health information could not have been retained by the person receiving it (Kempfert and Reed 2011; Boerner 2009).

Based on the findings of the investigation into the potential breach, an organization will make a determination regarding if the issue falls into the breach notification process or not and will take the proper steps to notify the affected individuals.

One of the changes in the 2013 final Omnibus Rule is the elimination of the limited data set exception that was within the preamble of the 2009 interim breach notification rule. If a limited data set is improperly used or disclosed outside the scope of the data use agreement, a breach investigation would need to be completed to determine the risk to the information and if there is low probability that the protected health information was compromised (Kastel 2013). Each of these cases would require a full investigation with documentation created and maintained similar to any other data breach investigation. An investigation process of a potential data breach is usually led by the HIPAA Privacy Officer or HIPAA Security Officer. If deidentified information is improperly used or disclosed, it would not be considered a data breach if it was deemed deidentified in one of the two approved methodologies discussed earlier in the chapter.

Patient's Privacy Rights with Research

Just as with other aspects of creating, maintaining, and storing PHI, patients have defined rights that apply to the use and disclosure of patient information for research purposes. When research is being conducted, it is important that the covered entity or business associate assure compliance with the Privacy and Security Rules as they relate to patient rights. Two specific areas of patient rights are impacted by research: access to protected health information and accounting of disclosures.

Access to Protected Health Information

Under the final HIPAA Privacy Rule, patients are allowed to have access to protected health information created by a covered entity or a business associate if it is within the designated record set. Research information and data that are collected and created may be considered part of the designated record set of a covered entity if the information within the research records is used to assist in making medical decision for a patient (HHS-NIH 2014). Based on this information, patients would have access to the research records that are maintained if they support the decisions for patient care. A covered entity should evaluate and establish a process for granting access to research records if a patient requests a copy. Additionally, if these records are stored and maintained electronically, a healthcare organization must be prepared to disclose an electronic copy of the patient information if the research records are part of the designated record set (HHS-NIH 2014). This information should be addressed within the organization's uses and disclosures of protected health information policy and procedure.

The one exception to access to research records is if a patient is part of a **clinical trial**. During a clinical trial while the research is in progress, the organization may suspend access to the records due to the fact that the individual cannot know if he or she is part of the placebo or controlled group (HHS-NIH 2014). In this scenario, documentation would need to exist regarding temporary restriction to the information and the covered entity or business associate would need to inform the participant of the temporary denial of access to that information (HHS-NIH 2014). Once the clinical trial has been concluded and is no longer active, the temporary suspension to access of those records would be eliminated and the patient would have access to those records.

Accounting of Disclosures for Protected Health Information

Another patient right that is impacted by research is the right to an accounting of disclosures. Under HIPAA's Privacy Rule, an individual is able to request a report of where his or her PHI has been disclosed for the previous six years, or a shorter time period if requested, which is referred to as an **accounting of disclosure**. An accounting of disclosures does not need to be maintained if the disclosure was made for the following reasons:

- For treatment, payment, or healthcare operations
- Under a valid authorization for disclosure
- To an individual about himself or herself
- As part of a limited data set where a data use agreement is established
- Prior to April 14, 2003 (HHS-NIH 2014)

If a patient requests an accounting of disclosures, the healthcare organization or covered entity must respond to the request within 60 days. The report must include at a minimum (1) date the disclosure was made; (2) name and address of person or entity receiving the PHI; (3) brief description of the PHI disclosed; and (4) brief statement of the purpose of the disclosure (HHS-NIH 2014). If the covered entity or business associate has made multiple disclosures to the same person or entity for the same purpose, the accounting can be listed once on the report with the initial date of the disclosure, the frequency or number of disclosures, and the last date of the disclosure (HHS-NIH 2014). If the disclosure of information for research purposes falls into the definition of accounting of disclosures, the covered entity must assure that the disclosure for research purposes is included in a patient's accounting for disclosure.

Review Exercises

Instructions: Choose the best answer.

1. True or False: The HIPAA Omnibus Rule allows for authorization of future research studies through compound authorizations.

2. What are the main sections of the HIPAA Security Rule?
   a. Technical, administrative, physical and system-wide safeguards
   b. Physical, technical, administrative, and organizational safeguards
   c. Administrative, organizational, technical, and privacy safeguards
   d. Organizational, technical, physical, and system-wide safeguards

3. Which of the following does not establish requirements for human subjects research?
   a. Centers for Medicare and Medicaid Services
   b. HIPAA Privacy Rule
   c. Food and Drug Administration
   d. None of the above

4. Which of the following are the two methods of deidentification described by the HIPAA Privacy Rule?
   a. Expert determination and limited data sets
   b. Expert determination and safe harbor method
   c. Safe harbor method and data use agreements
   d. Data use agreements and limited data sets

5. True or False: A covered entity is not allowed to create a unique list for deidentified patient data for the purpose of internal reidentification.

6. What are two patient rights under the HIPAA Privacy Rule as it relates to the use of PHI and research?
   a. Access to protected health information and accounting of disclosures
   b. Access to protected health information and deidentification
   c. Accounting of disclosures and amendment to protected health information
   d. Accounting of disclosures and deidentification

7. True or False: With the final HIPAA Omnibus Rule of 2013, if an unauthorized use or disclosure of protected health occurs with a limited data set, a breach investigation needs to be completed.

8. Which of the following is not one of the 18 identifiers that must be removed for the safe harbor method of deidentification?
   a. Health plan beneficiary numbers
   b. Device identifiers and serial numbers
   c. Web universal resource locators (URLs)
   d. Medical record report name

9. Which of the following are some common features designed to protect confidentiality of health information contained in patient medical records?
   a. Locks on medical record rooms
   b. Passwords to access computerized record
   c. Rules that prohibit employees from looking at records unless they have a need to know
   d. All of the above

10. What type of protected health information is protected by the HIPAA Security Rule?
    a. Paper
    b. Electronic
    c. Oral communication
    d. All of the above

References

Amatayakul, M. 2002. United under HIPAA: A comparison of arrangements and agreements. *Journal of AHIMA* 73(8): 24A–24D.

American Health Information Management Association. 2013. Analysis of Modifications to the HIPAA Privacy, Security, Enforcement, and Breach Notification Rules under the Health Information Technology for Economic and Clinical Health Act and the Genetic Information Nondiscrimination Act; Other Modification to the HIPAA Rules. http://library.ahima.org/xpedio/groups/public/documents/ahima/bok1_050067.pdf

American Health Information Management Association. 2012. Appendix A: Authorization Checklist—Required Elements. http://library.ahima.org/xpedio/groups/public/documents/ahima/bok1_049362.hcsp?dDocName=bok1_049362

American Health Information Management Association. 2001. Final Rule for Standards for Privacy of Individually Identifiable Health Information: What the Rule Covers. http://library.ahima.org/xpedio/groups/public/docments/ahima/bok1_001146.hcsp?dDocName=bok1_001146

American Health Information Management Association/Healthcare Information and Management Systems Society HIE Privacy and Security Work Group. 2011. The Privacy and Security Gaps in Health Information Exchanges [white paper]. http://library.ahima.org/xpedio/groups/public/documents/ahima/bok1_049023.pdf

Boerner, C. 2009. Breach notification, new regulations, and HIPAA privacy and security. *Journal of Health Care Compliance* 11(6):25–26, 69.

Department of Health and Human Services. n.d. Summary of the HIPAA Security Rule. http://www.hhs.gov/ocr/privacy/hipaa/understanding/srsummary.html

Department of Health and Human Services. 2013. Research. http://www.hhs.gov/ocr/privacy/hipaa/understanding/special/research/

Department of Health and Human Services. 2003. Business Associates. http://www.hhs.gov/ocr/privacy/hipaa/understanding/coveredentities/businessassociates.html

Department of Health and Human Services. 2012. Guidance Regarding Methods for Deidentification of Protected Health Information in Accordance with the Health Insurance Portability and Accountability Act (HIPAA) Privacy Rule. http://www.hhs.gov/ocr/privacy/hipaa/understanding/coveredentities/De-identification/hhs_deid_guidance.pdf

Department of Health and Human Services. 2015. Notice to the Secretary of HHS: Breach of Unsecured Protected Health Information. https://ocrportal.hhs.gov/ocr/breach/wizard_breach.jsf?faces-redirect=true

Department of Health and Human Services–National Institutes of Health. 2014. How Can Covered Entities Use and Disclosure Protected Health Information for Research and Comply with the Privacy Rule? http://privacyruleandresearch.nih.gov/pr_08.asp

Dimick, C. 2010. No harm done? Assessing risk of harm under the federal breach notification rule. *Journal of AHIMA* 81(8):20–25.

Gunn, P.P., A.M. Fremont, M. Bottrell, L.R. Shugarman, J. Galegher, and T. Bikson. 2004. The Health Insurance Portability and Accountability Act Privacy Rule: A practical guide for researchers. *Medical Care* 42(4):321–327.

HIPAA. 1996. Health Insurance Portability and Accountability Act of 1996. In *Pub. L. No. 104-191, 110 Stat. 1936.*

Kastel, G.M. 2013. HITECH Final Rule Results in Significant Changes to HIPAA Provisions. http://www.faegrebd.com/19470

Kempfert, A.E. and B.D. Reed. 2011. Health care reform in the United States: HITECH Act and HIPAA privacy, security, and enforcement issues. *FDCC Quarterly* 61(3):240–273.

Key Health Alliance. n.d. Healthcare Data Analytics Portal. http://www.khareach.org/portal/data-analytics

LaTour, K.M., S. Eichenwald Maki, and P.K. Oachs. 2013. *Health Information Management: Concepts, Principles and Practice*. Chicago, IL: AHIMA.

US Food and Drug Administration. 2014. Institutional Review Boards Frequently Asked Questions—Information Sheet. http://www.fda.gov/RegulatoryInformation/Guidances/ucm126420.htm

Warner, D. 2013. Regulations Governing Research (2013 update). American Health Information Management Association. http://bok.ahima.org/doc?oid=300270#.VL1fOkfF-So

Williams, E.D. 2005. *Federal Protection for Human Research Subjects: An Analysis of the Common Rule and Its Interactions with FDA Regulations and the HIPAA Privacy Rule*. Washington, DC: Library of Congress, Congressional Research Service.

Chapter 3

Introduction to Data Analytics: Tools, Techniques, and Data

David Marc, MBS, CHDA and Ryan Sandefer, MA, CPHIT

Learning Objectives

- Explain the principles of the data analytics process
- Distinguish open source and free software
- Identify the criteria of open source software
- Differentiate primary and secondary data analysis
- Explain the principles of the open government initiative

Key Terms

Data analytics
Open Government Initiative
Open source software
Primary data analysis
Secondary data analysis

Healthcare is an increasingly data-driven enterprise. According to one estimate, the amount of healthcare data collected in 2012 was approximately 500 petabytes, "or the equivalent of the contents of 10 billion four-drawer file cabinets. By 2020 this amount will likely increase to 25,000 petabytes, or the equivalent of the contents of 500 billion file cabinets" (Roski et al. 2014). This massive amount of data is being looked at to address the issue of rising healthcare costs and issues related to poor-quality outcomes. In order to leverage the value of these data, organizations need to be able to analyze the data using a variety of techniques.

Data analytics is defined as "the task of transforming, summarizing, or modeling data to allow the user to make meaningful conclusions. Data analysis may be characterized as turning data into information that may be used for operational decision making" (White 2013). Data analysts have the knowledge and expertise to "acquire, manage, analyze, interpret, and transform data" (White 2015).

A critical component of data analytics is the ability to aggregate data across multiple sources in order to gain value. This aggregation requires software and statistical knowledge. Others call this big data analysis and define it as "technologies (for example, database and data mining tools) and techniques (for example, analytical methods) that a company can employ to analyze large scale, complex data for various applications intended to augment firm performance in various dimensions" (Kwon et al. 2014).

Data analysis can be either primary or secondary. That is, data can either be analyzed for the primary reason that they are collected (for example, a lab test) (**primary data analysis**) or they can be analyzed for any other reason (for example, clinical quality measures). This text deals solely with **secondary data analysis**. Data analysis can also be divided into two main categories—descriptive and inferential statistics. Descriptive statistics relate to the distribution of the data, and inferential statistics relate to a variety of techniques that can be used to draw conclusions regarding the population of interest based upon a sample of data. Data analysis can be further broken down into exploratory data analysis that can be used to identify patterns in data and also predictive modeling that uses historical data to predict future outcomes (White 2013). This textbook will employ all of these types of analysis.

There are a variety of ways to approach data analysis; however, this text will focus on a six-step process (similar to the CRISP-DM process described in chapter 1) within a typical analysis project:

1. Problem understanding: Understand the goals and objectives or the project and develop a research question; identify the data that will be used to answer the research question and develop hypotheses
2. Data extraction: Extract or obtain relevant data to answer the research question
3. Data preparation: Prepare the extracted data for a formal analysis
4. Descriptive statistics: Apply basic descriptive statistics to summarize the data in the data set
5. Statistical analyses: Use inferential statistics to answer the research question and make conclusions regarding the proposed hypotheses
6. Dissemination: Summarize findings and disseminate results (Williams 2011; Azevedo 2008)

Each of these six steps will be discussed in detail in the remainder of the chapter.

This book focuses on three main areas of data analysis using an integrated, problem-solving approach: relational databases using MySQL, data preparation using Excel, and data analysis and statistics using RStudio. The book integrates the three main areas through the lens of conducting research projects using secondary data sources. Chapters walk readers through each step of the process in an effort to address a research problem.

Problem Understanding

The US federal government is a major generator of data, including healthcare data, and the government understands the potential of using these data for improving the performance of federal operations. "Federal agencies spent about $4.9 billion on Big Data resources in fiscal 2012 and the annual amount of such spending is expected to grow substantially through 2017" (Higgins 2013).

A major component of this effort is making federal data available to the American public for analysis. President Barack Obama has signed the "Memorandum for the Heads of Executive Departments and Agencies: Transparency and Open Government," which outlined the "Open Government Directive" (Sunstein 2011). There are myriad reasons for and benefits of making these data available. For example,

> Smart disclosures can help consumers to find and use relevant data, including data about the effect of their own past choices and those of others, to make decisions that reflect their individualized needs, and to revise and improve those decisions over time or as new circumstances arise.... Smart disclosure initiatives can help promote innovation, economic growth, and job creation in the market for consumer tools. Smart disclosure of consumer data yields other benefits, including allowing consumers to monitor more easily the accuracy and use of the information that companies hold on them. (Sunstein 2011)

A major component of the **Open Government Initiative** is to publish government information online. The initiative aims to "increase accountability, promote informed participation by the public, and create economic opportunity; each agency shall take prompt steps to expand access to information by making it available online in open formats" (Orszag 2009). The program required each federal agency to publish three high-quality data sets online within 45 days of the directive. The data sets could not have been previously available in downloadable format and were required to be made available on Data.gov (Orszag 2009).

As of January 5, 2015, there are 138,377 data sets published by 90 federal agencies and subagencies. On the associated HealthData.gov website, there are 1,676 data sets categorized as "health" related. The utility of these data sets is ultimately endless. Software developers can use the data to develop and test websites and mobile applications, consumers can use the data to better understand their communities and healthcare providers, and researchers can use the data for any number of projects.

For the purpose of this book, numerous publicly available data sets have been obtained from the Centers for Medicare and Medicaid Services, US Census, Office of the National Coordinator for Health Information Technology, Environmental Protection Agency, Centers for Disease Control and Prevention, and the Minnesota Department of Health. These disparate data sets have been aggregated into one relational database that is used for all analyses included.

Data Extraction

Once a problem is identified, it is critical to obtain data that allows a researcher or analyst to make meaningful conclusions regarding the questions that are posed. Data are available in many formats, and there is an increasing amount of data made available in the public domain. In healthcare, data are often stored in relational databases for efficiency purposes (it is more efficient to link related fields than to have redundant data), and therefore in order to make the data useful for analysis they must be extracted from these data storage systems, like a MySQL database. In an effort to combine these two areas (public data and relational databases), this textbook has been constructed around using a MySQL database populated with publicly available data.

Data can be stored in MySQL databases in multiple formats. Databases consist of multiple tables, each table containing different attributes. Each attribute of a table can be stored in different data formats. The tables are synonymous to a spreadsheet of data, and the attributes are synonymous to the columns within a spreadsheet. Table 3.1 describes some of the most common data types contained in MySQL databases.

For the purposes of this textbook, chapters 6 through 16 involve a formal research question that involves extracting data from this database using MySQL Workbench and MySQL queries. The queries range from simple to complex. Each chapter demonstrates the process for identifying the elements that are

Table 3.1. Common MySQL data types and descriptions

Data Type	Description	Example
Character Data		
CHAR	Contains binary data of variable length up to 64 kilobytes. When you enter variables of this type into columns, you must insert them as character strings.	F (for female)
VARCHAR	Contains character string data with a length of n, where n is a value from 1 to 255.	Attested (for physicians who have attested for meaningful use)
TEXT	Contains text data of variable length up to 64 kilobytes.	Duluth (for city name)
Numeric Data		
INT	Specifies an integer value, where n indicates the display width for the data. You might experience problems with MySQL if the data column contains values that are larger than the value of n. Values for INT can range from −2147483648 to 2147483647.	150 (for number of hospital discharges)
BIGINT	Specifies an integer value, where n indicates the display width for the data. You might experience problems with MySQL if the data column contains values that are larger than the value of n. Values for BIGINT can range from −9223372036854775808 to 9223372036854775808.	2000 (for number of uninsured individuals by county)
DOUBLE	Specifies a decimal number where there are numbers before and after a decimal point. Values can range from approximately −1.8E308 to −2.2E308 and 2.2E308 to 1.8E308.	0.04 (for hospital readmission ratio)

Source: SAS n.d.

required to answer the posed research question and explains the queries that are used to extract the information from tables within the MySQL database.

Data Preparation

After the data are extracted from a data source, a process is typically required to prepare them for analysis. This process includes identifying any erroneous values that exist in the data in an effort to normalize the data set. It is critical to identify and remove these values from the data set because of the impact that they can have on the analysis. For example, if there are numerical values included in the data set that represent nonnumeric measures, such as 9999.99 representing unknown, it is very important to remove them as they could significantly impact statistics such as mean, median, standard deviation, and so on. Similarly, a nonnumeric value included in a numeric data set can cause problems, such as "not available" or "NA." If these values are not removed, the results of the analysis may be impacted negatively.

In addition to normalizing the data, data that are extracted from databases often need to be transformed to make them either meaningful or more useful for interpreting the results. For example, rather than comparing 30 different types of physician specialties, an analyst may consider combining types of specialties into much fewer and more meaningful groups that can be used for drawing comparisons. This would require recoding the data.

There are a variety of techniques for preparing data for analysis. For the purpose of this textbook, data that are extracted from MySQL is prepared using Microsoft Excel. Erroneous or filler data is removed in multiple chapters by using Excel functions or Excel's find and replace feature. Data are recoded in Excel using Excel functions (such as IF or find and replace). Figures 3.1 and 3.2 illustrate how Excel's IF function can be used to recode a data set related to hospital readmissions in an effort to categorize those hospitals that are higher than the national average regarding readmission rates as "Higher than Average" and those that are lower than the national average as "Lower than Average." This recoding also allows us to convert the NULL values from

Figure 3.1.　Using Excel to recode readmission data—raw data

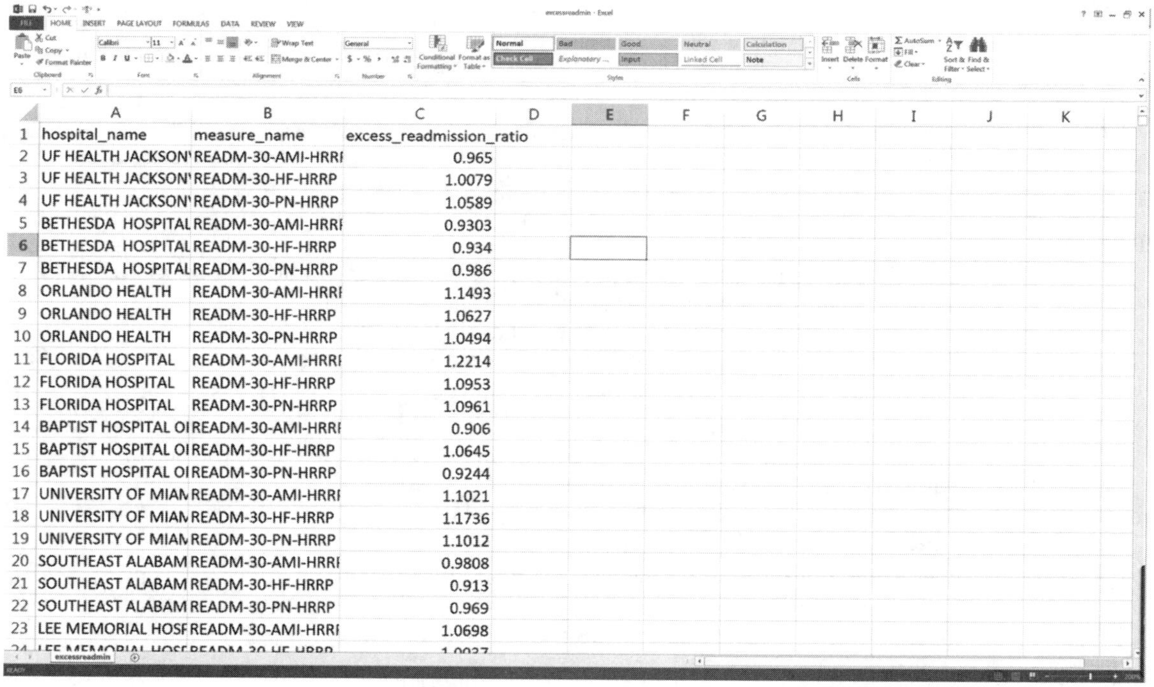

Source: Used with permission from Microsoft.

Figure 3.2. Using Excel to recode readmission data—recoded data using IF function

hospital_name	measure_name	excess_readmission_ratio	Readmission Recoded
UF HEALTH JACKSON	READM-30-AMI-HRRP	0.965	Lower than Average
UF HEALTH JACKSON	READM-30-HF-HRRP	1.0079	Higer than Average
UF HEALTH JACKSON	READM-30-PN-HRRP	1.0589	Higer than Average
BETHESDA HOSPITAL	READM-30-AMI-HRRP	0.9303	Lower than Average
BETHESDA HOSPITAL	READM-30-HF-HRRP	0.934	Lower than Average
BETHESDA HOSPITAL	READM-30-PN-HRRP	0.986	Lower than Average
ORLANDO HEALTH	READM-30-AMI-HRRP	1.1493	Higer than Average
ORLANDO HEALTH	READM-30-HF-HRRP	1.0627	Higher than Average
ORLANDO HEALTH	READM-30-PN-HRRP	1.0494	Higher than Average
FLORIDA HOSPITAL	READM-30-AMI-HRRP	1.2214	Higer than Average
FLORIDA HOSPITAL	READM-30-HF-HRRP	1.0953	Higer than Average
FLORIDA HOSPITAL	READM-30-PN-HRRP	1.0961	Higer than Average
BAPTIST HOSPITAL OI	READM-30-AMI-HRRP	0.906	Lower than Average
BAPTIST HOSPITAL OI	READM-30-HF-HRRP	1.0645	Higer than Average
BAPTIST HOSPITAL OI	READM-30-PN-HRRP	0.9244	Lower than Average
UNIVERSITY OF MIAN	READM-30-AMI-HRRP	1.1021	Higer than Average
UNIVERSITY OF MIAN	READM-30-HF-HRRP	1.1736	Higer than Average
UNIVERSITY OF MIAN	READM-30-PN-HRRP	1.1012	Higer than Average
SOUTHEAST ALABAM	READM-30-AMI-HRRP	0.9808	Lower than Average
SOUTHEAST ALABAM	READM-30-HF-HRRP	0.913	Lower than Average
SOUTHEAST ALABAM	READM-30-PN-HRRP	0.969	Lower than Average
LEE MEMORIAL HOSF	READM-30-AMI-HRRP	1.0698	Higer than Average
LEE MEMORIAL HOSF	READM-30-HF-HRRP	1.0037	Higer than Average

Source: Used with permission from Microsoft.

"NULL" to blank cells. Rather than having a range of numeric values related to each hospital's readmission rate, recoding the data allows us to create two groups for comparison.

Descriptive Statistics

Once the data have been extracted, normalized, and transformed, they are ready for analysis. The first task of the data analyst should be to become comfortable with the data set that is being analyzed, including the particular variables of interest. Conducting descriptive statistics is a method for providing an overall summary of the data. Descriptive statistics are defined as "a set of statistical techniques used to describe data such as means, frequency distributions, and standard deviations" and "they provide statistical information that describes the characteristics of a specific group or a population" (AHIMA 2014). By conducting these analyses that describe the different data elements at a high level, it is possible to determine:

- If there are issues with the data such as abnormal distribution (in other words, are the data skewed in some way)
- If there are discernable differences in the data that assist with understanding the problem being addressed or potentially modifying the question of interest

There are a variety of descriptive statistics that can be conducted depending on the type of data being analyzed. Table 3.2 summarizes the most common data types and associated analyses for each.

In the use cases provided in this book, the prepared data from Excel will be imported into RStudio for analysis. Within the RStudio environment, users will be asked to produce a variety of data summaries such as mean, median, mode, standard deviation, and quartiles. In addition to describing the data in statistical summary formats, users will also be asked to create a variety of data visualizations to describe the data. These data visualizations include boxplots, histograms, scatterplots, and barplots.

Table 3.2. Data types and descriptive statistics

Data Type	Description	Example	Appropriate Descriptive Statistics
Nominal	Categorical data where the categories are mutually exclusive but do not have natural order	Gender, HCPCS, department, or unit	Frequency counts, proportions, mode
Ordinal	Categorical data where the categories are mutually exclusive and they do have a natural order	Patient satisfaction scores, severity scores, trauma center level, surveys measured on a Likert scale	Frequency counts, proportions, mode, range
Interval	Naturally numeric data where the distance between two values has meaning, but multiplying values and zero value has no interpretation	Temperature, pH level, dates	Mean, median, standard deviation, range
Ratio	Naturally numeric data where zero has an interpretation and the values may be doubles or multiplied by a constant and still have meaning	Charges, length of stay, age	Mean, median, standard deviation, range, geometric mean, coefficient of variation

Source: LaTour et al. 2013, 527.

Statistical Analysis

The next step in the process is to conduct statistical analyses to test for significance, using a variety of inferential statistics as well as data mining and exploratory data analysis techniques to help answer research questions. Table 3.3 describes the statistical procedures used in this book, including their definitions, comparative measure, and each chapter that employs the specific statistical procedure.

Dissemination

The final step in the analytics process is to disseminate the findings. Once the statistics have been calculated, it is important to interpret the results and draw conclusions. Each chapter included in part II of this textbook includes a discussion section where the authors interpret the data and draw conclusions about the importance of the findings. One important aspect of drawing conclusions and disseminating findings is visualizing the data to improve understanding. Throughout this textbook, data visualizations are created with RStudio to assist in highlighting and presenting results. The data visualizations include boxplots, barplots, scatterplots, and other advanced visualization techniques such as dotplots and heat maps. Table 3.4 provides an example of data visualizations, including the chapter where the data visualization is created.

Open Source and Free Software

Open source software is also used in this textbook. **Open source software** is

> Software that can be freely used, changed, and shared (in modified or unmodified form) by anyone. There are a variety of benefits of using open source technology, including customization, lower cost, and the community of users that support the product. Open source software is made by many people, and distributed under licenses that comply with the open source definition. (OSI 2015)

Table 3.3.   Overview of statistical procedures

Procedure	Definition	When to Use	Chapter(s) That Employ the Statistic
One-sample *t*-test	Assesses whether the means of a group is statistically different from a population mean	Appropriate when comparing a sample statistic (mean) to a known population statistic (mean)	3
Two-sample *t*-test	Assesses whether the means of two groups are statistically different from each other	Appropriate when comparing the means of two groups	8
One-way ANOVA	Assess whether the means (variance) of two or more groups are statistically different from each other	Test used to determine the differences among two or more means when there is a single factor	10, 11
Two-way ANOVA	Assess whether the means (variance) of two or more groups are statistically different from each other	Test used to determine the differences among two or more means when there are multiple factors	8
Simple linear regression	Statistical technique that uses an independent variable to predict the value of a dependent variable	Appropriate when using one quantitative predictor variable to predict one quantitative dependent variable	8, 10, 13, 14
Multiple linear regression	Statistical technique used to quantify the relationship between an outcome and multiple explanatory variables	Appropriate when using multiple quantitative predictor variables to predict one quantitative dependent variable	16
Simple logistic regression	Probability modeling technique that uses multivariate data (quantitative and categorical) for predicting the odds or likelihood of a binary dependent variable.	Appropriate when there are numerous predictor variables predicting a binary response (dependent) variable)	9
Chi-Square	Used to test for relationships between categorical variables	Appropriate when the data are categorical, the observations are independent, the groups are mutually exclusive, and there must be at least five expected frequencies in each categorical variable	7
Exploratory data analysis	Aims to depict data graphically to help identify outliers, detect trends and patterns, and suggest hypotheses for formal testing	Appropriate when visualizing data to suggest hypotheses to test, rather than formally testing hypotheses	6
Decision tree analysis	Data mining technique that uses characteristics of the data—"roots," "branches," and "leaves"—to predict outcomes or decisions	Appropriate when attempting to predict future events and when deploying models.	15

Table 3.4. Data visualizations

Data Visualization Type	Description	Sample
Boxplot	Charts the median, 25th percentile, 75th percentile, mean, minimum, and maximum values. If the value is 1.5× the IQR (75th percentile–25th percentile) it is considered an outlier and is shown as a point outside the whisker.	
Barplot or histogram	Charts the frequency of data points (y-axis) based upon a particular measure of interest (x-axis).	
Scatterplot	Plots a point for two different numeric variables for each observation of interest.	
Dotplot	Similar to a histogram, plots the frequency of observations for a given variable in a data set.	

(Continued)

Table 3.4. Data visualizations (Continued)

Data Visualization Type	Description	Sample
Heat map	Plots all data points as a cell for two given variables of interest and, depending on frequency of observations in each cell, provides color to visualize high or low frequency.	
Correlation matrix	Creates a table of numeric variables and, depending on measure of correlation between the variables, the color changes to represent strength.	

Source: Samples used with permission from RStudio.

Open source software is used throughout this textbook with R statistical software and MySQL Workbench. In addition to requiring that the software source code is available, the Open Source Initiative, an organization that reviews and approves open source software, requires that 10 criteria must be met for an organization to be deemed "open source." These criteria are

1. Free redistribution: The license shall not restrict any party from selling or giving away the software as a component of an aggregate software distribution containing programs from several different sources. The license shall not require a royalty or other fee for such sale.

2. Source code: The program must include source code, and must allow distribution in source code as well as compiled form. Where some form of a product is not distributed with source code, there must be a well-publicized means of obtaining the source code for no more than a reasonable reproduction cost, preferably downloading via the Internet without charge. The source code must be the preferred form in which a programmer would modify the program. Deliberately obfuscated source code is not allowed. Intermediate forms such as the output of a preprocessor or translator are not allowed.

3. Derived works: The license must allow modifications and derived works, and must allow them to be distributed under the same terms as the license of the original software.

4. Integrity of the author's source code: The license may restrict source-code from being distributed in modified form only if the license allows the distribution of "patch files" with the source code for the purpose of modifying the program at build time. The license must explicitly permit distribution of software built from modified source code. The license may require derived works to carry a different name or version number from the original software.

5. No discrimination against persons or groups: The license must not discriminate against any person or group of persons.

6. No discrimination against fields of endeavor: The license must not restrict anyone from making use of the program in a specific field of endeavor. For example, it may not restrict the program from being used in a business or from being used for genetic research.

7. Distribution of license: The rights attached to the program must apply to all to whom the program is redistributed without the need for execution of an additional license by those parties.

8. License must not be specific to a product: The rights attached to the program must not depend on the program's being part of a particular software distribution. If the program is extracted from that distribution and used or distributed within the terms of the program's license, all parties to whom the program is redistributed should have the same rights as those that are granted in conjunction with the original software distribution.

9. License must not restrict other software: The license must not place restrictions on other software that is distributed along with the licensed software. For example, the license must not insist that all other programs distributed on the same medium must be open-source software.

10. License must be technology-neutral: No provision of the license may be predicated on any individual technology or style of interface. (OSI 2015)

The R statistical software is considered an open source technology; the code is made available and can be modified by developers. There are currently thousands of packages that have been developed by the R developer community. MySQL Workbench is also considered open source technology. This application is used for housing this textbook's relational database and is used in most book chapters.

Unlike open source software, free software is developed and owned by a person or organization that holds the copyright to the product but the product is made freely available for download and use. There is a growing amount of health data analytics free software available for use by individuals. The major difference between open source software and free software is the ability to customize the software by having access to the source code.

Review Exercises

Instructions: Choose the best answer.

1. Which of the following is not a component of the data analytics process?
   a. Software testing
   b. Dissemination
   c. Data extraction
   d. Data preparation

2. If you are attempting to identify if the average hospital readmission rate for a particular hospital in Duluth, MN, is different than the state of Minnesota's average hospital readmission rate, which of the following statistical procedures is most appropriate?
   a. Two sample *t*-test
   b. One sample *t*-test
   c. One-way ANOVA
   d. Simple linear regression

3. What type of graph is shown here?

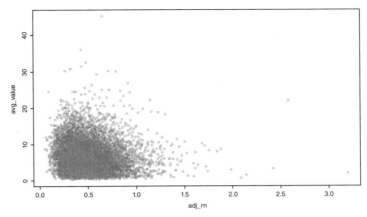

a. Barplot
b. Scatterplot
c. Dotplot
d. Boxplot

4. True or False: Data stored in the DOUBLE format within MySQL databases are character data.

5. True or False: Boxplots are able to provide the median, mean, and maximum values on one chart.

References

AHIMA. 2014. *Health Data Analysis Toolkit*. Chicago, IL: American Health Information Management Association.

Azevedo, A.I.R.L. 2008. KDD, SEMMA and CRISP-DM: A parallel overview. Proceedings of the IADIS European Conference on Data Mining, Amsterdam, The Netherlands, July 24–26.

Higgins, J.K. 2013. Feds to spend big on big data. *E Commerce Times*. http://www.ecommercetimes.com/story/77690.html

Kwon, O., N. Lee, and B. Shin. 2014. Data quality management, data usage experience and acquisition intention of big data analytics. *International Journal of Information Management* 34(3):387–394.

LaTour, K.M., S. Eichenwald Maki, and P.K. Oachs. 2013. *Health Information Management: Concepts, Principles and Practice*. Chicago, IL: AHIMA.

Open Source Initiative. 2015. Open Source Initiative. http://opensource.org

Orszag, P.R. 2009. Memorandum for the Heads of Executive Departments and Agencies. Washington, DC: Executive Office of the President Office of Management and Budget. https://www.whitehouse.gov/sites/default/files/omb/assets/memoranda_2010/m10-06.pdf

Roski, J., G.W. Bo-Linn, and T.A. Andrews. 2014. Creating value in health care through big data: Opportunities and policy implications. *Health Affairs* 33(7):1115–1122.

SAS. n.d. Data Types for MySQL. Cary, NC: SAS Institute. http://support.sas.com/documentation/cdl/en/ds2ref/68052/HTML/default/viewer.htm#p0rwlzs0gt9isyn1h5t4z1oekt5x.htm

Sunstein, C.R. 2011. Memorandum for the heads of executive department and agencies. Washington, DC: Executive Office of the President Office of Management and Budget. https://www.whitehouse.gov/sites/default/files/omb/memoranda/2011/m11-15.pdf

White, S. 2013. *A Practical Approach to Analyzing Healthcare Data*, 2nd ed. Chicago, IL: AHIMA.

White, S. 2015. *Certified Health Data Analyst (CHDA) Exam Preparation*. Chicago, IL: AHIMA.

Williams, G. 2011. *Data Mining with Rattle and R: The Art of Excavating Data for Knowledge Discovery*. New York: Springer.

Chapter 4

Introduction to MySQL

Piper Svensson-Ranallo, PhD

Learning Objectives

- Explain the difference between a database and a database management system (DBMS)
- Summarize key relational database concepts
- Interpret the entity-relationship diagram (ERD) and UML diagram
- Use MySQL to retrieve and update data from the textbook database
- Explain the role of the data dictionary in managing a database and use the textbook data dictionary to guide data retrieval

Key Terms

Attribute
Cardinality
Data dictionary
Database
Database management system (DBMS)
Entity
Entity-relationship diagram
Flat file database
Model
MySQL Workbench
Relation
Relational database
Structured Query Language (SQL)
Tuple
Unified Modeling Language (UML) model

This chapter provides a brief introduction to databases—what they are and why they are used. It also discusses how a database differs from other strategies for storing data and will present some common design approaches. The focus is on one specific type of database called a relational database.

This chapter introduces different ways to create a graphical representation, or model, of a database; and discusses the symbols (and their meanings) used in these models. The entity relationship diagram (ERD) is the type of model most commonly used to create a visual image of a database. Another document commonly used to describe a database is called a data dictionary and it plays an essential role in ensuring that the data in a database are truly meaningful. Following background information on relational databases, examples are given demonstrating how queries can be generated using the textbook database using a language called structured query language (SQL).

Relational Databases

A database is a structured collection of data related to a specific domain. For example, common database software is Microsoft Excel. A spreadsheet is a specific kind of database called a **flat file database**. Some of the disadvantages of this way of storing data include the following:

- Multiple users cannot access and modify the file simultaneously.
- It can be hard to keep track of versions in single flat files.
- Flat files do not support large volumes of data well.
- It is hard to pull data out of these files programmatically.

An example of a flat file database that was created using Microsoft Excel is shown in figure 4.1. This database has rows and columns. The rows represent a single record or **tuple**, which is an ordered set of elements. A record in an Excel spreadsheet is the ordered set of data contained in each row. The columns represent the individual details, or attributes, of the record. The first three records in the Excel file show that it is difficult to know what the record (row) is based on. Is this a record about patients or diagnoses? Is this a record about medications? The rows in this database are based on the specific medication that a patient is taking for a given diagnosis. This inability to determine the basis of the record is one of the primary disadvantages of flat file databases.

Another disadvantage of a flat file database is that the number of columns tends to expand over time as more pieces of information are added to the database. Flat file databases tend to contain large amounts of redundant data. For example, the patient ID, patient gender, and patient diagnosis need to be reentered for each new medication prescribed for the diagnosis. Whenever redundant information appears in a database, errors have to be fixed in multiple locations. For example, if the name of a medication was inadvertently misspelled, all occurrences of the medication would need to be updated in the database. Large-scale changes to data in flat file databases are very time intensive. Finally, if there is the need to limit user access to certain columns of data, this is difficult to manage in a flat file database as one would need numerous versions of the database saved for each user.

Description of Relational Databases

Relational databases were designed to avoid the limitations of database architectures like flat file types. The term *relational* refers to the specific way in which data are stored in the database. This way of storing data is based

Figure 4.1. Flat file type clinic database

Patient Id	Gender	Diagnosis	Medication	Dose
1	F	Major Depressive Disorder, Recurrent	paroxetine	20 mg
1	F	Major Depressive Disorder, Recurrent	aripiprazole	10 mg
1	F	Major Depressive Disorder, Recurrent	olanzapine	20 mg
2	M	Borderline Personality Disorder	paroxetine	40 mg
2	M	Borderline Personality Disorder	quetiapine	400 mg
3	M	Major Depressive Disorder, Recurrent		
4	M	Bipolar Disorder I, Mixed Features	aripiprazole	15 mg
5	F	Panic Disorder	paroxetine	20 mg
5	F	Panic Disorder	clonazepam	4 mg
6	M	Generalized Anxiety Disorder		
7	F	Borderline Personality Disorder	paroxetine	20 mg
7	F	Borderline Personality Disorder	gabapentin	200 mg

Rows (records, tuples)

Columns (attributes, fields)

on relational theory (Codd 1970). Relational theory specifies that the data for any database can be thought of very simply in terms of three things: the entities used to store data, the attributes of those entities, and the relations between them. In the relational model, **entities** are the nouns, or real world things, about what is used to store data. In the flat file database example shown in figure 4.1, the entities are patients, diagnoses, and medications. **Attributes** are the adjectives that describe the entities. Patients, for example, have attributes such as name, gender, race, and date of birth. Medications have attributes such as name, dose, brand, and route. Entities also have relations to each other. **Relations** are the verbs that describe how the entities are related. For example, patient *acquires* a disorder, a disorder is *treated* by a medication, and a medication is *consumed* by a patient.

When representing entities, attributes, and relations on a schematic known as an entity relation model, specific symbols are used for each database component. Figure 4.2 displays the various symbols. An entity is represented with a square; an attribute is represented with an oval; a relation is represented with a diamond. Later in the chapter how these symbols are used to develop a model for visualizing a relational database is explored.

Entities

A database is a collection of data related to a specific topic or domain. In the database for this textbook, the domain is *Quality of Healthcare in the United States*. The database can be understood as falling in this domain because all of the data are publicly available and published by federal agencies for reporting on the quality of healthcare in the United States. A relational database takes a specific approach to managing data in a domain. The first step is to identify the major entities in the domain. Entities are groups of data that represent things that exist in the real world. In the textbook domain, examples of entities include *geographic region, hospitals, nursing homes, hospital-associated infections*, and *patient deaths*. These entities are depicted in figure 4.3.

Figure 4.2.   Symbols used to depict database components

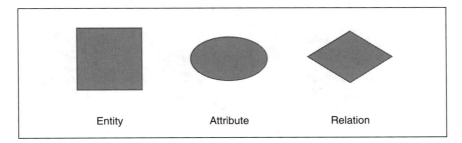

Source: Chen 1976.

Figure 4.3.   Entities in the domain

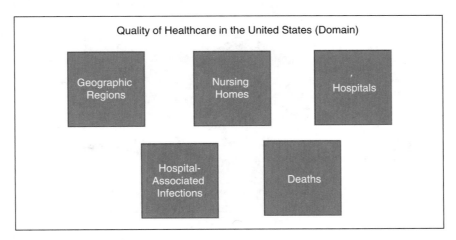

Attributes

Attributes are adjectives that describe the characteristics of the entity. For example, all patients have a name, gender, and date of birth. These attributes are intrinsic features of the patient—it is hard to think of an entity of this type that does not have these attributes as defining characteristics. Most patients also have an address, phone number, and at least one significant person who is intimately involved in their life (a guardian, a significant other, or a close friend). These features are not intrinsic attributes of the patient, and some of them can be thought of as distinct entities with specific relations to the patient entity, rather than attributes of the patient.

In the domain covered in this textbook, geographic information is an important attribute of most entities. This is because the domain covers a large geographic area, and healthcare quality may vary by geographic region. The attributes are depicted in figure 4.4.

Relations

Relations are the verbs that describe the way two entities relate to each other. For example, a patient *ingests* a medication, a medication *treats* a condition, and a provider *orders* a medication. These relations are shown in figure 4.5.

Figure 4.4.   Attributes of entities in the domain

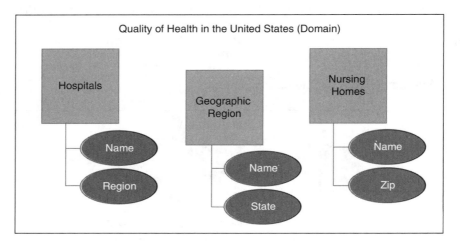

Figure 4.5.   Relations between entities in the domain

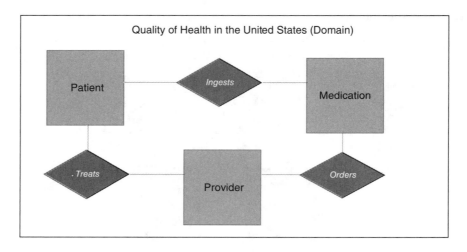

Database Diagrams

Databases are detailed and complex entities. They can have hundreds of tables, thousands of fields, and billions of rows of data. Like any complex entity, it can be easier to understand a database if there is a visual representation of it. Visual representations of databases are typically called **models**. A model helps to create an image of the overall database. A model also presents the individual pieces of the database and how these pieces fit together. It is a single source that contains all the essential information needed to understand the database.

Models give a standard way to depict and focus on the relevant information about a specific type of real-world entity, and the process of creating a model is called modeling. When it comes to databases, there are two modeling terms that are relevant. The first is ERD, and the second is **Unified Modeling Language (UML) model**. An ERD offers a visualization of the entities of a database—what attributes belong to each entity and how each entity is related. A UML model is a standard notation that can be used for depicting entities, attributes, and relations, and is used for many diagrams including an ERD.

Entity Relationship Diagrams

An **entity-relationship diagram** (ERD) is a diagram that depicts the entities and relationship between entities in a given domain. As stated previously, a database is a structured collection of data related to a specific domain. Typically, an ERD is created to represent not just the domain, but the database itself. When developing an ERD, early versions of the model may contain entities, attributes, and relationships that may not become part of the final database. However, the final ERD for a database is often the very specification that is used to build the physical database. When an ERD is converted into physical databases, the entities become tables and the attributes become columns. The relations between tables are implemented as keys in each of the two tables they connect. Keys, discussed in detail later in the chapter, are specially chosen columns in a table that help define its relationship to both to the tuple (row) and to other tables.

The diagram in figure 4.6 is one section of the larger ERD for the database used in this textbook. This ERD was generated using the ERD modeling software included with MySQL Workbench. MySQL Workbench has a design module that can aid in the development of a database. Essentially, users can create an ERD, which can be forward engineered into a database. Using the UML model notations, entities appear as squares, the attributes appear as line items within the square, and relationships appear as lines with symbols at either end of them. Some columns have a small key icon next to them, and others have a diamond icon. Columns with the key icon next to them are primary key (PK) columns, and those with red diamond icons next to them are foreign keys (FKs).

Tables and Columns

Relational databases typically create a separate table for each entity. There are four entities shown in figure 4.6 including, hospital_general_information, ipps_2011, hcahps, and readmission_reduction. If there are different instances of a specific entity in the domain that are different enough, a table for each type of entity can be created. An example of an entity that is often implemented as two different entities in a database is a patient visit. Visits to a hospital ambulatory clinic are different enough from an inpatient visit that two tables can be created: one for inpatient visits (admissions) and a separate table for outpatient visits (office visits).

Tables contain columns, or fields. The columns in a table are the attributes of the entity that the table represents. Columns in the hospital_general_information tables shown in figure 4.6 are the important attributes that describe a hospital. These attributes include the name of the hospital, address, city, state, phone number, the type of hospital, ownership type, and an indicator as to whether the hospital offers emergency services.

Relationship Cardinality

Cardinality refers to the type of relationship one table has with another table. More specifically, cardinality explains which number of records in one table can be associated with which number of records in another.

Figure 4.6. Part of the ERD for the textbook database

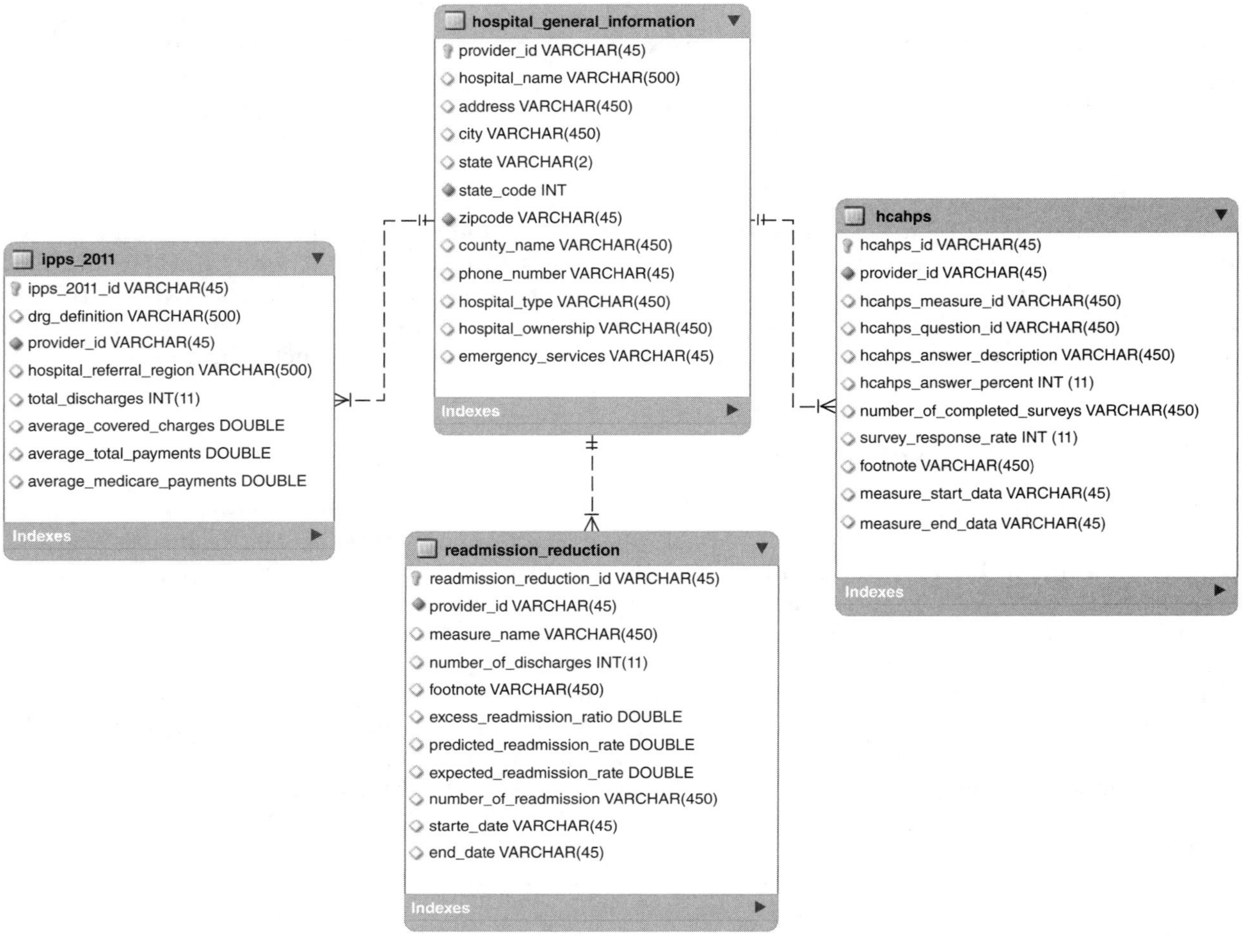

There are three basic types of relationships that can exist between two tables and are depicted with specific notations on an ERD (see figure 4.7). These are

1. One-to-one
2. One-to-many
3. Many-to-many

A one-to-one relationship means that each record in the first table is associated with one—and only one—record in the second table. Similarly, each record in the second table is associated with only one record in the first table. An example of a one-to-one relationship is the relationship between a patient table and the patient–spouse table. These kinds of relationships are rare in databases. In general, when a one-to-one relationship exists, one of the tables is extended to include the columns in the other. In the case of the patient–spouse table, a spouse column would be added to the patient table. This takes the entity "spouse" and turns it into an attribute of the patient entity. If, however, there were multiple pieces of data to store about each patient's spouse, a separate spouse table could be created.

A one-to-many relationship is a relationship in which each record in the first table is associated with many records in the second table. Each record in the second table, however, is associated with only one record in the first table. An example of a one-to-many relationship is patients and phone numbers. A patient may have many phone numbers (a home phone number, a work phone number, and a cell phone number). However, any given phone number is associated with only one patient. One-to-many relationships are

Figure 4.7. Relationship cardinality

Symbol	Meaning
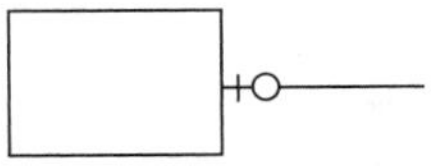	Zero or one
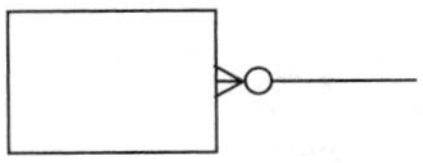	Zero, one, or many
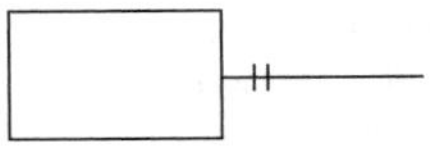	One and only one
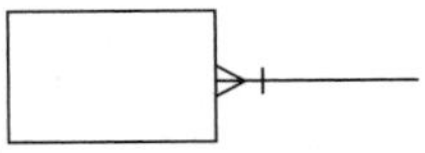	One or many

implemented by adding a column from the table on the "one side" of the relationship to the table on the "many side" of the relationship. In the example of patients and phone numbers, a column would be added to store the patient id in the phone number table.

A many-to-many relationship is one in which each record in the first table is associated with many records in the second table. Similarly, each record in the second table is associated with many records in the first table. An example of a many-to-many relationship is the relationship between patients and diagnoses. Each patient may have many diagnoses, and each diagnosis may be given to many patients. Many-to-many relationships between entities are very common. They are more complicated to implement in a database than one-to-many relationships. One-to-many relationships are implemented by adding a column from one table to the other table. Many-to-many relationships, however, require an entirely new table to manage the relationship. The relationship between patients and medications may be a many-to-many relationship. That is, a patient may have zero, one, or many medications. Similarly, a medication may be given to zero, one, or many patients. In order to manage this relationship, a third table needs to be created to store each patient–medication combination. This table will have a one-to-many relationship to the patients table, and a one-to-many relationship with the medications table. This type of table is commonly referred to as an intermediate table.

An intersect table was used in the textbook database and is shown in figure 4.8. The ep_provider_paid_ehr table includes information about providers that were paid for attesting for Meaningful Use under the electronic health record (EHR) incentive program. Many providers were paid once and some were paid more than once. The national_downloadable_file table includes information about each individual provider including their name, medical school, type of specialty, and the organization they are associated with. Some providers are listed more than once since they can be associated with more than one organization. Because a single provider may occur more than once in the ep_provider_paid_ehr table and the national_downloadable_file table there exists a many-to-many relationship. The provider_intersect table was added as an intermediate table to manage the many-to-many relationship that exists between these two tables and generate two one-to-many relationships.

Relationships between tables are depicted in models using a line with a symbol at each end. The line is either dashed or solid (more on that later) and runs between the related tables. Figure 4.7 depicts the symbols commonly used in ERD models. Note that this diagram depicts each line with a symbol at only one end. In an ERD, the symbol is placed at both ends of the line connecting the tables. Figure 4.6 shows several examples of one-to-many relationship that exist in the database used in the textbook. As shown, there is a one-to-many relationship between the hospital_general_information and hcahps tables. That is, one hospital can have one or many rows of data in the hcahps table.

Every relationship between tables is actually two relationships—the relationship of the first table to the second table, and the relationship of the second table to the first table. For example, in the relationship between the Patients and the PrimaryCareProviders table in the diagram in figure 4.9, the symbols are shown on both sides of the line joining the two tables. The "zero or one" symbol is on the PrimaryCareProvider side of

Figure 4.8. An intermediate table

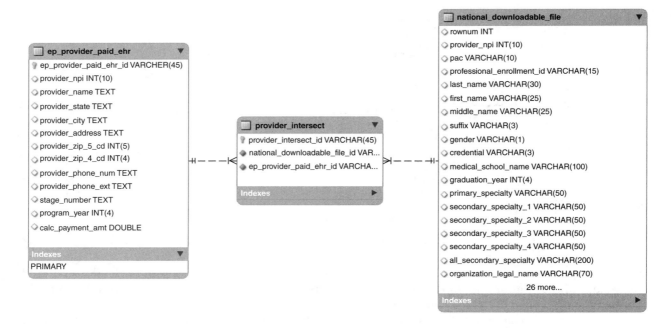

Figure 4.9. Reading the relationship between two tables

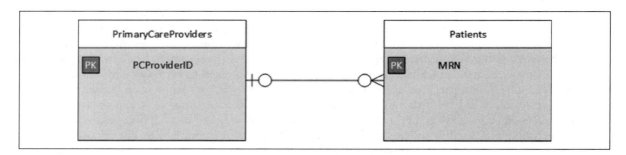

the relationship, and the "zero, one, or many" symbol is on the Patients side of the relationship. There are two relationships depicted here: the first shows how many patients a given primary care provider can have, the second shows how many primary care providers a given patient can have.

To read the relationship from the PrimaryCareProviders table to Patients table in figure 4.9, start at the PrimaryCareProvider table and follow the line to the symbol at the Patients table end of the line. At the Patients table, the symbol on the line represents zero, one, or many, which shows that each record in the PrimaryCareProvider can be related to zero, one, or many records in the Patients table. That is, a given primary care provider may have no patients, one patient, or many patients in this database. Next, read the relationship from Patients to PrimaryCareProviders, starting with the Patients table and following the line to the symbol at the PrimaryCareProvider. This symbol nearest the PrimaryCareProvider tables represents that each record in the Patients table may have either no record or one record in the PrimaryCareProvider table. That is, one patient will have only one primary care provider, but may have none.

Primary Keys

Every table in a database must have a primary key (PK). The PK is the column (or columns) that uniquely identify a record in the table. Because this column uniquely identifies the entire record, the

Figure 4.10. Primary keys

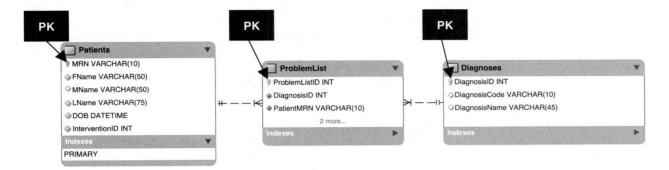

Figure 4.11. The relationship between a primary key (PK) and a foreign key (FK)

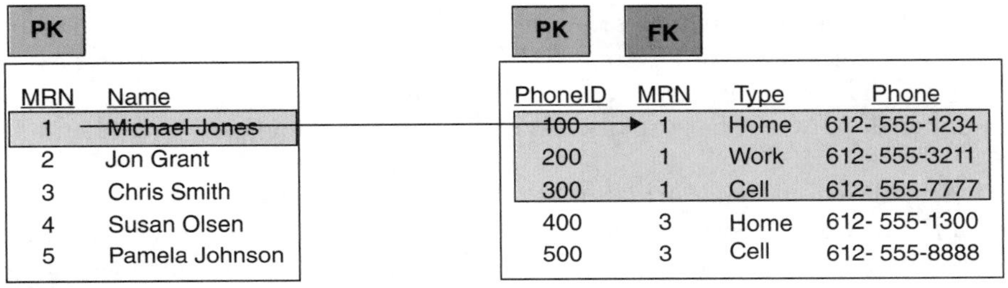

value in the PK column must be unique. Shown in figure 4.6, the PK for the Patients table is the medical record number (MRN). Each patient is given a unique MRN. The system will not allow a record to be added to the Patients table when the MRN already exists in the table. This is because the database uses the value in the MRN column to identify that particular record, or tuple. A PK cannot contain a NULL value. Some value must be entered into the column in order to create a new record.

In MySQL, PKs are identified in the data model by a golden colored key icon. Figure 4.10 shows that the MRN is the PK for the Patients table. Similarly, ProblemListID is the primary key in the ProblemList table, and DiagnosisID is the primary key in the Diagnosis table.

Foreign Keys

Foreign keys (FKs) are essential to implementing a relationship between tables. An FK is a column in one table that holds the primary key value of the table to which it is related. An FK always points to the PK in another table. If the PK in one table exists as an FK in another table, it creates a relationship between the two tables. Earlier, the example of patients and phone numbers was used as an instance of a one-to-many relationship. The way these two tables are related is by putting a column in the phone number table to store the patient ID of the patient to whom each number is related. The patients table is related to the phone number table by creating an FK column in the phone number table (see figure 4.11). This FK column contains the value of the PK for the record in the patients table to which the phone number record is related.

The Data Dictionary

A **data dictionary** is an essential tool for effectively managing and using the data in a database. A data dictionary is a structured way of documenting the data stored in a database. Data dictionaries vary in content. At minimum, a data dictionary includes the names and definitions of all entities and attributes in the database. It includes important metadata such as data type, data length, keys, and constraints. A data dictionary often includes information about the source of the data, as well as the information about any conversions or transformations the data undergo as they move from the original system to the current database.

The primary goal of creating and actively maintaining a data dictionary is to ensure that data are defined consistently and standardized throughout the system. The American Health Information Management Association (AHIMA) emphasizes the central role a data dictionary plays in improving the reliability, dependability, and trustworthiness of data use (AHIMA 2012). The data dictionary provides a source for the definition of each data element within the database, its format, and the relationship between different fields and tables. It is critical for working with data stored within the system. Figure 4.12 provides an example of the data dictionary from this textbook's database.

The data dictionary shown in figure 4.12 displays the name of the database table, a description of the table of data, and the names, data types, definition, and key information for each column of data in the table. Two tables of data are displayed. The first is the hospital_general_information table. The description states that the table contains general information on hospitals that have been registered with Medicare. The information includes a unique identifier for the hospital, name, address, city, state, zip code, county name, phone number, type, ownership type, and an indicator of offering emergency services for each hospital. The PK is the provider_id, which is a unique identifier for each hospital using the CMS Certification Number (CCN). There are two PKs including the state_code and zipcode for each hospital. The second table is called hcahps, which offers a list of hospital ratings for the Hospital Consumer Assessment of Healthcare Providers and Systems (HCAHPS) survey regarding patient experiences during inpatient hospital stays. The table includes information about the questionnaire item, the answers, the percentage and number of patients that provided specific answers, and the start and end dates of the collection period.

The data dictionary shown in figure 4.12 can be used to understand some of the data that are shown in the ERD diagram in figure 4.6. This way, when an individual is developing a query he or she can understand the definitions of each data element as well as how these data elements may be related.

Introduction to MySQL and the Textbook Database

Now that the basic concepts and components of relational databases have been introduced, the next part of the chapter will focus on a discussion of MySQL Workbench, the software that is used for working with this textbook's database.

MySQL and MySQL Workbench

MySQL Workbench is a software that allows the user to talk to a MySQL database. MySQL Workbench is not the database itself. Instead, it is an application installed on a client computer. This software allows the user to connect to, visualize, and communicate with any MySQL database (see figure 4.13). The database that is connected could be running on the same computer that MySQL Workbench is running. More often, though, it will be running on a dedicated server somewhere else. A MySQL server is just a computer with MySQL **database management system (DBMS)** software installed on it. A DBMS is software that allows the user to create and manage databases. Most DBMSs allow the user to create things other than just databases. For example, virtually all DBMSs provide tools to allow administrators to create logins, as well as rules about which databases these users can access. Each MySQL DBMS can have potentially hundreds of individual MySQL databases. For example, if a DBMS is thought of as a big island in an ocean, the individual databases would be the towns or villages on this island.

As stated earlier in the chapter, a **database** is just a structured collection of data stored in a single file. For example, a hospital has a MySQL DBMS installed on a server. On this server, a user may want to create one database to store information specific to each department. In this case, the server is running the DBMS, and the databases contain the collection of data files related to what the user wants to track for each department.

Figure 4.12. Part of the data dictionary for the textbook database

Table name: hospital_general_information

Description: General information on hospitals that have been registered with Medicare

Source: https://data.medicare.gov/data/hospital-compare

Column Name	Data Type	Definition	Key
provider_id	varchar	Unique identifier for each hospital, which corresponds to the hospital's CMS Certification Number (CCN)	PK
hospital_name	varchar	Name of the hospital	
address	varchar	Address for the hospital	
city	varchar	Name of the city where the hospital is located	
state	varchar	Abbreviated name of the state where the hospital is located	FK
state_code	int	FIPS code for the state where the hospital is located	FK
zipcode	varchar	Zip code for the hospital	
county_name	varchar	Name of the county where the hospital is located	
phone_number	varchar	Phone number for the hospital	
hospital_type	varchar	The type of hospital including Acute Care Hospital, Critical Access Hospital, Children's	
hospital_owernship	varchar	The ownership type for the hospital including Government Federal, Voluntary nonprofit—Private, Government-Hospital District or Authority, Voluntary nonprofit—Other, Proprietary, Government—State, Voluntary nonprofit—Church, Government—Federal, Government—Local, Physician, Tribal	
emergency_services	varchar	An indicator as to whether the hospital offers emergency services. Values include Yes or No.	

Table name: hcahps

Description: A list of hospital ratings for the Hospital Consumer Assessment of Healthcare Providers and Systems (HCAHPS). HCAHPS is a national, standardized survey of hospital patients about their experiences during a recent inpatient hospital stay.

Source: https://data.medicare.gov/data/hospital-compare

Column Name	Data Type	Definition	Key
hcahps_id	varchar	Unique identifier for the hcahps table data	PK
provider_id	varchar	Unique identifier for each hospital, which corresponds to the hospital's CMS Certification Number (CCN)	FK
hcahps_measure_id	varchar	Abbreviated name for each of the HCAHPS survey items	
hcahps_question	varchar	Description of the HCAHPS survey items including communication with hospital staff, responsiveness of hospital staff, pain management, communication about medicines, discharge information, cleanliness of hospital environment, quietness of hospital environment, and transition of care.	
hcahps_answer_description	varchar	Description of the answers that are available for each HCAHPS survey item	
hcahps_answer_percent	int	The percent of patients that answered with the respective hacahps_answer_description for each hcahps_question	
number_of_completed_surveys	varchar	A description of the range of the number of patients that completed the HCAHPS survey	
suvey_response_rate	int	The percentage of patients that completed the HCAHPS survey	
footnote	varchar	A description explaining why data may be missing for some records	
measure_start_date	varchar	The date when the collection of HCAHPS survey data began	
measure_end_date	varchar	The date when the collection of HCAHPS survey data ended	

Figure 4.13. How the MySQL Workbench application relates to the MySQL database

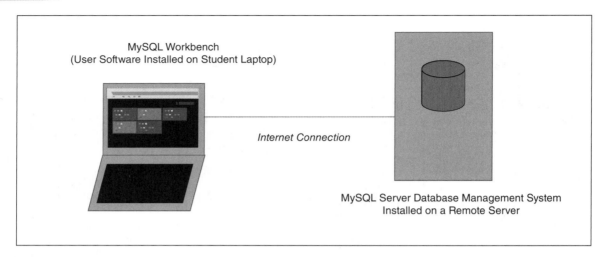

Structured Query Language

MySQL Workbench uses **Structured Query Language (SQL)** language for working with databases. SQL is the universal language of databases. No matter what database is used, an understanding of American National Standards Institute (ANSI) standard SQL, with only minor modifications, provides the ability to communicate with virtually any database in the world. All SQL databases are selective about the exact words used, as well as the order of these words. One way to become good at SQL is to memorize a few general rules about how to form good SQL sentences and practice implementing these general rules.

Anytime a user talks to a database, the user is asking it to do something for him or her. All database requests fall into one of four general categories: create, retrieve, update, and delete (CRUD) (Heller 2007). When it comes to databases, these are the only four things the user can ask the database to do. Although some requests can be far reaching, a user can only ask the database to create, retrieve, update, or delete something. This simplifies the process of learning the language, because it allows the user to create a few general SQL templates that can be used over and over. Not only can the user create a general template for each type of request, but he or she can also create a master template on which all four of the specific templates can be based.

An SQL statement can be as simple as a few words, or span your entire screen. No matter how simple or complex your SQL statement, all queries follow the same basic structure. And just like the English language is made of words formed from only 26 letters, any query imaginable can be written with about 30 basic keywords. The next section will discuss the structure of an SQL statement, starting with a simple statement and gradually reviewing more complex statements. As these examples are introduced, the most important (and commonly used) keywords in the language will be presented.

Retrieving Data
A complete SQL statement consists of a minimum of two SQL keywords: SELECT and FROM. These key words allow the user to specify the minimum information the database needs in order to retrieve data. The SELECT keyword is used to specify which column(s) contain the data to retrieve. The FROM keyword is used to specify the name of the table (or tables) in which to find where the data live. The basic SQL statement is formatted as follows:

```
SELECT <name of one or more columns>
FROM <name of table>
```

To write the SQL statement, start with the keyword SELECT. This keyword SELECT tells the database to *retrieve* data, and what follows is the list of attributes (also known as columns) containing the data to

> Figure 4.14.   Example of a basic MySQL query

```
SELECT       hospital_name,
             address,
             city,
             state
FROM         hospital_general_information;
```

retrieve. If more than one attribute is retrieved, the name of attribute is specified after the SELECT statement with a comma separating each attribute name. The comma tells the database that what follows is the name of another attribute. After the names of the attributes that will be retrieved have been listed, the keyword FROM is used next to tell the database the name of the table (or tables) where the listed attributes can be found.

For example, to know the hospital name, address, city, and state of all hospitals in the database, the first thing to do is to determine the name of the table that contains the hospital data. The next thing is to determine the name of each attribute that holds the hospital data desired for retrieval: hospital name, address, city, and state. The ERD and data dictionary is used to determine the name of the table and attributes. When reviewing the ERD data dictionary provided online with this textbook, the hospital data are stored in a table called hospital_general_information. Looking at the columns in this table (figure 4.14), the names of the columns are hospital_name, address, city and state.

Notice that a comma is included after each attribute in the SELECT statement except the last one. In a SELECT clause, the comma tells the database that the next item in the list is another attribute. The keyword FROM after the last field in the list tells the database that there are no more attributes (so a comma is not necessary). After the FROM statement, the name of the table where these attributes are found is listed. The query is terminated with a semicolon. The semicolon tells the database that the query is done and the data can be retrieved.

Filtering Data

There are several ways to filter, or limit, the data one wants to retrieve. The simplest (and most common) way to filter data is to use the WHERE clause. The WHERE clause allows the user to include conditions that must be met in order to include the data in the results. The WHERE clause always comes immediately after the FROM clause:

```
SELECT <name of one or more attributes>
FROM <name of table>
WHERE <conditions that must be met to include the data>
```

For example, the name of the hospital, address, city, and state for all hospitals in the database that are in the state of California can be retrieved by adding a WHERE clause to the query. An SQL statement, or query, has already been provided in figure 4.14 to retrieve these fields from the database. In order to limit the results to those hospitals in the state of California, a WHERE clause needs to be added. It's important that when using the WHERE clause, users specify the exact criteria. If the incorrect criteria are provided, no results may be retrieved. For instance, when reviewing the data dictionary, the attribute for state in the hospital_general_information table is written with uppercase letters as an abbreviation. Therefore, in the WHERE clause the state of California must be specified as 'CA' rather than 'California' or 'ca'. If 'CA' is not specified, zero observations will be returned. An example of the query is shown in figure 4.15.

Notice the condition state = 'CA'. For each record in the patient table, the query engine will determine whether the value in the state field meets the condition (is equal to 'CA'). If the condition is true, the record will be retrieved and included in the final data set. If the condition is false, it will not be retrieved, and will not

Figure 4.15.   Example of a MySQL query with WHERE clause

```
SELECT          hospital_name,
                address,
                city,
                state
FROM            hospital_general_information
WHERE           state= 'CA';
```

Figure 4.16.   Types of WHERE clause operators

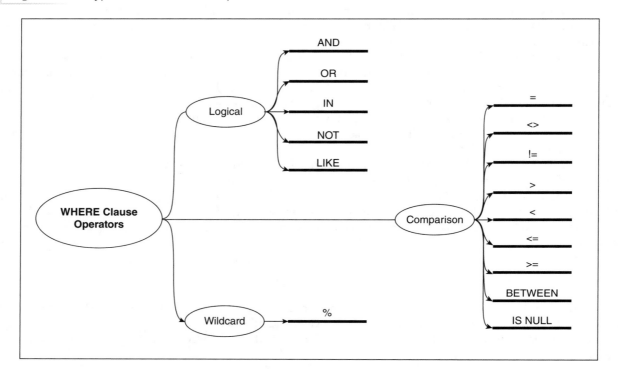

Figure 4.17.   Using the MySQL wildcard operator

```
SELECT DISTINCT  hospital_name,
                 hospital_ownership
FROM             hospital_general_information
WHERE            hospital_ownership  LIKE  '%government%';
```

appear in the result set returned by the query. In this example, the equality operator (the = sign) is used in the condition. This is a commonly used operator for the WHERE clause, but other operators are also commonly used. Figure 4.16 displays the types of operators that can be used in a WHERE clause.

Figure 4.17 shows the use of the wildcard operator. The SQL statement in figure 4.16 returns the hospital name and ownership status for all hospitals containing the string "government" as the ownership status.

In the WHERE clause, the wildcard operator (%) is used along with the logical operator LIKE to specify that the query should return all observations when the hospital_ownership includes the word "government." The hospital_ownership can take on the following values:

- Government—federal
- Voluntary nonprofit—private
- Government—hospital district or authority
- Voluntary nonprofit—other
- Proprietary
- Government—state
- Voluntary nonprofit—church
- Government—federal
- Government—local
- Physician
- Tribal

When the WHERE clause specifies that observations will only be returned when hospital_ownership status contains the word "government," this limits observations to those hospitals that have an ownership status of the following:

- Government—federal
- Government—hospital district or authority
- Government—state
- Government—federal
- Government—local

Joining Tables

When data are retrieved from a relational database, the data most often reside in more than one table. In order to retrieve data from multiple tables, how the tables are to be joined must be specified. In SQL, the keyword JOIN is used to join tables. This keyword is used within the FROM clause. The FROM clause is where all tables containing columns from which we want data are specified. The general format of a query with a JOIN is as follows:

```
SELECT <name of one or more columns>
FROM <name of table 1>
JOIN <name of table 2>
   ON<table 1 column> = <table 2 column>
WHERE <conditions that must be met to include the data>
```

The keyword JOIN must be used anytime more than one table is used in the query. The JOIN is specified between each of the table names. If a query is executed where specific attributes are returned from the hospital_general_information table, the FROM clause looks like this:

```
FROM hospital_general_information
```

However, if there are attributes returned that are found in more than one table, the FROM clause will be followed by a JOIN. For instance, if a query is executed where specific attributes are returned from the hospital_general_information table and the readmission_reduction table, the FROM clause looks like this:

```
FROM  hospital_general_information
JOIN  readmission_reduction
  ON hospital_general_information.provider_id = readmission_reduction.
     provider_id
```

Oftentimes, novice SQL programmers will list the tables they want to join with a space or comma between the table names. This syntax is NOT correct. The names of the tables must be separated using the keyword JOIN.

The keyword JOIN is rarely used without using the keyword ON. The keyword ON is used to specify the columns used to relate the two tables. For example, there is an attribute named provider_id in the hospital_general_information table and the readmission_reduction table. This field contains the provider ID of the hospital. The provider_id is the PK in the hospital_general_information table and a FK in the readmission_reduction table. When the hospital_general_information and readmission_reduction tables are joined, the field that links these tables needs to be specified. To do this, the keyword ON is used immediately following the name of second table.

The method for listing attributes after the SELECT statement is also different when a JOIN is included in the query. If two tables are joined together, and there will be attributes returned from both of those tables, the attributes need to be listed with the table name and attribute name in the SELECT statement. The name of the table where the attribute is found is listed first, followed by a period, and ends with the name of the specific attribute. For instance, if the hospital name is to be returned from the hospital_general_information table and the number of readmission is to be returned from the readmission_reduction table, the attributes would be specified after the SELECT statement as follows:

```
SELECT      hospital_general_information.hospital_name,
            readmission_reduction.number of readmissions
```

An example of a MySQL query that returns the hospital name, address, city, state, readmission measure name, and number of readmissions for that measure is shown in figure 4.18.

The query in figure 4.18 can be added to by returning observations that meet certain criteria by adding a WHERE clause. The hospital name, address, city, state, and number of readmissions can be returned for only those hospitals located in the state of California by adding a WHERE clause (figure 4.19).

The query shown in figure 4.19 can be expanded by joining three tables and returning attributes that are available in each of the joined tables. For instance, patient satisfaction survey results can be added to the query by adding attributes related to the question name and percentage that responded to the answer located in the hcahps table. These attributes include hcahps_question and hcahps_answer_percent, respectively. Refer to the ERD in figure 4.6—it shows that the hcahps table is related to the hospital_general_information table. Therefore, when the hcahps table is joined in the query, the ON statement will relate the PK from hospital_general_information to the matching FK in the hcahps table, which is provider_id. In addition, the readmission_reduction table will be joined to the hospital_general_information table. Also, data will only be returned for those hospitals located in the state of California. The resulting query is shown in figure 4.20.

When comparing figures 4.19 and 4.20 it is apparent that any number of tables can be joined to the SQL statement by simply repeating the same standard JOIN syntax. One thing to note about joining tables is that it is not necessary to include a column from the table in the SELECT clause when joining a table. Sometimes a table is included in a FROM clause simply to limit the data that are retrieved from other tables using a WHERE clause.

Aggregating Data

Sometimes more than just the raw data contained in the table are needed; for example, to see how many hospitals are located in each state or the maximum number of readmissions in a particular state. To retrieve any of these types of summaries from data retrieved from a database, the data needs to be aggregated using an aggregate function. The general syntax is as follows:

Figure 4.18.   Example of a MySQL query with a JOIN

```
      SELECT        hospital_general_information.hospital_name,
                    hospital_general_information.address,
                    hospital_general_information.city,
                    hospital_general_information.state,
                    readmission_reduction.number_of_readmissions
      FROM          hospital_general_information
      JOIN          readmission_reduction
   ON               hospital_general_information.provider_id=
            readmission_reduction.provider_id;
```

Figure 4.19. Example of a MySQL query with a JOIN and WHERE

```
SELECT          hospital_general_information.hospital_name,
                hospital_general_information.address,
                hospital_general_information.city,
                hospital_general_information.state,
                readmission_reduction.number_of_readmissions
FROM            hospital_general_information
JOIN            readmission_reduction
ON              hospital_general_information.provider_id=
        readmission_reduction.provider_id
WHERE           hospital_general_information.state= 'CA';
```

Figure 4.20. Example of a MySQL query with multiple JOINs and a WHERE

```
SELECT          hospital_general_information.hospital_name,
                hospital_general_information.address,
                hospital_general_information.city,
                hospital_general_information.state,
                readmission_reduction.number_of_readmissions,
                hcahps.hcahps_question,
                hcahps.hcahps_answer_percent
FROM            hospital_general_information
JOIN            readmission_reduction
ON              hospital_general_information.provider_id=
        readmission_reduction.provider_id
JOIN            hcahps
ON              hospital_general_information.provider_id=hcahps.provider_id
WHERE           hospital_general_information.state= 'CA';
```

```
SELECT <name of one or more columns>,
    FUNCTION (<name of column>)
FROM <name of table 1>
JOIN <name of table 2>
ON <table 1 column> = <table 2 column>
WHERE <conditions that must be met to include the data>
GROUP BY <name of one or more columns>
```

The data are aggregated using the keywords GROUP BY, followed by the name of the column to aggregate (or group the data). GROUP BY tells the query engine to calculate the aggregate function specified in the SELECT clause for each unique value in the GROUP BY column. For example, a query can be generated that lists the hospital name and the state it is located in for each hospital in the database using the query shown in figure 4.21. The first few rows of the results of the figure are shown in figure 4.22.

From these data, the number of hospitals that are in each state can be computed. This can be done using software other than MySQL workbench, such as MS Excel. However, to save time, this same activity can be done within MySQL workbench. Instead of retrieving a list of hospital names and the state name where those hospitals are located, a query can be run that shows the total number of hospital for each state. The hospital name needs to aggregate the data based on the state and both the state and count of hospitals in the state need to revealed. The COUNT function can be used to aggregate the hospital name. The GROUP BY function is used to group the count of each hospital by the state. The resulting query is shown in figure 4.23, and the first few rows of results from the query are shown in figure 4.24.

Figure 4.21.   Example of a MySQL query without aggregation

```
SELECT          state,
                hospital_name
FROM            hospital_general_information;
```

Figure 4.22.   The first few rows of results of the MySQL query shown in figure 4.21

	state	hospital_name
▶	AL	BIRMINGHAM VA MEDICAL CENTER
	AL	VA CENTRAL ALABAMA HEALTHCARE SYSTEM - MONTGOMERY
	AL	TUSCALOOSA VA MEDICAL CENTER
	AZ	PHOENIX VA MEDICAL CENTER
	AZ	VA S. ARIZONA HEALTHCARE SYSTEM
	AZ	VA NORTHERN ARIZONA HEALTHCARE SYSTEM
	AR	FAYETTEVILLE AR VA MEDICAL CENTER
	AR	VA CENTRAL AR. VETERANS HEALTHCARE SYSTEM LR
	CA	FRESNO VA MEDICAL CENTER - VA CENTRAL CALIFORNIA
	CA	VA LONG BEACH HEALTHCARE SYSTEM
	CA	VA N CALIFORNIA HEALTHCARE SYSTEM

Filtering Based on Aggregate Values

The previous section introduced the GROUP BY clause. This clause is used to aggregate data and calculate an aggregate value for some field. In figures 4.23 and 4.24, the total number of hospitals for each state was calculated, by using the COUNT function. Just as the WHERE clause is used to limit the results of the data set based on the value in some field, the HAVING clause can be used to limit the results of the data set based on an aggregate value. The following is the SQL syntax for this type of query:

```
SELECT <name of one or more columns>,
    FUNCTION (<name of column>)
FROM <name of table 1>
JOIN <name of table 2>
  ON <table 1 column> = <table 2 column>
WHERE <conditions that must be met to include the data>
GROUP BY <name of one or more columns>
HAVING <conditions based on aggregate values>
```

In the previous example, the total number of hospitals for each state was calculated by using the COUNT function. In figure 4.25, the HAVING clause will be used to limit the results of this query to only those states having 20 or more hospitals. The first few results of the query are shown in figure 4.26.

Functions

MySQL includes a number of functions. Functions are used to manipulate and convert the data. Functions are also used to perform calculations. For instance, the COUNT function was used previously to count the number of hospitals in each state. Different functions are used for different tasks. The diagram in table 4.1 shows the different classes of functions that are available and summarizes the various functions that are available in MySQL.

Figure 4.23. Example of a MySQL query with aggregation

```
SELECT          state,
                COUNT(hospital_name)
FROM            hospital_general_information
GROUP BY        state;
```

Figure 4.24. The first few rows of results of the MySQL query shown in figure 4.23

state	COUNT(hospital_name)
AK	21
AL	93
AR	78
AS	1
AZ	78
CA	346
CO	79
CT	32
DC	9
DE	7
FL	187

Figure 4.25. Example of a MySQL query with aggregation

```
SELECT          state,
                COUNT(hospital_name)
FROM            hospital_general_information
GROUP BY        state
HAVING          COUNT(hospital_name)>20;
```

Figure 4.26. The first few rows of results of the MySQL query shown in figure 4.25

state	COUNT(hospital_name)
AK	21
AL	93
AR	78
AZ	78
CA	346
CO	79
CT	32
FL	187
GA	136
IA	118
ID	42
IL	181

Table 4.1. Types of MySQL functions

Function Type	Key Word	Meaning
Aggregate functions	COUNT( )	Return the number of records
	SUM( )	Return the arithmetic sum of values
	MIN( )	Return the minimum value
	MAX( )	Return the maximum value
	AVG( )	Return the average of the values (excludes NULLs)
Mathematical functions	TRUNCATE( )	Truncate the number of decimal places
	MOD( )	Return the remainder
	ROUND( )	Round a number
	POWER( )	Return the argument raised to the specified power
Date and time functions	DATEDIFF( )	Subtract two dates
	HOUR( ), MINUTE( ), SECOND( )	Extract the hours, minutes, or seconds
	DAY( ), WEEK( ), MONTH( ), YEAR( )	Extract the day, week, month, or year
	DATE( ), TIME( )	Extract the date or time part of date-time
	CURDATE( ), CURTIME( )	Return the current date or time
	NOW( )	Return the current date and time
	SYSDATE( )	Return the time at which the function executes
	DATE_ADD( )	Add time intervals to a date value
	DATE_SUB( )	Subtract time intervals to a date value
	STR_TO_DATE( )	Convert a string to a date
Data type functions	CONVERT( )	Convert a string value to a different character set
	CAST( )	Cast a value as a certain type
String functions	CHAR_LENGTH( )	Return number of characters
	CONCAT( )	Return a concatenated string
	INSTR( ), LOCATE( ), POSITION( )	Return the position of the first occurrence of substring
	SUBSTR( ), SUBSTRING( )	Return a specified substring
	TRIM( ), RTRIM( ), LTRIM( )	Remove leading and trailing spaces
	UCASE( ), UPPER( )	Transform strings to uppercase
	LCASE( ), LOWER( )	Transform strings to lowercase

Review Exercises

Instructions: Choose the best answer.

1. When working with databases, entities can be considered which of the following?
   a. Verbs
   b. Adverbs
   c. Nouns
   d. Adjectives

2. The AND statement is considered what type of WHERE clause operator?
   a. Wildcard
   b. Logical

    c.   Comparison
    d.   All of the above

3. A data dictionary is critical for which of the following elements when using data from databases?
   a. Reliability
   b. Trustworthiness
   c. Dependability
   d. All of the above

4. True or False: MySQL workbench is considered a database.

5. True or False: Foreign keys are the columns of data within a database that uniquely identify a record in the table.

References

AHIMA. 2012. Managing a Data Dictionary. *Journal of AHIMA* 83(1):48–52.

Chen, P.P. 1976. The entity-relationship model: Toward a unified view of data. *ACM Transactions on Database Systems* 1(1):9–36.

Codd, E.F. 1970. A relational model of data for large shared data bank. *Communications of the ACM* 13(6):377–387.

Heller, M. 2007. REST and CRUD: The impedance mismatch. *Developer World, InfoWorld.* http://www.infoworld.com/article/2640739/application-development/rest-and-crud–the-impedance-mismatch.html

Introduction to R

David Marc, MBS, CHDA and Ryan Sandefer, MA, CPHIT

Learning Objectives

- Describe the basic functionalities of the R Statistical Package
- Construct data summaries and graphical presentations
- Identify common analytical packages for statistical analysis in healthcare

Key Terms

Argument
Boxplot
Function
Histogram
Object
Operator
Vector

R is a widely adopted statistical programming language. R is referred to as a language because users carry out tasks by specifying instructions using a common set of rules with varying words and phrases. When these words and phrases are processes within the R environment, the computer translates that information to carry out the instructions that the user supplied. In that way, the user is supplying instructions using a language the computer can understand and these instructions are then translated into an action.

R is considered an interpreted language, not a compiled language. This means that each command typed on the keyboard can be interpreted and processed without having to develop a complete computer program. There are a variety of different interpreted computer programming languages including PHP and Python. Some examples of a compiled language include C, Visual Basic, and Fortran.

Although R is a programming language, the syntax is relatively easy to learn and use. With just a few lines of code, one can develop complex statistical models. However, to really get a handle on what R can do, the user does need to have basic knowledge of statistics and mathematics. Learning the R language itself will come with practice.

The R Interface

Opening the base R program (denoted by the ℞ or ℞ icon), the user will find a surprisingly limited and simple design to the interface. Notice a window labeled "R Console" (figure 5.1). The R console is where the code that is typed in is processed. To run a command in the R console simply type in a command, hit enter, and the output will be shown below the text entry.

Figure 5.1. The base R interface

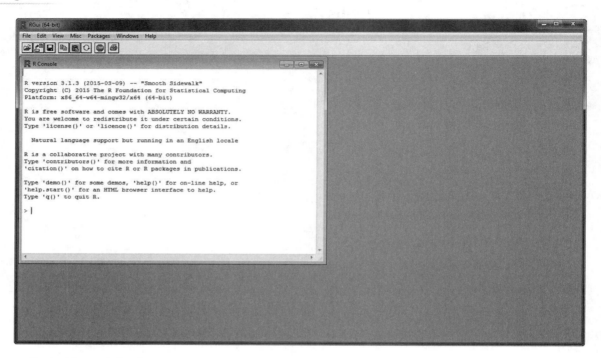

Source: Used with permission from R.

Figure 5.2. Basic mathematics in the R console

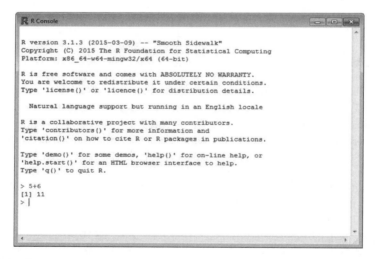

Source: Used with permission from R.

For instance, if one wanted to calculate the solution to the math problem 5 plus 6, he or she can type 5+6 into the R console, hit enter, and directly below the text entry the output of 11 will appear (figure 5.2). Also notice that a [1] appeared before the 11. The [1] indicated the line number of the output. Also note that R is case-sensitive. Many of the functions stored in R must be entered with all lowercase characters (such as the mean, standard deviation, and summary functions). However, there are several functions that do require a mix of lowercase and uppercase characters (for example the TukeyHSD function). The user needs to make certain that he or she is using the correct case sensitivity for all functions. The most common errors in R are due to incorrect use of lowercase and uppercase characters.

One issue with running code directly within the console is that everything typed directly into the console will be erased if R is closed down. In most situations, the user will want to save the R code being used so that the next time R is opened the previously used R code can be loaded to rerun, edit, or add to the analysis. An alternative method for running code is to type the code into a scripting window. The scripting window is a separate window where one can enter code. The R code entered in the scripting window can be saved. The output, however, is not saved with the R code (this will be discussed further later in this chapter). When the content is saved in the scripting window, it is stored in a text file. That text file can be loaded back into R for later use. A scripting window can be opened by clicking File > New script. The scripting window can be arranged within the R viewer under Windows > Tile Vertically. The resulting view is shown in figure 5.3.

Code can be written in the scripting window and that code processed in the console. The output will still appear in the console. If one was to write 6+7 into the scripting window, that line of code could be processed by placing the cursor somewhere on the same line where 6+7 was written (before, after, or within the text) and either clicking the ▣ icon listed in the upper left-hand side of the screen or using a keyboard shortcut. If Windows is the operating system, the keyboard shortcut is Ctrl+R; if using a Mac OSx, the keyboard shortcut is Command+Enter. The result will be as shown in figure 5.4.

As shown, 6+7 was processed in the console, and the resulting output of 13 was provided. To save the content in the scripting window, click into the scripting window and go to File > Save As. The user will have to select a location on his or her computer to save the resulting text file. These R scripts can be reopened by going back into R and going to File > Open script.

Each time R is opened for a new session, the previous R console will be deleted. Therefore, the user will need to rerun the code to see the output each time R is restarted. If one wants to see the output again, the fastest way to rerun all of the code stored in the scripting window is by highlighting the code and clicking the run icon or using the keyboard shortcut.

The Basics of Coding in R

Terms often found using R include vector, function, objects, operators, and arguments.

Vector

The first term to be familiar with is a **vector**. A vector is simply a list of items. A vector may include numbers, characters, words, sentences, or a combination.

Vectors can be created using the concatenate function, which is denoted by the lowercase letter c. Concatenate refers to the function of combining individual items into a list or series. For example, to create a vector of numbers, where each number represents the amount of money in a piggy bank over a period of five days, the concatenate function can be used to generate the following vector:

```
c(2, 6, 8, 10, 12)
```

This means that on day one, the piggy bank had two dollars. On day two, the piggy bank had six dollars. On day three, eight dollars, and so on.

If the vector contains letters or words, quotation marks must be used around each letter or word. The reason for the quotation marks is to inform computers to interpret each item in the list as text. For instance, to create a list of names for each member living in the household, the following vector can be generated:

```
c("Greg", "Henry", "Emily", "Susan")
```

Function

A **function** is a command that executes specific processes on either a vector or object of data. An example of a function is a mean. The mean function will find the average of a specified list of numbers. All functions need to be written with parentheses. Within those parentheses, a vector or object is specified. The function will only be processed on the content within the parentheses. For instance, to find the average of money in the piggy bank, using the list of numbers 2, 6, 8, 10, 12, use the mean function as such:

```
mean(c(2, 6, 8, 10, 12))
```

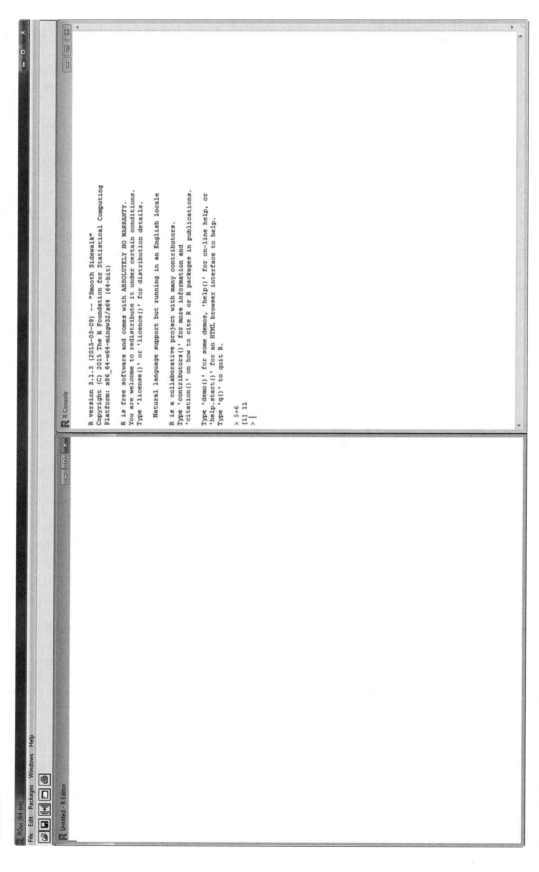

Figure 5.3. The base R interface shown with a scripting window on the left-hand side and the R console on the ride-hand side

Source: Used with permission from R.

Figure 5.4. Demonstration of using the R scripting window to process a mathematical function. The output from that function is shown in the R console

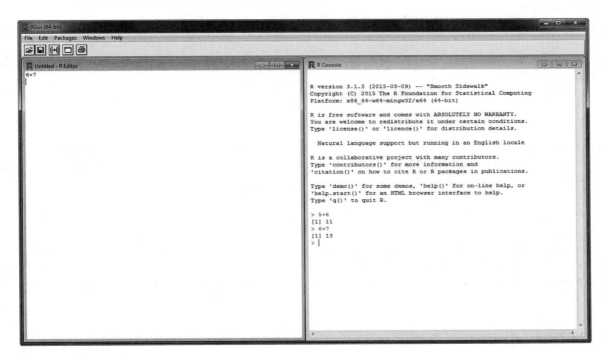

Source: Used with permission from R.

Table 5.1. Common numeric functions and their descriptions

Function	Description
min(x)	Minimum value
max(x)	Maximum value
sum(x)	Sum of all values
mean(x)	Average of all values
median(x)	Median of all values
length(x)	Number of values in a list
sd(x)	Standard deviation of all values
summary(x)	Returns the minimum, first quartile, median, mean, third quartile, and maximum values

Notice that the concatenate function is still included, because the vector still needs to be created. From there, the mean function is able to calculate the average of the numbers listed in the specified vector.

Table 5.1 is a list of the common numeric functions and their descriptions (the x would be replaced by a vector or object).

Objects

When using R, data, variables, functions, and results are often stored in the active memory of the computer in the form of **objects**. Each object is assigned a name. The name is assigned either by R or by the user. For instance, R comes preloaded with data sets. These data sets are stored as objects, and the name of these objects are assigned by R. A user can create his or her own objects by assigning a vector to a name that he or she specifies. Users can manipulate the stored objects with functions and operators. For instance, if a user wanted to store the numerical vector created previously to the object name "data," the following can be done using variable assignment:

```
data<- c(2, 6, 8, 10, 12)
```

Essentially, R takes that vector that is concatenated using the "c" function and then stores the list to the object named "data." From here, the user can manipulate the object "data." For instance, if the user wanted to calculate the mean of the object, he or she can do the following:

```
mean(data)
```

The output from mean(data) will be 7.6, which is the same output from mean(c(2, 6, 8, 10, 12)). The only difference is that rather than typing the vector within the parentheses of the mean function, the name of an object that was assigned as that vector is typed instead.

Operators

Common **operators** use arithmetic or logic. Operators are symbols that express specific actions or criteria. For instance, the plus sign (+) is an arithmetic operator to calculate the sum of objects while the greater than sign (>) is a logical operator that can calculate whether one object is greater than another object. Operators will be discussed later in this chapter.

Arguments

A function may also have specific arguments. **Arguments** can be objects that are modifiable by the user in order to alter the way a function works. For instance, if using the mean function on a list of numbers that contained values that were not available (NAs), the output NA would result. The reason the output will be NA is because one cannot take the mean of a value that is not available. However, if an argument called na.rm=TRUE within the parentheses of the mean function was included, the NAs will be ignored in the list of numbers thereby allowing one to calculate the mean. The purpose of na.rm is to indicate whether NA values should be stripped before the computation of the mean proceeds.

The following line of code will give the output of NA because the user is telling R to take the mean of vector of numbers that contains NAs:

```
mean(c(2, 6, 8, NA, 10, 12))
```

Most likely, the output of NA is not desired. If the goal is to calculate the mean of a vector of numbers by ignoring the NAs, the user can implicitly specify that the NAs should be ignored from the list of numbers by adding the argument na.rm=T to the mean function:

```
mean(c(2, 6, 8, NA, 10, 12), na.rm=T)
```

With na.rm=T included within the parentheses of the mean function, the desired output of 7.6 is now received.

To learn about the specific arguments of each function, one can use the help function if connected to the Internet. For example, to learn more about the mean function, a single question mark (?) can be used before the function name, mean. The help menu will be accessed by running the following line of code:

```
?mean
```

The help menu will automatically appear, as shown in figure 5.5.

The first thing listed in the help menu is a Description of the function. Next is a programmable explanation for the way the function works listed under Usage. The Usage section also displays the default arguments. For instance, by default na.rm is equal to FALSE, meaning the NAs are not stripped from a list of numbers by default:

```
mean(x, trim = 0, na.rm = FALSE)
```

Figure 5.5.   An example of the help menu. This example shows the help menu for the mean function

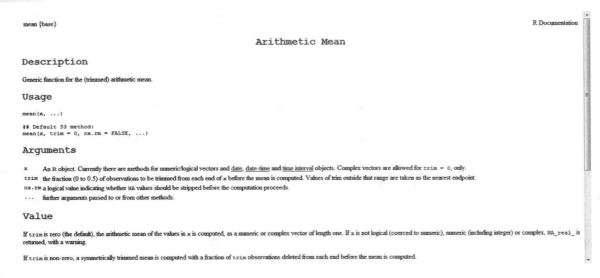

Source: Used with permission from R.

The Arguments section offers further explanation of each available argument. X is the object of data for which one wants to calculate the mean. The object could be a vector or the name of the stored vector. For instance, the user can take the mean of the object "data" since it already has an assigned vector to that name "data."

The next argument is trim, which can take on a value from 0 to 0.5. The purpose of the trim argument is to remove a percentage of values from the vector. Therefore, if trim=0.2 is specified, this would remove 20 percent of the highest and 20 percent of the lowest observations from the data set. The only time one may want to use the trim attribute is to remove an equal number of outliers at the high end of the distribution and the low end of the distribution.

The last argument is na.rm, which is a logical value (meaning it can be either TRUE or FALSE). As a reminder, the purpose of na.rm is to indicate whether NA values should be stripped before the computation of the mean proceeds. If TRUE, NA values will be stripped. If FALSE, NA values will not be stripped.

Additional information on how some arguments are handled is often listed under the Value section. Also, the References supporting the function are provided, as well as related functions listed under the See Also section. Often there are examples included at the end of the help documentation.

R versus RStudio

Base R can be cumbersome to navigate. This is particularly true when creating many graphics and needing to access the help menu. An alternative graphical user interface (GUI) was designed to assist users in managing their R code and output. The name of the alternative GUI is RStudio. RStudio functions in the same way as base R. That is, there is a scripting window, a console, and the same keyboard shortcuts are used.

Open RStudio from the Start window. Once RStudio opens, go to File > New File > R Script to open a scripting window. The scripting window in RStudio holds the same function of the scripting window in base R. The purpose of the scripting window is to offer users a place to enter R scripts where they can be saved and later reloaded. The results are shown in figure 5.6.

The window panes include

A. R scripting
B. Saved objects
C. Help menu as well as any graphics that are created
D. R console

Arithmetic Operators

As described previously, R can process basic arithmetic. Table 5.2 shows examples of the common mathematical operators that can be used in R.

Logical Operators

Logical operators are used to specify criteria when analyzing data. Table 5.3 provides a list of the most common logical operators.

Often the user wants to specify criteria when analyzing a vector. For instance, assume one wanted to recreate in RStudio the data set called "data" from before and return all values in the object when the values are greater than or equal to eight. In RStudio, enter the following code into the scripting window: data<- c(2, 6, 8, 10, 12) to recreate the data set. The following code, using brackets and within those brackets the specific criteria with the logical operators, returns all values greater than or equal to eight:

```
data[data>=8]
```

Figure 5.6. Description of the RStudio user interface

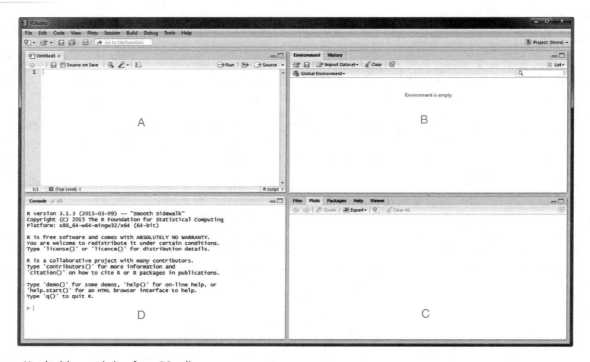

Source: Used with permission from RStudio.

Table 5.2. Common mathematical operators used in R

Operator	Description	Example
+	Addition	5+9
−	Subtraction	9–3
*	Multiplication	3*2
/	Division	6/2
^ or **	Exponentiation	4^2

Table 5.3. Common logical operators used in R

Operator	Description
<	Less than
<=	Less than or equal to
>	Greater than
>=	Greater than or equal to
==	Exactly equal to
!=	Not equal to
!x	Not the value x
x | y	Either the value x or the value y
x & y	Both the value x and the value y

This code will be processed where values will be returned from the object when those values from the object "data" are greater than or equal to eight.

The user can also use a function in combination with the logical operators. Here, one can use the length function, which counts the number of items in a vector. For instance, if the user wanted to know how many numbers in the object "data" are greater than or equal to eight, he or she can use the length function and do the following:

```
length(data[data>=8])
```

The value that is returned is 3, since there are three numbers in the object "data" that are greater than or equal to eight.

To count the number of values in the object "data" that are equal to eight, use two equal signs as the operator (==). It is important to use two equal signs. One equal sign does variable assignment. In this way, one equal sign has the same function as <-. Remember <- is used to assign data to a named object (for example, data<-c(2, 6, 8, 10, 12)). Two equal signs are interpreted as equality. That is, two equal signs are a logical argument that tests whether an object is equal to another object. Therefore, to count the number of times the value 8 occurs in the vector, the user would want to use the following code:

```
length(data[data==8])
```

The number 1 will be returned in the output, since there is only one value in the list that is equal to eight.

Graphical Functions

In addition to numeric functions, graphs are another way to summarize data. R supports a variety of graphical outputs. Two of the most common graphs that are used in R are histograms and boxplots.

Histogram

The first graph is a **histogram**. A histogram can be used to see how frequent different numbers or groups occur in a vector. For example, create a new numeric vector and assign the vector to an object called "graphs." In the RStudio interface, run the following script in the scripting window (if there are already scripts written in the scripting window, simply enter the following information at the bottom of the scripting window. Many different scripts can be written in a single scripting window):

```
graphs<- c( 2, 3, 3, 3, 4, 4, 4, 4, 4, 4, 5, 5, 5, 6)
```

After running this script, the object "graphs" can be used to make a histogram with the hist function:

```
hist(graphs)
```

Running this hist function will produce the graph shown in figure 5.7.

As shown in the histogram in figure 5.7, the frequency of each value is depicted based on the values in the object called "graphs." A histogram is a common method for describing the distribution of data.

Boxplot

The second common graph is a **boxplot**. A boxplot is a way to graphically summarize the range and center of data. To create a boxplot of the object "graphs," run the following script:

```
boxplot(graphs)
```

The result is shown in figure 5.8.

Figure 5.7.   Example of a histogram

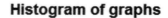

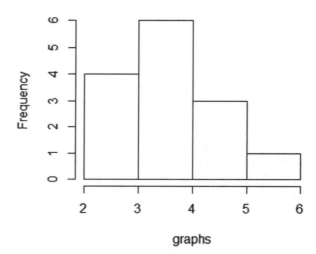

Source: Used with permission from RStudio.

Figure 5.8.   Example of a boxplot

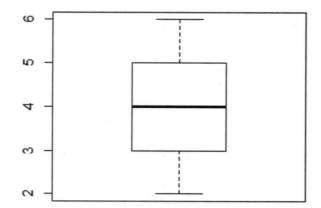

Source: Used with permission from RStudio.

Function	Description
barplot	Creates a barplot of an object
plot	A generic function for plotting R objects; can be used for generating scatterplots and line graphs
dotchart	Draws a Cleveland dot plot of R objects
pie	Generates a pie chart of the frequency of items in a R object

Table 5.4. List of other graphical functions in R

The boxplot provides a great deal of information in a single plot. The lower whisker is drawn at the minimum value, the bottom of the box is drawn at the value of the first quartile, the bold middle line is the median, the top of the box is the value of the third quartile, and the upper whisker is the maximum value. R is capable of producing many other graphics. For a list of other graphics that R supports, see table 5.4.

Combining Vectors

Commonly, vectors need to be combined. For instance, to compare the average of a number between two groups, the user may want to combine two vectors. One of the vectors may contain the name of the groups, while the other may contain the numeric values. The two most common ways of combining vectors include combining two vectors as distinct rows or combining two vectors as distinct columns. In order to take a closer look at both methods, create two vectors and save them as the objects, v1 and v2. Create the two vectors by running the following scripts on separate lines in the RStudio scripting window:

```
v1<-c("A", "A", "A", "B", "B", "B", "C", "C", "C")
v2<-c(1, 2, 3, 4, 5, 6, 7, 8, 9)
```

To run each line of code, the user can either highlight both lines and use the keyboard shortcut to run the scripts (ctrl+R for Windows users or command+enter for Mac OSx users) or place the cursor on the first line of code, use the keyboard shortcut to run the script, then use the keyboard shortcut a second time to run the next line of scripts. Notice that each time the keyboard shortcut is used to run the line of code, the cursor will move to the next line.

Arranging the Two Vectors

Typically, the user will want the data stored as columns. However, there may be circumstances where one would prefer that the data are stored as rows. If we wanted to combine each vector whereby v1 is in one row and v2 is in a second row, we can use the rbind function. One thing to note is that the rbind function will only work if the two vectors are of the same length. If one vector has more numbers than does the second vector, they cannot be combined. To use the rbind function, run the following script:

```
rbind(v1,v2)
```

More commonly, the user will want to arrange the data in columns. The reason a columnar arrangement is preferred is because R interprets each column of data as a vector. Those column names, which become vectors of data, can be used as the R objects for functions. Therefore, to combine each vector whereby v1 is in one column and v2 is in a second column, use the cbind function. Similar to rbind, the cbind function will only work if the two vectors are of the same length. To use the cbind function, run the following script:

```
cbind(v1,v2)
```

The combined vectors can also be saved as a new object using variable assignment. This is a very common practice in R. The reason one may want to save the two columns as a single R object is because vectors will then be presented together and meaningful statistics can be generated based on the relationship between the two vectors. To do this, save the cbind of vector v1 and v2 to the object named "combined."

```
combined<- cbind(v1,v2)
```

Common Ways for Summarizing the Relationship between Two Vectors

Frequently, it is important to examine the relationship between two vectors. For instance, to compare the mean of a numeric value between two groups, one would have to combine two vectors to evaluate this relationship.

For example, assume that vector v1 is a variable that specifies a person. Looking at the letters contained in v1, there are three people: A, B, and C. The column v2 is time in minutes. Notice that there were nine times recorded. Each group was timed on three different occasions based on how fast they could complete the task of folding a paper airplane. The tapply function can be used to calculate the average time it took each person to fold a paper airplane. The combination of a numeric vector and vector that contains a label is an example of what is sometimes called a ragged array. The tapply function will summarize the numeric vector at each level of the label vector based on a specified function. The following is an example:

```
tapply(v2, v1, mean)
```

In this case, the tapply function is going to summarize v2 (time in minutes) at each level of v1 (the letters for each person) and apply the mean function. Therefore, the output shows the average time in minutes it takes persons A, B, and C to fold a paper airplane: person A averaged 2 minutes, person B averaged 5 minutes, and person C averaged 8 minutes.

To use the tapply function, the user must always specify the quantitative variable as the first argument, then the grouping variable as the second argument, and finally the function as the third argument. All of the functions specified in table 5.1 can be used with tapply. Graphical functions should be avoided, however, as the output produces two graphs with the last graph overwriting the first.

Graphs can also be used to summarize data based on the relationship of two vectors. A tilde (~) is used to explain one variable based on the levels of another variable. To create a boxplot for each of the three individuals, use the following code:

```
boxplot(v2~v1)
```

The resulting output will generate the graph in figure 5.9.

Figure 5.9. Example of a boxplot comparing the differences between three groups

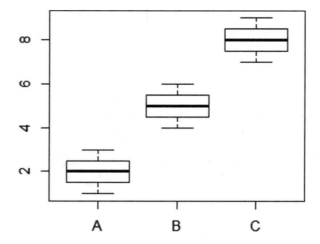

Source: Used with permission from RStudio.

A box is drawn based on the data for each individual. These results allow one to quickly see that person A took the least amount of time folding a paper airplane and person C took the most amount of time. These graphs are an easy way to summarize the relationship between the vectors of data.

Loading Data into RStudio

Data are often provided to an analyst in the form of a spreadsheet (including formats such as XLSX, CSV, TXT). Up to this point, R objects have been created by assigning vectors a name. The import function in RStudio can automatically create R objects based on individual columns of data that are found in a spreadsheet. In order to import a spreadsheet of data into RStudio, the file needs to be saved in the CSV or TXT file format. The reason that the file needs to be saved in one of these formats is due to encoding restrictions that other file formats may have on the import feature.

In part II of this text, a CSV file of data will be created to answer a research question. This spreadsheet is derived from a MySQL query, which is explained further in chapter 7. For example, in chapter 7, the name of the spreadsheet is "Ep_attest." Using the spreadsheet of data from that chapter, one can import the data into RStudio. Figure 5.10 displays the first step in the process for importing the CSV file. Click *Import Dataset* and choose the "From Text File" option in the drop down window. Navigate to the CSV file that was saved, highlight the file, and click "Open."

Figure 5.10. Importing a CSV file into RStudio—Step 1

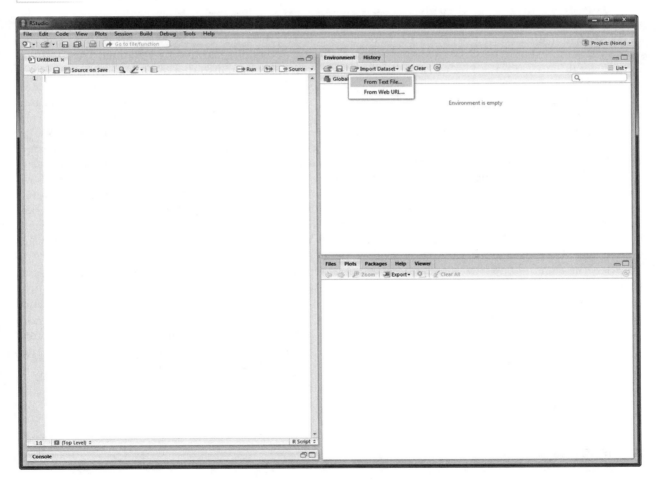

Source: Used with permission from RStudio.

Figure 5.11.   Importing a CSV file into RStudio—Step 2

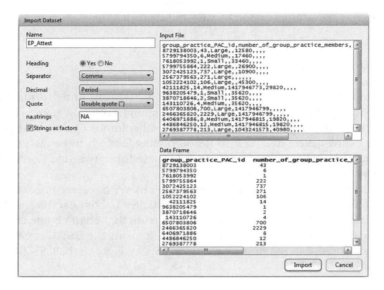

Source: Used with permission from RStudio.

Figure 5.11 shows the second step in the import process. Make sure that the *Name* of the data set matches the CSV file (for example, in chapter 7 it will be titled "Ep_Attest"). The *Heading* option should be "Yes" to indicate that the first row of data includes column labels. Since a CSV file is being imported, the *Separator* option should be set as "Comma" since each field of data is separated by a comma. The *Decimal* option should be "Period" to indicate that the numeric data is formatted so that any number that includes a decimal includes a period. The *Quote* option should be "Double Quote" to indicate that double quotations are used around any field with text. The *na.strings* option should be listed as NA to fill in blank values with the letters "NA." The *Strings as factors* checkbox should be checked to import all text as a character rather than attempt to convert the text to a number. After double-checking these settings, click "Import."

Figure 5.12 shows the final step in the importing process. After importing the data, the data will become viewable in the upper left quadrant of the RStudio application window. For data sets that are particularly large (exceeding 10,000 rows), the user will not be able to view the entire data set. The reason for this is to conserve the memory of the computer and prevent the computer from crashing. In the upper right quadrant, the user will see the data set that was imported into RStudio, including a summary of the size of the data set (number of observations and number of variables). If more than one data set has been imported, or assigned R objects, all of those objects will be listed in this window. After importing the data, the R scripts that were used by RStudio will be shown in the R console window.

After the data are imported into RStudio, the first step is to attach the data set. The reason that the data set needs to be attached is to create the column names into R objects in order to make them easier to work with in RStudio. Without the use of the attach function, the only way to work with the data by the column names is to specify the name of the data frame followed by a dollar sign and the name of the column. For example, if a data set named "AllData" was imported into RStudio and there was a need to call out the column "Age," without attaching the data, a user would be required to use the following script: AllData$Age. If the data set is attached, a user can simply call the column by its name: Age. For example, to attach the data in chapter 7, the following R Script will be in the console:

```
attach(EP_Attest)
```

R Packages

The versatility of R is a result of the extensive packages that are available. These packages are created and maintained by the R Foundation for Statistical Computing. Individuals can contribute packages, which are

Figure 5.12.   Importing a CSV file into RStudio—Step 3

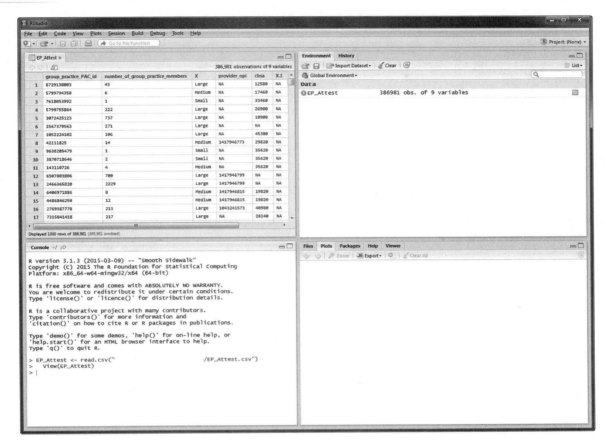

Source: Used with permission from RStudio.

vetted and tested by the R Development Core Team before they are released to the public. Hundreds of R packages have been developed to carry out a variety of analytical tasks. Throughout this book, the reader will become familiar with several of these packages including ggplot2 and dplyr, To see the extensive list of R packages (which is constantly growing), visit the r-project.org webpage.

Review Exercises

Instructions: Choose the best answer.

1. What function would be used to determine how many items are in a vector?
   a. count
   b. length
   c. tapply
   d. c

2. What is the purpose of the concatenate function?

3. True or False: When the na.rm=TRUE attribute is used with the mean function, any NAs in a vector will be ignored when calculating the mean.

4. Choose the correct R script to return the number of items in the vector called "data" that are equal to 3.
    a. length(data[data==3])
    b. length(data[data=3])
    c. length([data==3])
    d. length([data=3])

5. Describe the purpose of the attach function when importing data into RStudio.

References

R Core Team. 2014. R: A Language and Environment for Statistical Computing. R Foundation for Statistical Computing, Vienna, Austria. http://www.R-project.org/
RStudio. 2014. RStudio: Integrated Development Environment for R [Computer software]. Boston, MA.

Part II

| Chapter 6 | # Exploratory Data Analysis and Data Visualization of MS-DRGs |

David S. Pieczkiewicz, PhD

Learning Objectives

- Differentiate the economic impact of MS-DRGs on healthcare delivery
- Summarize the analytical techniques used to evaluate coded healthcare data
- Demonstrate the use of exploratory data analysis and data visualization techniques for presenting aggregate data

Key Terms

Bar chart
Data visualization
Exploratory data analysis (EDA)

Analysts have been depicting data graphically for hundreds of years. Two early examples are the *Commercial and Political Atlas* and the *Statistical Breviary*, published in 1786 and 1801, respectively, by William Playfair, a Scottish political economist and pioneer in data visualization (figure 6.1). While historians debate whether Playfair himself or earlier analysts first created different statistical graphics, these two works are credited with widely promoting the use of such designs as bar, line, and pie charts, in much the same forms as people use them today. With dozens of illustrations in each book, Playfair's graphics are remarkable, not just for historical reasons, but because of the sheer amount of work it must have taken to manually compile the data required—and then draw every figure by hand.

By the 1960s, computers were increasingly used to work with data. While memory and storage space were still at a premium, it was already feasible to turn repetitive calculations over to computers, freeing analysts from manual or mechanical number crunching. However, early computers did not have graphical user interfaces, or anything meaningful in the way of computer graphics. If analysts wanted to chart their data, it was still a painstaking process of drawing artifacts such as bar charts and scatterplots by hand, even if a computer helped with calculations. If computer programs did create "graphics," they were often in the form of strategically-placed dashes, asterisks, and periods typed out, one character at a time, by line printers.

By the 1970s and 1980s, however, computer graphics were becoming more prevalent, and it became feasible to make charts and graphs an integral part of the analytic process. At this time, American mathematician and statistician John Tukey was formative in the development of **exploratory data analysis (EDA),** and published an influential book by the same name in 1977. In this book and other work, Tukey argued that too much emphasis was being placed on testing statistical hypotheses and not enough on visualizing data to suggest hypotheses to test (Tukey 1977). The EDA approach to analysis aims to depict data graphically to help identify outliers, detect trends and patterns, and suggest hypotheses for formal testing. The EDA ideas of Tukey and those who extended his work were critically important in the creation of modern statistical software such as R, especially with respect to its graphics capabilities.

Figure 6.1.   Line chart from the *Commercial and Political Atlas*

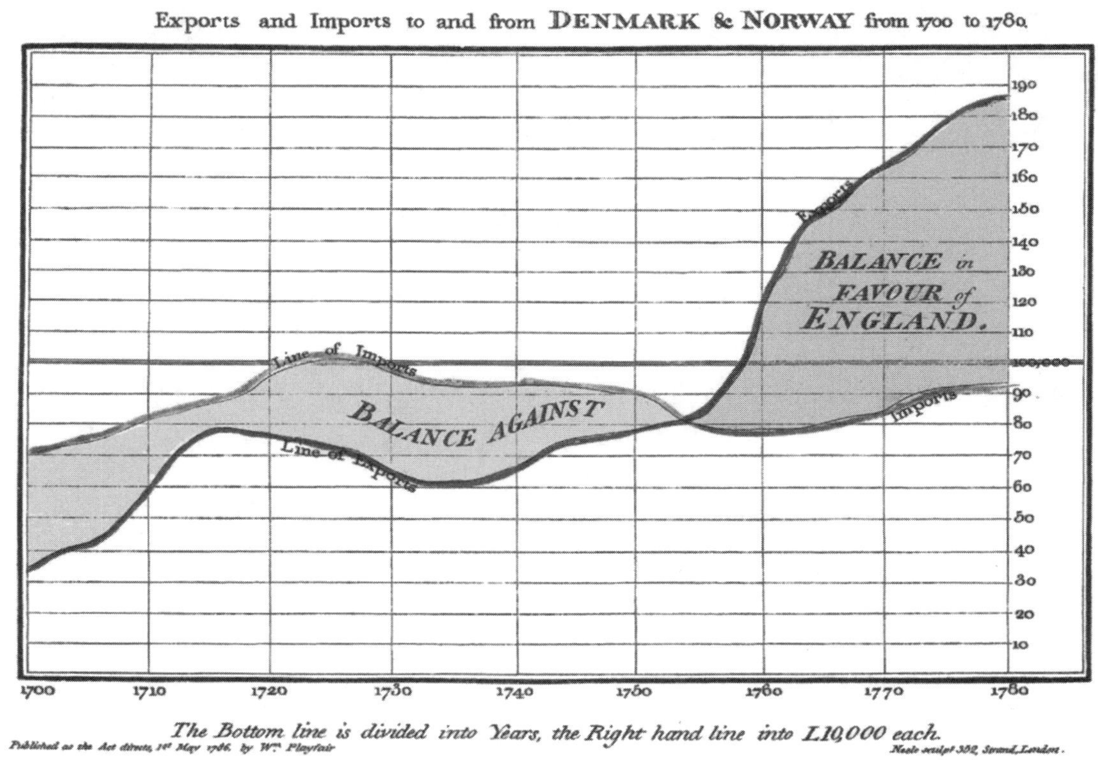

Source: Playfair 2005.

Research Question and Hypothesis

The primary purpose of EDA is to obtain an understanding of the data to address the broad question, "What is going on here?" EDA offers an understanding of data without formal modeling or hypothesis testing. The derivation of patterns can illustrate stories with the data. In this way, EDA is often adopted as an initial phase for gaining an understanding of the data in order to develop further research questions that are accompanied by formal hypotheses.

The research questions posed during EDA are typically broader and less defined. The questions are meant to direct the data exploration to determine if possible patterns exist. The data for this chapter explore the following research question:

Do payments from non-Medicare sources differ in interesting, meaningful ways by MS-DRG, state, or both? If so, how?

Checklist

To answer the research question, a specific process of data acquisition, preparation, and discovery is required. The following steps are explained in this chapter:

1.   Extract data sets from MySQL
     a.   SELECT the appropriate columns of data

2. Data preparation with Microsoft Excel
   a. Rename column headers to make analysis easier
3. Import the data into RStudio
   a. Manipulate R data frames using dplyr package
4. Conduct data visualization procedures:
   a. Use ggplot package to explore data visually
   b. Develop research hypotheses based upon results

The Analysis

This chapter examines the inpatient component of the Medicare Provider Utilization and Payment Data, provided by the Centers for Medicare and Medicaid Services (CMS 2014). This data set provides hospital-specific, aggregated charges for the 100 most frequently billed hospital discharges in the years 2011 and 2012. The discharges are coded and categorized using the Medicare Severity-Diagnosis Related Group (MS-DRG) system. The data set covers more than 3,000 US hospitals, and represents more than seven million discharges—more than 60 percent of hospital discharges under the Medicare Inpatient Prospective Payment System (IPPS).

Hospitals set their own rates for the care they provide. While their total charges are billed to Medicare, the IPPS provides set amounts that Medicare will pay for each discharge MS-DRG. Along with any patient deductibles and third-party payments, the total amount that is actually paid to a hospital for its services may be much less than what was originally billed. As part of their agreements with Medicare, hospitals must accept the total payments they are given, whatever the amount. Any charges in excess of what is paid are not paid by any other party, including the patient.

The Medicare Provider Utilization and Payment Data breaks down these numbers, recording for each hospital/MS-DRG combination the total number of discharges, the average charges billed, the average total amount of money that was paid to the hospital, and the average total amount of money that was paid by other means, such as deductibles and third-party payments. These numbers are of obvious interest, because they can show how much different hospitals charge for care, as well as how much Medicare and others will actually pay for different conditions.

Step 1: Data Extraction

Two data sets must be extracted from the MySQL database. One data set represents IPPS data from FY2011 and the other from FY2012. Figure 6.2 shows the two MySQL queries that were used for extracting the two data sets. The first query selects all columns of data from the table ipps_2011. The * shown after the SELECT statement is used for returning all columns of data in the specified table. Also, the hospital name is derived from the hospital_general_information table. Therefore, the hospital_general_information table must be joined to the ipps_2011 table. The second query selects all columns of data from the table ipps_2012 and the hospital name from the hospital_general_information table.

To execute each query, place the cursor on the line of the query you want to process. Click the 🔧 icon to execute the script where your cursor is placed. After executing each query, export the data to a CSV file (save the files as ipps_2011.csv and ipps_2012.csv). You will have a separate CSV file for each query. For detailed instructions regarding exporting data from MySQL Workbench to CSV format, see chapter 4.

Figure 6.2. SQL script and returned data for combining three data sets

```
SELECT
  ipps_2011.*, hospital_general_information.hospital_name,
  hospital_general_information.state
FROM
  ipps_2011
JOIN
  hospital_general_information ON ipps_2011.provider_id =
  hospital_general_information.provider_id;
```

(Continued)

Figure 6.2.   SQL script and returned data for combining three data sets *(Continued)*

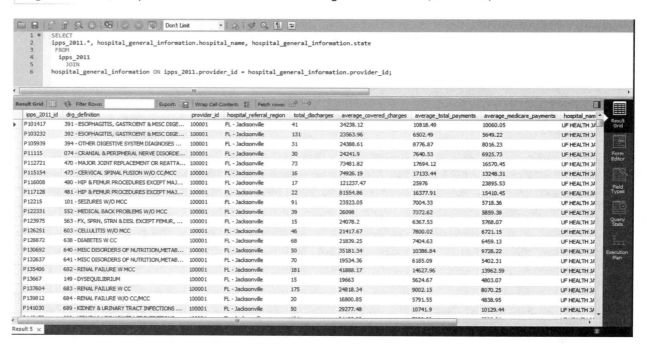

```
SELECT
  ipps_2012.*, hospital_general_information.hospital_name,
  hospital_general_information.state
FROM
  ipps_2012
JOIN
  hospital_general_information ON ipps_2012.provider_id =
  hospital_general_information.provider_id;
```

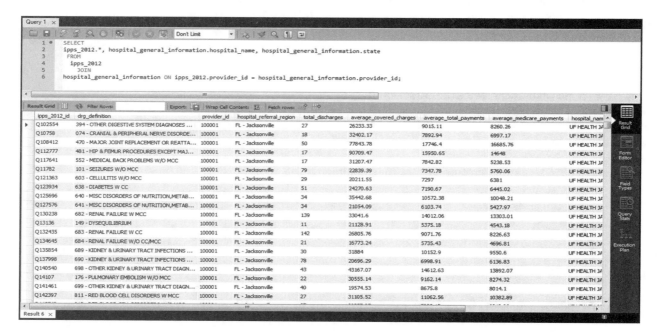

Step 2: Data Preparation

Much of the work in this chapter will be done from within RStudio, but a few preliminary steps will be easier in Microsoft Excel. Start by loading the CSV files into Excel and examining them. The general structure for each is the same: a listing where each row is an individual hospital. The following columns should appear:

- ipps_2011_id or ipps_2012_id: The MS-DRG code number and its description, in all capital letters. You will frequently see references to different conditions or procedures with or without complication or comorbidity (CC) or (major complication or comorbidity) MCC.
- drg_definition: The code number assigned to an individual inpatient hospital.
- provider_id: The unique identifier provided by the Centers for Medicare and Medicaid Services to all Medicare-certified hospitals.
- hospital_referral_region (HHR): A regional market area for specialized consultative care, where caring for a patient may require the use of a major referral center in that region. There are 306 different HRRs, and some may cross state borders, so that a hospital in one state may be part of another state's HRR, depending on the location of different referral centers. Each HRR is named using a state, coupled with the name of a city in that state.
- total_discharges: The number of patients discharged from the hospital under the given MS-DRG for that year.
- average_covered_charges: The average charge for a given MS-DRG at a particular hospital. This is the amount that is billed, though it may not be the total amount paid.
- average_total_payments: The average amount that is actually paid by Medicare and other parties for a given MS-DRG.
- average_medicare_payments: The average amount that is paid by Medicare itself. Note that this amount is a subset of the previous field, average total payments.
- hospital_name: The name of the hospital that reported the measured data for the specific MS-DRG code.
- state: The state where the hospital is located.

Preparing the data for analysis is a major component of every analytics project. This section describes how to prepare the data in a way that makes it easier to analyze in RStudio.

Renaming Column Headers in Excel

When we import this data into RStudio, these column header names will become the names of different fields in a data frame. RStudio will do the best job it can of working with names that have spaces in them, but it would be better to make each of these field names shorter now, while in Excel, rather than changing them in RStudio (or worse, typing long field names in RStudio each time we want to use them). Table 6.1 contains the names to use when renaming the column headers. Note that the discharge, charge, and payment fields are appended with "_h", which will stand for "hospital." To rename column headers in Excel, simply click each individual cell, highlight the contents, delete the content, enter the new column name, and click return. Repeat this process for each column header. These header changes should be made in both the ipps_2011.csv and ipps_2012.csv files.

Step 3: Import the Data

Once these changes have been made to the column headers, save the files and then import both the 2011 and 2012 IPPS data sets into RStudio (for a detailed description of how to import data into RStudio, see Loading Data into RStudio in chapter 5). When importing the data into RStudio, you may be required to specify that the data has a header row. To do so, ensure that the radio button for yes is selected in the import window listed after the Heading option. When importing, name the data frames drg2011_h and drg2012_h, respectively. While both data sets are large, they should fit comfortably in your RStudio environment. After the data are

Table 6.1.   Original and revised column names within Excel

Original Name	Revised Name
ipps_2011_id	ipps_2011_id
ipps_2012_id	ipps_2012_id
drg_definition	drg
provider_id	pid
hospital_referral_region	hrr
total_discharges	discharges_h
average_covered_charges	avgcovcharges_h
average_total_payments	avgtotpayments_h
average_medicare_payments	avgmcpayments_h
hospital_name	name
state	state

imported into RStudio, open an R scripting window. The R scripting window is where you will enter the R code in order to analyze the data. To open a new R scripting window, go to File > New File > R Script. This will add a new tab to the upper-left quadrant of RStudio. By default, the title of the tab is Untitled1.

Step 4: Data Visualization

Once the data files are imported into RStudio, a few additions can be made to make the sets easier to work with and potentially more informative. While these changes can be made using base R commands, we will use an R package called dplyr to make the syntax easier to write and understand. The name dplyr is a play on the phrase "data frame pliers" and is a collection of tools to help perform common data manipulation tasks, such as reshaping, combining, and summarizing data sets. As with any other package, dplyr needs to be installed and then loaded into R to make it available for use. The following two commands, run separately, will do this:

```
install.packages("dplyr")
library(dplyr)
```

You may see messages about certain other commands being "masked." All this means is that some built-in functions, such as filter(), intersect(), and so on, are being replaced with functions in dplyr that have the same name. This is intended and is nothing to be concerned about.

As noted previously, the full data sets show information at the hospital level. If we wanted to obtain measures at the state level, we will need to compact the data—totaling the number of discharges for all hospitals in the state and making averages of the charges and payments. The following commands will do this for the drg2012_h set:

```
drg2012_h <- group_by(drg2012_h, drg, state)

drg2012_s <- summarize(drg2012_h, discharges_s=sum(discharges_h),
avgcovcharges_s=weighted.mean(avgcovcharges_h, discharges_h),
avgtotpayments_s=weighted.mean(avgtotpayments_h, discharges_h),
avgmcpayments_s=weighted.mean(avgmcpayments_h, discharges_h))
```

The first command will change the drg2012_h data frame slightly, using dplyr to mark the data set as being grouped by one or more variables. In this case, the data set should be grouped by drg, and then within each drg, by each state. Strictly speaking, this command does not change the underlying data themselves, but sets them up for the following command, which creates a new data frame called drg2012_s. (As might be expected, this data frame will contain data at the state level.) The summarize() function takes the original data frame (drg2012_h) and collapses it, creating a new data frame where each line is a single state (not hospital) within a given MS-DRG. The drg and state variables are kept, since they are grouping variables, but everything else is removed. However, we are adding four new variables, which will replace the ones that were dropped:

- **discharges_s**: The number of discharges for each state. This is defined in the command as the sum of all of the discharges_h for each of the hospitals in each state and MS-DRG combination.
- **avgcovcharges_s**: The average charge for a given MS-DRG in a given state. This is defined in the command as taking the hospital-level figures and averaging them by state. Since each hospital has a different number of discharges, we need to calculate a weighted average to obtain an accurate overall mean. This is done through the weighted.mean() function, which takes the variable we want to average as the first argument, and the weighting variable as the second argument.
- **avgtotpayments_s**: The average amount that is actually paid by Medicare and other parties for a given MS-DRG. Like avgcovcharges_s, this is calculated at the state level using a weighted average, using the number of discharges at each hospital as weights.
- **avgmcpayments_s**: The average amount that is paid by Medicare itself. Like avgcovcharges_s and avgtotpayments_s, this is calculated at the state level using a weighted average, using the number of discharges at each hospital as weights.

The same commands for the drg2011_h data set should be run as well, making sure to replace drg2012_h with drg2011_h in each command. We will now have two data frames for each year, one being at the hospital level and one at the state level. One more pair of data frames needs to be created, this time aggregating the data further to the MS-DRG level. The following commands will do this:

```
drg2012_s <- group_by(drg2012_s, drg)

drg2012_d <- summarize(drg2012_s, discharges_d=sum(discharges_s),
avgcovcharges_d=weighted.mean(avgcovcharges_s, discharges_s),
avgtotpayments_d=weighted.mean(avgtotpayments_s, discharges_s),
avgmcpayments_d=weighted.mean(avgmcpayments_s, discharges_s))
```

This time, we are creating another collapsed data set, where each record contains information on discharges, charges, and payments, averaged for each MS-DRG. As you should notice from the summarize() function, we are again taking the sum (across each state within a given MS-DRG) of discharges and weighted averages of the charges and payments. The same commands should be run with the drg2011_s data frame, again replacing drg2012_s with drg2011_s.

Each of the six data sets that were created should appear in your Environment window as follows: drg2011_d, drg2011_h, drg2011_s, drg2012_d, drg2012_h, and drg2012_s. Once this preparation work is done, we are almost ready to explore the data visually within RStudio.

Next, EDA principles are used to explore the Medicare charge data that were extracted and manipulated. We will create several graphical displays of the data, which will reveal some interesting patterns that can then be explored with more formal statistical hypothesis testing. We will use the graphics capabilities of the R package ggplot2, which provides powerful and easy-to-use functionality to visualize data. Unlike more traditional graphics toolkits, ggplot2 uses principles from the theory of the Grammar of Graphics (the "gg" in ggplot2) to provide a consistent syntax for describing charts and graphs of many different forms (Wilkinson 2005). The Grammar of Graphics provides a consistent way of specifying any **data visualization** as a series of mappings from variables to graphical elements. For example, a scatterplot of human heights and weights can be specified by mapping height to the *x*-axis and weight to the *y*-axis, and specifying a point to represent individual data elements. Other variables can be mapped to additional features, such as mapping sex to point color. While ggplot2 uses slightly different terminology and commands to produce graphics than many other toolkits, it is not difficult to understand the basics; we will discuss these as we perform our exploratory analyses.

There are many possible questions that we could explore in the Medicare cost data we have prepared, but we will restrict ourselves to just one area for simplicity. Recall the three monetary figures tracked in the data:

average charges billed by the hospitals, average payments made by Medicare and other sources, and the average component of those payments from Medicare itself. Hospital charges at different locations, or for different MS-DRGs, are one area of interest, as are the amounts that Medicare pays. (CMS makes some adjustments to the rates it provides for different MS-DRGs depending on geographic location, for instance.) We will concentrate, however, on the payments made to the hospital that are not from Medicare, but are instead from deductibles, co-pays, and payments made by third parties for the coordination of benefits. While not perfect (since the data do not break down the payments further), this component of the total payments can be a good proxy for the overall financial burden on patients and non-Medicare parties. From this, we can create a working research question:

> Do payments from non-Medicare sources differ in interesting, meaningful ways by MS-DRG, state, or both? If so, how?

Note that this is a *research question*, which provides an impetus for our analyses. It is not the same as making one or more formal statistical hypotheses. In the EDA approach, we will explore the data graphically, and then see if we can formulate hypotheses as we go.

First, however, we will need to extract the non-Medicare payment component from the total payments. This is simply the average total payments field(s), minus the Medicare payments field(s). Using the mutate() function from dplyr, we can add a new field to each of our three data frames to hold this new amount. As you would expect, there will be different amounts at the hospital, state, and MS-DRG levels.

```
drg2012_h <- mutate(drg2012_h, paymentdiff_h = avgtotpayments_h -
avgmcpayments_h)

drg2012_s <- mutate(drg2012_s, paymentdiff_s = avgtotpayments_s -
avgmcpayments_s)

drg2012_d <- mutate(drg2012_d, paymentdiff_d = avgtotpayments_d -
avgmcpayments_d)
```

The same commands should be run for the 2011 data set, substituting 2011 for 2012 as appropriate. Finally, be sure to install and load the ggplot2 package so that we can visualize the data with the following command:

```
install.packages("ggplot2")
library(ggplot2)
```

Now we are finally ready to analyze the data. First, we need to get an idea of how the non-Medicare payments vary by MS-DRG, without examining state- or hospital-level measures. For this, we will use the drg2012_d data frame (we will restrict our explorations at the moment to the 2012 data). What we will have, essentially, is a list of 100 numbers representing the amount paid from non-Medicare sources for different MS-DRGs. While there are a variety of ways we could graphically display these numbers, including numeric tables, a reasonable way to visualize them for comparative purposes is to build a simple **bar chart**; each MS-DRG will be a single bar in the chart and the heights of the bars will correspond to the mean of the non-Medicare payments. To help the comparison process, we will also order the bars from highest to lowest. It is better in this case to make a horizontally oriented bar chart so that the MS-DRG descriptions are all along the *y*-axis and are easier to read. The following commands will make such a chart:

```
diff_d <- ggplot(drg2012_d, aes(x=reorder(drg, paymentdiff_d),
y=paymentdiff_d))

diff_d + geom_bar(stat="identity") + coord_flip()
```

The first command creates what will become our chart, which we are calling diff_d (payment difference at the MS-DRG level). In the ggplot() function, the first argument tells R to use the drg2012_d data frame for the data. The aes() function ("aes" stands for *aesthetic*—in this case, appearance) specifies that the *x*-coordinate in the graph should be the MS-DRG descriptions, which will become the different bars, and the y-coordinate should be represented by the MS-DRG-specific payment difference we calculated. The x-coordinate also uses the reorder() function, which takes the MS-DRG descriptions, and orders their appearance in the graph by the payment difference. Here, the MS-DRG with the highest payment difference will be the first bar, followed by the MS-DRG with the next highest payment difference, and so on.

Note that typing this command on its own does not do anything visible in R. An object called diff_d is created in memory, but no chart will appear. In ggplot terms, there is a graph object, but it cannot be rendered to the screen because a specific geom has not been defined for it. Put simply, a ggplot geom is a geometric object that helps define the visual appearance of the chart. Since we want a bar chart, we apply the bar geom in the next command. Many other geoms exist, including those that can create line charts, pie charts, and other types of charts and effects.

The second line will actually result in a visible chart. The syntax may look strange, as it looks like we are taking the new object and somehow adding quantities to it. In ggplot, however, the + sign can have special meanings. In this case, it takes a graph object and adds layers to a plot. These layers can be geoms, colors, or many other transformations. Here, we are applying the geom_bar() geom, resulting in a bar chart appearance for the overall graphic. Note that there is a single argument being used, stat="identity", which defines the way the bars are represented. By default, geom_bar() will chart the counts of different attributes (also called stat="bin"), to create a frequency histogram. For the purposes of this text, the bars will represent the actual payment difference values. By including stat="identity", we are telling ggplot not to apply any type of transformation to the data, and just use the actual values (that is, an identity transformation). Finally, we add the coord_flip() layer, which will swap the x- and y-coordinates before actually drawing the graph. This is the only way to create a horizontally-oriented bar chart; try removing the coord_flip() layer, or switching the x- and y-coordinates in the original ggplot() statement to see what happens instead.

You should obtain the chart in figure 6.3.

Using RStudio, click on the zoom 🔍 Zoom in the upper left part of the Plot window to show the chart in its own window. Then, enlarge the window to the full screen size to see as much detail as possible. We can see that most of the MS-DRGs have low average payments from non-Medicare sources, typically around $1,000. The upper 25 percent of the MS-DRGs exhibited higher payments, mostly ranging from a mean of about $1,500 to a mean of $2,750. The highest MS-DRG, however, is code 460, "spinal fusion except cervical without major complication or comorbidity." Spinal fusion procedures that do not involve the cervical (neck) vertebrae involve average non-Medicare payments of almost $4,000. An outlier has been found, but what does it mean?

Note that the chart, while legible, has a lot of distracting ink on it, in the form of the black bars. At different magnifications, the gaps between the bars can run together to make even more distracting white line patterns. We can apply a different geom to show the varying heights without all the black areas:

```
diff_d + geom_point(size=3) + coord_flip()
```

This command takes the same base chart and uses simple points with a 3-pixel radius to mark the tops of the bars. The resulting chart (figure 6.4), sometimes called a dotplot, is arguably much easier on the eyes, and this format will be used instead of a more traditional bar chart for a similar graphic later on.

Returning to the data themselves, we now want to examine the outlier MS-DRG identified earlier. Do different states see similar, high rates of non-Medicare payments for this particular MS-DRG, or are certain states pulling the average payment figure higher? We can find out visually with another bar (or dot) chart. Using the drg2012_s state-level data frame, we can create a similar plot, with different states on one axis, and the average payments for each state on the other axis. The commands are similar to the ones before, but we have one extra complication: We just want to see the state-level average payments for a particular MS-DRG, and not all MS-DRGs in the data set. To filter out the data and plot only what we want, we can use the filter() command from dplyr to first select which MS-DRG group we want data from, and go from there:

```
drg2012_s_fusion <- filter(drg2012_s,drg == "460 - SPINAL FUSION EXCEPT
CERVICAL W/O MCC")

diff_s_fusion <- ggplot(drg2012_s_fusion,aes(x=reorder(state,
paymentdiff_s), y=paymentdiff_s))

diff_s_fusion + geom_point(size=3) + coord_flip()
```

Figure 6.3.   Bar chart showing average payments from non-Medicare sources by MS-DRG for 2012

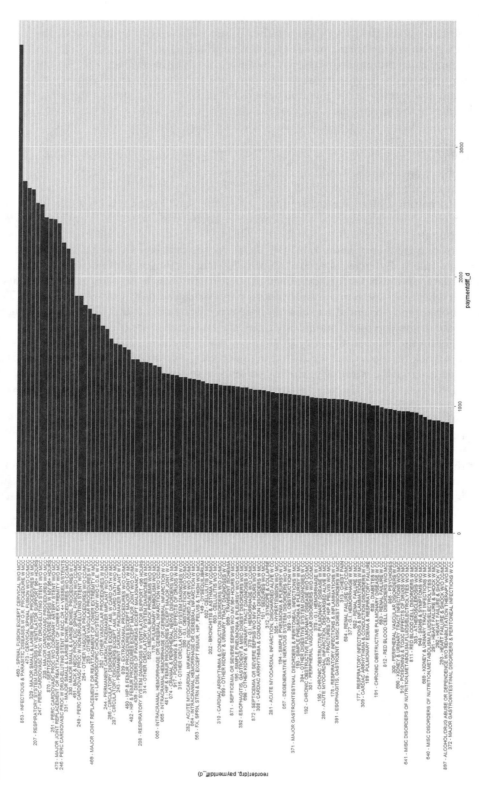

Source: Used with permission from RStudio.

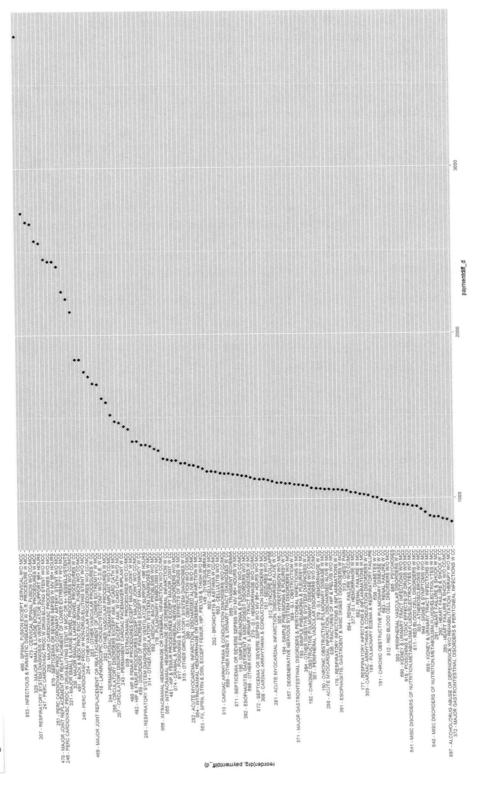

Figure 6.4. Dotplot showing average payments from non-Medicare sources by MS-DRG for 2012

Source: Used with permission from RStudio.

Here, filter() limits or subsets the data by creating a new data frame (drg2012_s_fusion) where only observations that have a drg value of "460 – SPINAL FUSION EXCEPT CERVICAL S/O MCC" are included. The long text string is the actual value of the drg variable. Note the use of double equal signs (==) to perform the match, rather than a single equal sign. The other two commands create a graphic from the new data frame, much as created in the previous example (see figure 6.5).

There appears to be a fairly even distribution of average payments by each state around the mean. Hawaii and Utah are at the upper tail of the distribution, but they do not appear to be outliers affecting the mean disproportionately. From this, we can informally deduce that noncervical spinal fusion procedures involve unusually high non-Medicare payments nationwide. We can then use statistical tests to formally test this and related hypotheses.

A reasonable question is whether we can discern state-level differences in other MS-DRGs with similar, high non-Medicare payments. We can construct similar charts substituting different MS-DRGs, but this can quickly become cumbersome. Fortunately, there are techniques to help visualize these data as a single graphic. We will create a heat map of the different non-Medicare payments, showing all possible states within all possible MS-DRGs. Imagine a spreadsheet where all the rows (or columns) are different MS-DRGs, and all the columns (or rows) are the various states. While a standard spreadsheet might put dollar values in each cell to show the payments, a heat map will represent the numbers as colored cells. We can specify that cells (combinations of MS-DRG and state) with higher average non-Medicare payments will be colored more brightly than those with lower average payments, thus showing where the "heat" is in the data.

Producing a heat map with ggplot is simple. We still specify which variables should be on the x- and y-coordinates, but instead of applying a bar or dot geom, we will apply a tile so that all the data will be arranged in a grid pattern. We can then specify that the brightness of the cell colors should be tied to the payment values. The following commands will create a heat map for the state-level non-Medicare payment data, using red as a base color:

```
diff_smap <- ggplot(drg2012_s, aes(x=state, y=drg, fill=paymentdiff_s))
diff_smap + geom_tile() + scale_fill_gradient(low="grey", high="red")
```

In the first command, we specify that the fill (internal) color of any geom elements we later request should be based on the value of paymentdiff_s. In the second command, we specify the tile geom, and also specify the color scale to use for the tiles. Scale_fill_gradient() is used to define the specific colors; here, the lowest non-Medicare payment value in the set should be gray, and the highest point should be bright red (the figure generated using your computer will appear with red. However, the image in the textbook will appear with dark gray rather than a red color). If we did not specify these limits, the default colors would be a very dark blue at the low end, brightening to a turquoise blue at the high end. Figure 6.6 is a representation of what will appear on your screen, with the darker gray cells representing the red cells on your screen. To best see the individual cells, be sure to zoom and expand the graphic to your maximum screen size.

Along the x-axis is each state, in alphabetical order. Along the y-axis, each MS-DRG appears in apparently reverse order. Just as it would for increasing numeric values, ggplot orders categories starting at the bottom of the axis. There are ways to change this ordering, but the default graphic is fine for our present purposes. You will see some lighter gray spaces in the heat map; these are where there were no data for a particular state and MS-DRG combination and ggplot did not place a tile, which reveals the underlying light gray background grid. Note the isolated bright red points, due to individual states having individual MS-DRGs with very high average non-Medicare payments. More broadly, we can also see horizontal bands of brighter color, corresponding to MS-DRGs with higher overall payments. For example, MS-DRG 460—the noncervical spinal fusion procedure—stands out compared to most other MS-DRGs. To a smaller extent, we can even see brighter vertical bands for some states, such as Hawaii and Nevada.

Finally, we will compare this payment data across time, to see if there were interesting patterns of increase or decrease in average non-Medicare payments between 2011 and 2012. To do this, we will take the state-level data from both the 2011 and 2012 data sets, combine them into a new data frame, and then calculate the difference in average payment between the two years. The following commands will do this:

```
diff2011 <- select(drg2011_s, drg, state, diff2011=paymentdiff_s)
diff2012 <- select(drg2012_s, drg, state, diff2012=paymentdiff_s)
diffchange <- inner_join(diff2011, diff2012, by=c("drg","state"))
diffchange <- mutate(diffchange, diff_change = diff2012 - diff2011)
```

Figure 6.5. Dotplot showing average payments from non-Medicare sources for noncervical spinal fusion by state for 2012

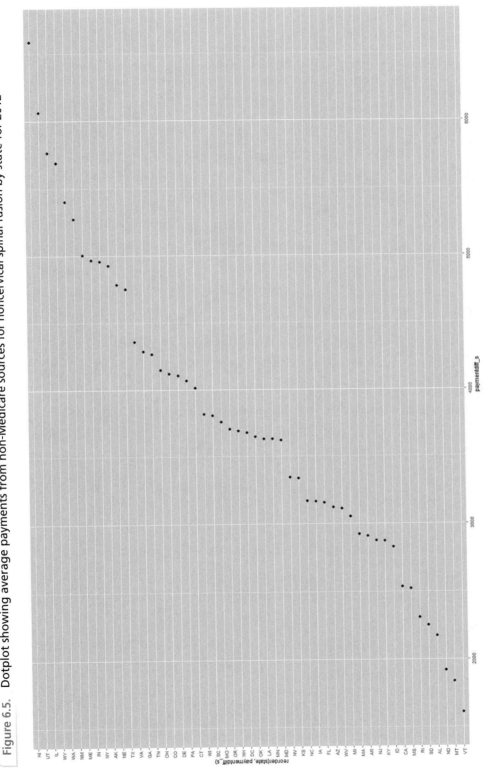

Source: Used with permission from RStudio.

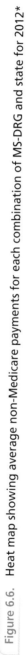
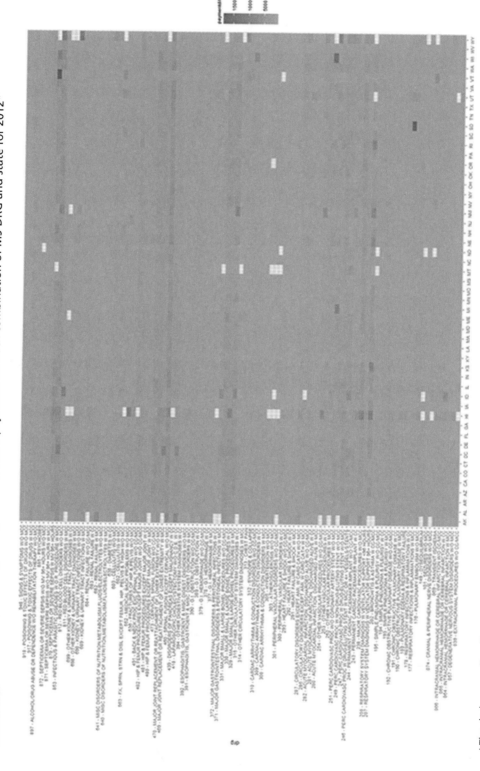

Figure 6.6. Heat map showing average non-Medicare payments for each combination of MS-DRG and state for 2012*

*The dark gray cells will appear as red on the computer screen.
Source: Used with permission from RStudio.

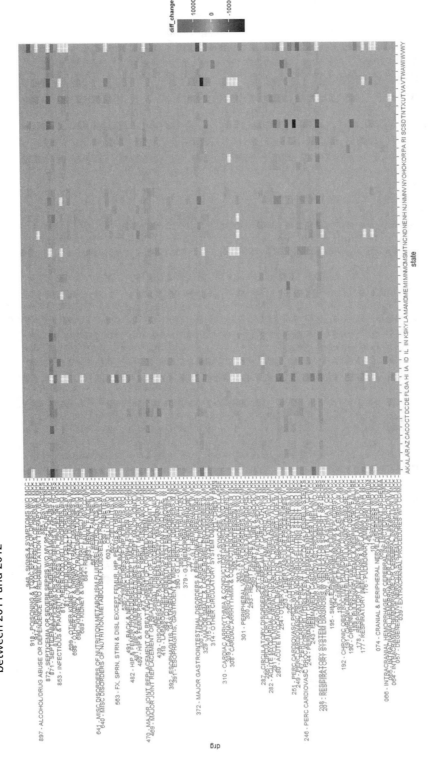

Figure 6.7. Heat map showing the difference in average non-Medicare payments for each combination of MS-DRG and state between 2011 and 2012*

*The dark gray cells will appear as red on the computer screen.
Source: Used with permission from RStudio.

The first two lines take the 2011 and 2012 state-level data sets, respectively, and derive new data frames from them. The select() function from dplyr will put selected variables into the new frames. We do not need all of the data from the original data frames, and just select the drg, state, and payment difference fields. Note that the payment variables are renamed according to their respective years. The third line uses dplyr's inner_join() function, which merges the two new data frames. The "by" clause specifies which fields to match. Since we want to match up each MS-DRG and state combination, we want to specify both fields. The inner_join() function also has the effect of only merging MS-DRG and state combinations that appear in both data sets; if a specific combination occurs in one year but not another (which can happen if a given MS-DRG falls into or out of the top 100 from one year to the next), it is not included in the resulting data frame. The last line changes the new data frame, adding a new field that provides the difference in average payments between the two years.

With this data preparation, we can create another heat map, using the change in average payments as a basis for the tile colors:

```
diffmap <- ggplot(diffchange, aes(x=state, y=drg, fill=diff_change))

diffmap + geom_tile() + scale_fill_gradient2(low="black", mid="grey",
high="red")
```

Figure 6.7 is a representation of what will appear on your screen, with the darker gray cells representing the red cells on your screen. You should recognize how the first line works from the previous heat map example. The second line also looks similar, but this time we are using a different color scale. Since some values might be positive and some negative, it would be nice to set a difference of zero to gray—then positive numbers in one color and negative numbers in another. The scale_fill_gradient2() command specifies these transitions; we give positive changes red values and negative changes black values.

As with the previous heat map, we can see horizontal stripes where there were stronger changes in some MS-DRGs than others. We can also see some vertical striping, indicating large changes at the state level. Individual black and red points on the computer screen (black and dark gray in the text) reveal specific MS-DRG and state combinations with large changes.

Discussion

With this visual information, we can start exploring specific MS-DRGs, states, and combinations. We can even drill down to the individual hospital level to see the patterns of non-Medicare payments. For example, we can ask if there are particular hospitals with much higher or lower charges. We can then use these observations to create formal hypotheses to test statistically, and support (or disprove) our intuitions by inspecting the graphics. This is the essence of EDA: using data visualization techniques to detect outliers, patterns of interest, and trends, in conjunction with statistical analyses.

Note that EDA is not the same as formal statistical testing. In fact, we did not perform any statistical tests in this chapter. The point, of course, is not to say that statistical analysis is unimportant—it is important. EDA, however, teaches that there are advantages to seeing the data with our own eyes, and that our visual observations can then drive the discovery and testing of statistical hypotheses. In that sense, exploratory analysis and statistical analysis can be, and should be, partners in the overall analytic process.

Conclusion

This chapter provided several examples of visualizing data with the ggplot2 package for R for analyzing multiple MS-DRGs across every state, but was not an exhaustive tutorial. We only scratched the surface of what is possible—ggplot2 has many other features and potential visualization types. Fortunately, ggplot2 has become extremely popular within the R community and there are a number of excellent resources available for learning more. A few of these resources include

- ggplot2.org: The ggplot2 home page, which features extensive documentation and links to other resources (Wickham 2013)
- *ggplot2: Elegant Graphics for Data Analysis*: Hadley Wickham, ggplot2's creator, has also written a definitive book on the package (Wickham 2009)

- Plotting with ggplot2: Parts I and II: A YouTube video offering a free tutorial (Peng 2013a, Peng 2013b)
- *R Graphics Cookbook*: A cookbook approach to choosing and creating graphics through extensive examples, most using ggplot2, but some using R's base graphics and other packages (Chang 2012)

This chapter also featured a fair amount of data manipulation using the dplyr package. While the dplyr package is much newer and does not have a published literature, the dplyr home page on GitHub (Wickham 2015) is a good source for information, as are the vignettes available within R. These vignettes show multiple examples of code with explanations and can be accessed with the command:

```
vignette(package="dplyr")
```

This will provide a list of different vignettes available for the dplyr package, and specific vignettes can be specified in subsequent commands. For example, the introductory vignette is available through the following command:

```
vignette(package="dplyr", topic="introduction")
```

The overall topic of data visualization is a large one, with many published books, research articles, and websites, among other sources. Key considerations include the purpose of data visualizations—should they enable exploratory work, as discussed in this chapter, or should they be used in published work to inform or persuade others? Appropriate techniques can vary between statistical and persuasive graphics since different audiences can have varying degrees of technical sophistication and understanding of the information being explored or related. In addition, the type of data is also important. Are the data continuous variables such as dollar figures, or categorical variables like MS-DRGs and states? Different combinations of different variables can suggest different visualization techniques.

Along with the original EDA text (Tukey 1977), there are many published books offering advice on creating statistical or persuasive graphics. For statistical graphics, one of the most recognized in the field is *The Visual Display of Quantitative Information* (Tufte 2001). While Tufte's book is more philosophical in nature than a how-to book, it remains one of the best texts available on how to think about data and visualize them effectively and responsibly. *Now You See It* (Few 2009) takes a more practical, EDA approach to quantitative data analysis. Another book by the same author, *Show Me the Numbers* (Few 2009), concentrates on using data visualization to convey information to others. Both texts provide concrete advice to make your own exploratory data analyses and reporting more effective and fruitful.

Review Exercises

Instructions: Choose the best answer.

1. Exploratory data analysis aims to accomplish which of the following?
   a. Depict data graphically to help identify outliers
   b. Detect trends and patterns
   c. Suggest hypotheses for formal testing
   d. All of the above

2. A data visualization technique that assigns color based upon data frequency is called a(n):
   a. EDA
   b. dplyr
   c. bar chart
   d. heat map

3. The package used to manipulate data frames such as reshaping, combining, and summarizing data sets is called:
   a. RStudio
   b. ggplot
   c. dplyer
   d. None of the above

4. An object that helps define the visual appearance of a chart is called a(n):
   a. geom
   b. aes
   c. gradient
   d. dotplot

5. The ggplot function that puts variables in descending order on a visualization is called:
   a. inner_join()
   b. aes
   c. reorder()
   d. coord_flip()

References

Chang, W. 2012. *R Graphics Cookbook*. Sebastopol, CA: O'Reilly Media.

Centers for Medicare and Medicaid Services. 2014. Medicare Provider Utilization and Payment Data: Physician and Other Supplier. http://www.cms.gov/Research-Statistics-Data-and-Systems/Statistics-Trends-and-Reports/Medicare-Provider-Charge-Data/Physician-and-Other-Supplier.html

Few, S. 2009. *Now You See It: Simple Visualization Techniques for Quantitative Analysis*. Berkeley, CA: Analytics Press.

Peng, R. 2013a. "Plotting with ggplot2: Part 1." https://www.youtube.com/watch?v=HeqHMM4ziXA

Peng, R. 2013b. "Plotting with ggplot2: Part 2." https://www.youtube.com/watch?v=n8kYa9vu1l8

Playfair, W. 2005. *Playfair's Commercial and Political Atlas and Statistical Breviary, Reprint Edition*. Cambridge, UK: Cambridge University Press.

Tufte, E.R. 2001. *The Visual Display of Quantitative Information,* 2nd ed. Cheshire, CT: Graphics Press.

Tukey, J.W. 1977. *Exploratory Data Analysis*. Boston, MA: Addison-Wesley.

Wickham, H. 2013. ggplot2. http://ggplot2.org

Wickham, H. 2009. *ggplot2: Elegant Graphics for Data Analysis*. New York, NY: Springer.

Wickham, H. 2015. dplyr. https://github.com/hadley/dplyr

Wilkinson, L. 2005. *The Grammar of Graphics*. Chicago, IL: Springer Science & Business Media.

Chapter 7

Evaluating Participation in the EHR Incentive Program

David Marc, MBS, CHDA and Ryan Sandefer, MA, CPHIT

Learning Objectives

- Describe the process of combining multiple data types for carrying out analytical procedures
- Explain how to use Excel for recoding variables for analysis
- Differentiate null and alternative hypotheses for statistical testing
- Demonstrate the use of chi-squared test to assess the relationship of healthcare practice characteristics to EHR adoption

Key Terms

Alternative hypothesis
Categorical data
Chi-squared goodness of fit test
Core-based statistical areas (CBSA)
Cross-tabulations (contingency table)
Dependent variable
Descriptive statistics
Filler
Independent variable
Null hypothesis
Zip code tabulation area (ZCTA)

Electronic health records (EHRs) have the potential to improve healthcare quality and reduce its cost (Blumenthal and Tavenner 2010). The HITECH Act's EHR Incentive Program that was included as part of the American Recovery and Reinvestment Act (ARRA) provided approximately $27 billion dollars to promote the adoption and meaningful use of EHR systems across the US healthcare delivery system, including hospitals, primary care providers, specialists, and other eligible professionals (Blumenthal 2009; Blumenthal and Tavenner 2010). The program provides monetary incentive payments to those hospitals and professionals who adopt certified EHR systems and use them to meet various measures related to technical functions and clinical and administrative processes.

The EHR Incentive Program has had a dramatic effect on EHR adoption in the United States. Since 2009, the rate of basic EHR adoption among office-based physicians has increased from 26 percent to 48 percent and the rate of basic EHR adoption among hospitals has increased from 9.4 percent to 59.4 percent (Furukawa et al. 2014; King et al. 2012). Basic EHRs are defined by capabilities, including "recording patient history and demographic information; maintaining patient problem lists; recording clinical notes; recording medication and allergy lists; viewing laboratory results; viewing imaging reports; and using computerized prescription ordering" (Furukawa et al. 2014).

Research has shown that while the adoption of EHR systems by eligible professionals has increased dramatically since 2009, there are gaps in adoption by practice size and provider specialty (McCullough et al. 2011; GAO 2012). According to research, primary care practices are significantly more likely than other specialties to have adopted basic EHRs and solo clinic practices are significantly less likely to adopt these systems (Furukawa et al. 2014). Research has shown that urban settings have a higher rate of adoption than their rural counterparts (McCullough et al. 2011; Casey et al. 2013). It is clear that rural providers are at risk for falling behind urban counterparts in regard to health information technology adoption and use, including using technology to improve clinical outcomes and decision making. Further analysis is needed to better understand the impact of meaningful use provider adoption and use of EHRs by specialty and geographic location.

The purpose of this chapter is to evaluate the adoption and meaningful use of EHRs by eligible professionals, including a comparative analysis of eligible providers by practice size and geographic location.

Research Question and Hypothesis

Is there a difference in the proportion of eligible professionals that attested for meaningful use when comparing practices by size or location?

A research question should include a dependent and independent variable. The **dependent variable** is the measured variable. The dependent variable for the proposed study is the proportion of eligible professionals that attested for meaningful use. The **independent variable** is the variable being used to compare groups. In the case of the proposed research question, there are two independent variables: practice size and location. The independent variables have more than one level. That is, the independent variable can be broken down into distinct groups. These groups can be compared using the dependent variable. Practice size has three levels: small, medium, and large. Location has two levels: rural and urban. Therefore, the analysis for answering the proposed research question will have two parts:

1. A comparison of the proportion of meaningful use attestation among small, medium, and large practices
2. A comparison of the proportion of meaningful use attestation between rural and urban locations

Given the research question, several hypotheses should be proposed and tested. The hypotheses should be stated as a null (H_0) and alternative (H_A). The **null hypothesis** states that we will observe the same measured outcome of our dependent variable for each level of our independent variable. The **alternative hypothesis** states that we will observe different measured outcomes of our dependent variable for each level of our independent variable. Because the research question is measuring meaningful use attestation rates for different groups (that is, practice sizes and locations), there are more than one set of hypotheses.

Hypotheses

$H1_0$: The average proportion of eligible professionals that attested for meaningful use is the same among small, medium, and large practices.

$H1_A$: The average proportion of eligible professionals that attested for meaningful use is not the same among small, medium, and large practices.

$H2_0$: The average proportion of eligible professionals that attested for meaningful use is the same between rural and urban geographic settings.

$H2_A$: The average proportion of eligible professionals that attested for meaningful use is not the same between rural and urban geographic settings.

Checklist

To answer our research question, a specific process of data acquisition, preparation, and discovery is required. The following steps will be explained in detail:

1. Extract data sets from MySQL
   a. SELECT the appropriate columns of data
2. Data preparation with Microsoft Excel
   a. Create a variable to categorize practice size as either small, medium, or large
   b. Create a variable to categorize practices as rural or urban
3. Import the data into R
   a. Calculate the proportion of providers in each group practice that attested
   b. Calculate the proportion of providers in each group practice that attested
4. Conduct descriptive statistics
5. Conduct statistical procedures: chi-squared goodness of fit test

The Analysis

Now that the research question and hypotheses is written, we have identified the data elements necessary to answer the research question, determined the appropriate statistical procedures for the project, and can begin the process for analyzing the data.

Step 1: Data Extraction

In order to carry out the analysis, the following data elements are needed:

- A list of all healthcare providers in the United States
- An indicator as to whether the provider attested for meaningful use
- An indicator as to whether the provider is in an urban or rural area
- An indicator as to the size of the group practice for which the provider works

Several tables of data need to be combined to obtain the needed data to answer the proposed research question. The first table is named ep_provider_paid_ehr and was made available by the Centers for Medicare and Medicaid Services (2014). The data set lists all of the providers that have successfully attested for meaningful use and received payment as of December 2014. Each unique provider is identified by their national provider identification number (NPI), which is a unique ID provided to all organizations and individual providers that are certified by Medicare. The data set also includes the location of the provider and the size of the provider's group practice.

The second data set is named national_downloadable_file and derived from the Physician Compare database that was created and made available by CMS (2015). This data set lists all of the providers in the United States who are eligible to bill to Medicare. Each unique provider is identified by their NPI. The NPI values from the national_downloadable_file data set can be mapped to the NPI values in the ep_provider_paid_ehr data set to display which providers have been paid for attesting to meaningful use. The data set also includes the location of the provider.

The third data set is named zip_to_cbsa and was published by the US Census Bureau (2011). The data set includes a crosswalk between the **core-based statistical areas (CBSA)** and **zip code tabulation area (ZCTA)**. A CBSA is defined as either metropolitan or micropolitan. A metropolitan area is an urban cluster with greater than 50,000 people. A micropolitan area is an urban cluster with 10,000 to 50,000 people. If an area is not included in a CBSA, that area is considered rural. The ZCTA is the general assigned zip codes for the United States Postal Services. The zip_to_cbsa data set can be mapped to the zip codes for each provider's practice location to determine if that practice is in a rural (not in a CBSA) or urban (metropolitan or micropolitan) location.

These data sets will be combined using MySQL scripts (as illustrated in figure 7.1). The scripts will be constructed so that only the following data elements are extracted: group practice PAC ID, size of group practice, the provider NPI for those that attested for meaningful use, and the CBSA (figure 7.1). In order to combine these tables, there are two additional tables that will be joined in the query. The provider_intersect table is used as an intermediate table (explained in Chapter 4) that is used to join the ep_provider_paid_ehr table to the national_downloadable_file table. The zipcode_table will be used to join the national_downloadable_file table to the zip_to_cbsa table. Note that you must alter a setting in MySQL so that the output shows all of the results rather than just showing the first 1,000 rows (see chapter 4).

Figure 7.1 shows the SQL script that combines the three required data sets and extracts only the relevant data elements. Because the ep_provider_paid_ehr table and the national_downloadable_file have a many-to-many relationship, the intermediate table called provider_intersect was used to join the two tables. A LEFT JOIN is used when adding in the ep_provider_paid_ehr table so that all the records from the national_downloadable_file are retrieved even when a match is not found in the ep_provider_paid_ehr table. A LEFT JOIN is also used when joining the zip_to_cbsa table to the zipcode_table so that all of the zip codes are retrieved even when a CBSA is not found for that zip code. This is important as not all zip codes have a CBSA if that zip code is associated with a rural area. The top section of the figure depicts the MySQL script that was used to obtain the data. The bottom section of the figure depicts the first few rows of the output that was derived from the query. Given the volume of data that is being retrieved, the query may take several minutes to process.

Export the data from MySQL Workbench and save the data in a CSV file and name the file "EP_Attest." Open EP_Attest.csv and you should see the following columns in Microsoft Excel:

- group_practice_PAC_id: Unique group practice ID assigned by the Medicare Provider Enrollment, Chain, and Ownership System (PECOS) to the group practice with which the individual professional works—will be blank if the address is not linked to a group practice
- number_of_group_practice_members: The number of providers working within the practice
- provider_npi: The national provider identifier (NPI)—will only be revealed if a provider in that practice attested for meaningful use
- cbsa: The total population living within the boundaries of the Census-based Core-Based Statistical Area

Step 2: Data Preparation

Data preparation is the most labor-intensive and, arguably, the most important step in the analytics process. The purpose of data preparation is to ensure the correct data—in the correct format—are used for the analysis.

Figure 7.1. SQL script and returned data for combining three data sets

```
SELECT DISTINCT
    national_downloadable_file.group_practice_PAC_id,
    national_downloadable_file.number_of_group_practice_members,
    ep_provider_paid_ehr.provider_npi,
    zip_to_cbsa.cbsa
FROM
    national_downloadable_file
        JOIN
    provider_intersect ON
    national_downloadable_file.national_downloadable_file_id =
    provider_intersect.national_downloadable_file_id
        LEFT JOIN
    ep_provider_paid_ehr ON
    provider_intersect.ep_provider_paid_ehr_id =
    ep_provider_paid_ehr.ep_provider_paid_ehr_id
    JOIN
    zipcode_table ON
    national_downloadable_file.zipcode =
    zipcode_table.zipcode
        LEFT JOIN
    zip_to_cbsa ON
    zipcode_table.zipcode = zip_to_cbsa.zipcode
    WHERE national_downloadable_file.group_practice_PAC_id<>'NA';
```

(Continued)

Figure 7.1.   SQL script and returned data for combining three data sets *(Continued)*

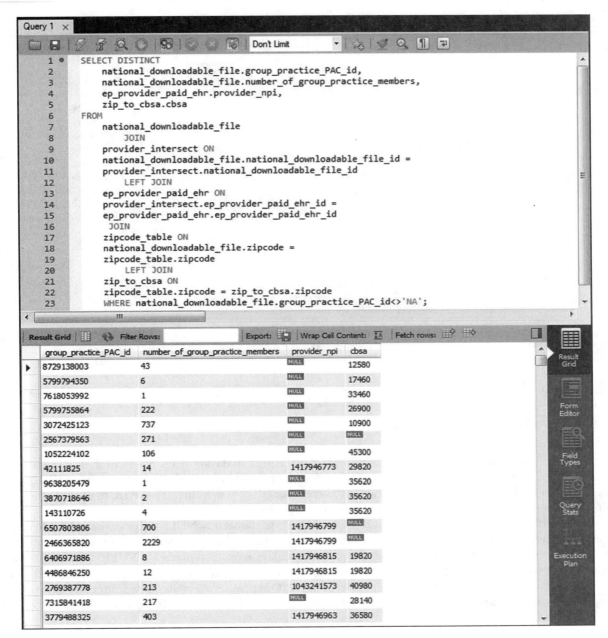

Removal of Erroneous Values

One of the first steps in data preparation is to carefully examine if the data include erroneous values or blanks. An erroneous value may be a value that was used as a **filler**. A filler is often used as a default value to indicate a blank field. For example, the value –1111.1 may be used to represent a blank field entry. It is best to eliminate the fillers from your data set because they often hold a numeric value.

For example, consider for a moment the impact of the filler –1111.1. Suppose you wanted to calculate the average length of stay for patients. When the average length of stay was unknown, assume that the value –1111.1 was entered. If we included five patients in the analysis and one of those patients were assigned the filler value for the length of stay, this would greatly impact the average length of stay value. Assume the

Figure 7.2. Finding and replacing NULL values using Microsoft Excel

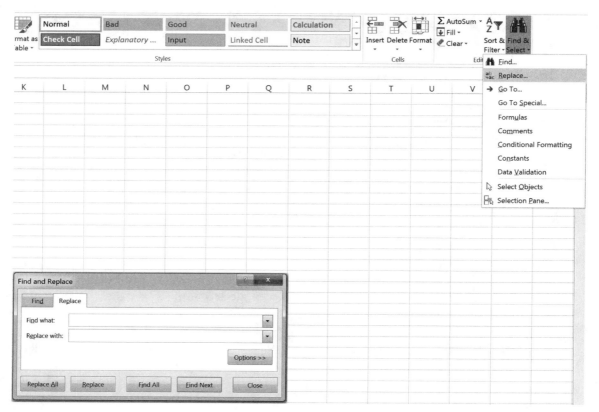

Used with permission from Microsoft.

five recorded length of stay values were the following (measured in days): 3, 12, 6, –1111.1, 4. If we were to calculate the average length of stay of these five patients, we would obtain the calculation of –217.22 days. The inclusion of the filler results in an erroneous average length of stay value. If we were to exclude the filler value, we would obtain a more appropriate calculation of 6.25 days.

In the data set created from the MySQL query, there are numerous NULL values. These NULL values should be removed in order to properly recode the data. To remove the NULL values, open the exported data set in Excel. Next, under the HOME tab, find the binoculars icon to replace all NULL values as blanks. Figure 7.2 demonstrates how to find and replace characters in Excel. To replace characters in Excel, click on the binoculars icon listed on the far right side of the HOME tab. Select Replace under the drop-down window. In the Find and Replace window, enter NULL in the Find what textbox. Keep the Replace with textbox blank. Click Replace All.

Recoding Data Fields

Second, certain data fields need to be recoded. Recoding is a data normalization step that can be adopted to convert a quantitative variable into qualitative groups (for example, converting distinct ages into age groupings). Also, recoding can be adopted to alter existing qualitative groupings (for example, sex coded as the numeric values as 1 for male and 2 for female can be recoded as the textual entries of "male" and "female").

In the data set for this analysis, three data fields need to be recoded: number_of_group_practice_members, provider_npi, and cbsa.

The number_of_group_practice_members field is currently formatted as a real number representing the total number of individual professionals affiliated with the group practice. This field will be recoded as a small, medium, or large practice to create groups to compare. To determine the groupings, a statistical method can be adopted to divide the providers into three distinct categories. One method for dividing the practices is to calculate the values at the 33rd and 66th percentile to determine the numbers that will be used to divide the data into the three categories. The value that is calculated at the 33rd percentile can be interpreted as the number where 33 percent of the providers have a practice size equal to or less than that number. Therefore, we can use this number to generate a rule to recode the data as small practices. Medium practices are defined as provider practice sizes that are greater than the number at the 33rd percentile but equal to or less than the number at the 66th percentile. Large practices have a practice size greater than the number at the 66th percentile.

The percentile values can be determined using the PERCENTILE function in Microsoft Excel (figure 7.3). The size of group practice variable can be recoded as small, medium, and large using the IF function in excel. The IF function is a rule to generate text when the size of group practice number falls below the 33rd percentile (small), between the 33rd and 66th percentile (medium), or greater than the 66th percentile (large); see figure 7.4. To calculate the 33rd percentile, in a cell (such as G2) enter the following formula =PERCENTILE(B:B,0.33). The formula will calculate the value at the 33rd percentile. The same can be done to get the value of the 66th percentile, in a cell (such as G3) enter the following formula =PERCENTILE(B:B,0.66). The value you should obtain for the 33rd percentile is 2 and the value at the 66th percentile is 31.

MS Excel's IF function can be used to recode the size of group practice variable into small, medium, or large groups (figure 7.4). Small practices are defined as those where the number of providers is less than or equal to 2. Medium practices include 3 to 31 providers. Any practice with greater than 31 providers is considered large. Insert a new column in MS Excel in the C column and label it "Size." Enter the formula in cell C2: =IF(B2<=2,"Small",IF(AND(B2>2,B2<=31),"Medium",IF(B2>31,"Large",""))). After adding the formula to cell C2, double-click the small square icon on the bottom-right of cell C2. This will fill in the rest of the cells with the formula input in cell C2. At this point, you can delete the table you created next to the data to determine the percentiles.

The second variable that needs to be recoded is provider_npi. This data field will be used to determine if a provider has attested for meaningful use. Currently, the provider_npi data field displays only the NPI number of the provider's that attested for meaningful use. For some of the providers listed in the data set, the provider_npi field is blank. The field is blank because these providers were not found in the ep_provider_paid_ehr table in the database. Therefore, this is an indicator that providers with a blank in the provider_npi field did not attest for meaningful use.

Figure 7.3. Using Microsoft Excel's percentile function

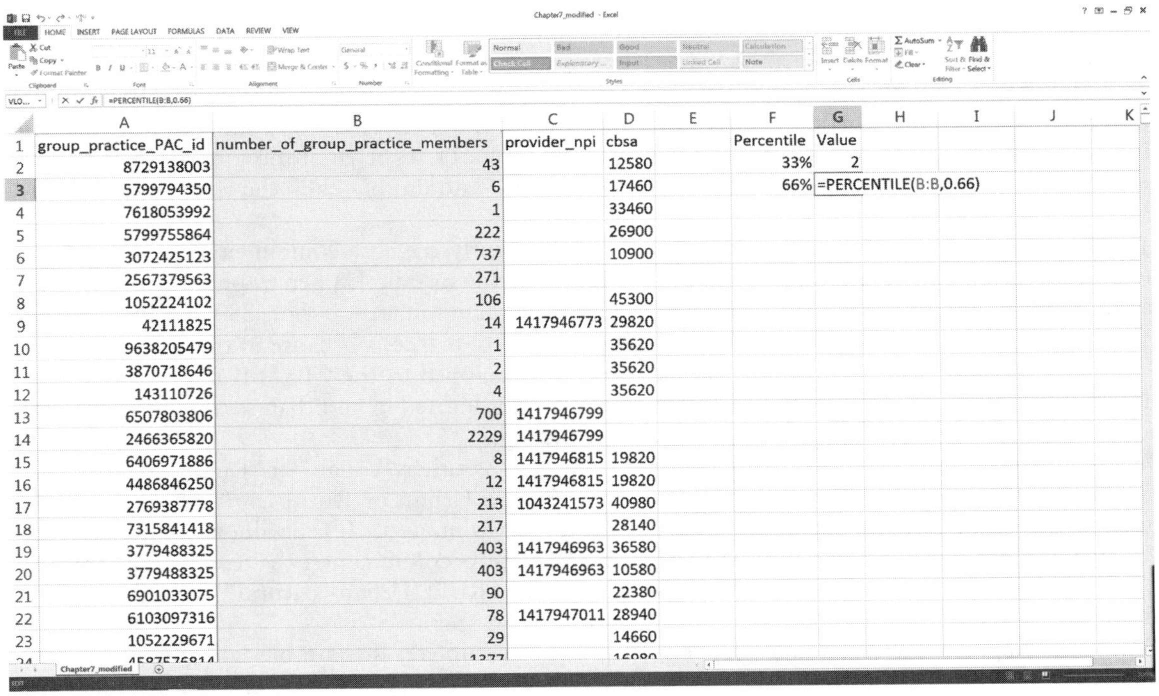

	A	B	C	D	E	F	G
1	group_practice_PAC_id	number_of_group_practice_members	provider_npi	cbsa		Percentile	Value
2	8729138003	43		12580		33%	2
3	5799794350	6		17460		66%	=PERCENTILE(B:B,0.66)
4	7618053992	1		33460			
5	5799755864	222		26900			
6	3072425123	737		10900			
7	2567379563	271					
8	1052224102	106		45300			
9	42111825	14	1417946773	29820			
10	9638205479	1		35620			
11	3870718646	2		35620			
12	143110726	4		35620			
13	6507803806	700	1417946799				
14	2466365820	2229	1417946799				
15	6406971886	8	1417946815	19820			
16	4486846250	12	1417946815	19820			
17	2769387778	213	1043241573	40980			
18	7315841418	217		28140			
19	3779488325	403	1417946963	36580			
20	3779488325	403	1417946963	10580			
21	6901033075	90		22380			
22	6103097316	78	1417947011	28940			
23	1052229671	29		14660			
24	[illegible]	[illegible]		[illegible]			

Figure 7.4. Using Microsoft Excel's IF function to recode data regarding practice size

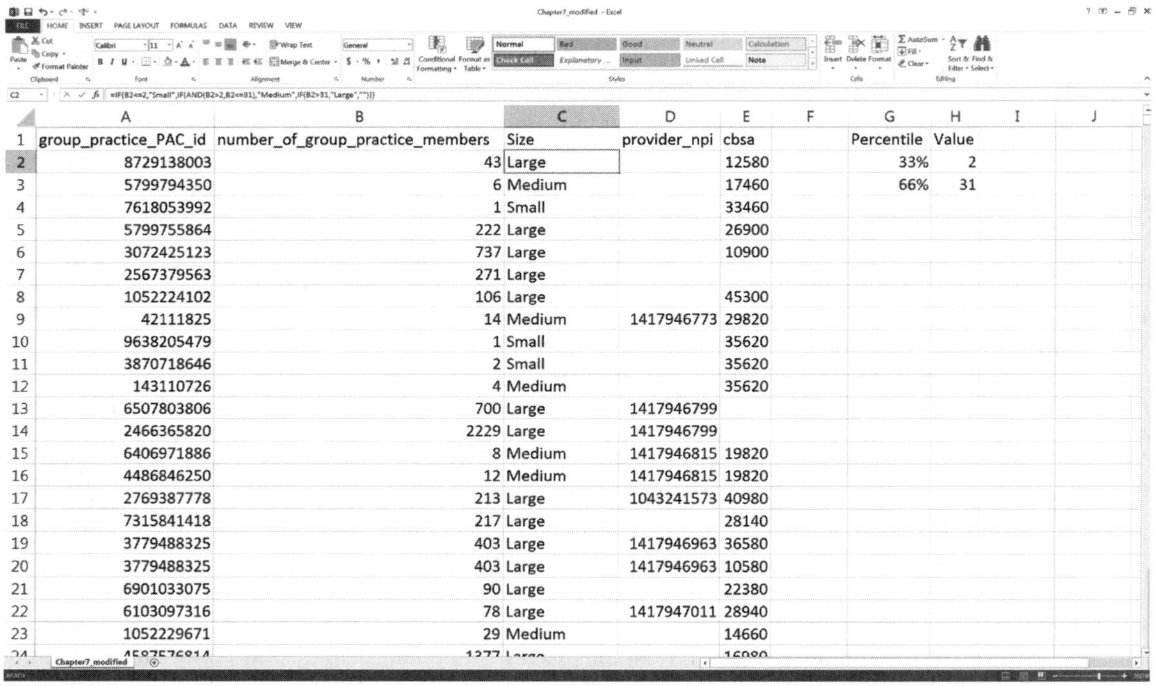

	A	B	C	D	E	F	G	H
1	group_practice_PAC_id	number_of_group_practice_members	Size	provider_npi	cbsa		Percentile	Value
2	8729138003	43	Large		12580		33%	2
3	5799794350	6	Medium		17460		66%	31
4	7618053992	1	Small		33460			
5	5799755864	222	Large		26900			
6	3072425123	737	Large		10900			
7	2567379563	271	Large					
8	1052224102	106	Large		45300			
9	42111825	14	Medium	1417946773	29820			
10	9638205479	1	Small		35620			
11	3870718646	2	Small		35620			
12	143110726	4	Medium		35620			
13	6507803806	700	Large	1417946799				
14	2466365820	2229	Large	1417946799				
15	6406971886	8	Medium	1417946815	19820			
16	4486846250	12	Medium	1417946815	19820			
17	2769387778	213	Large	1043241573	40980			
18	7315841418	217	Large		28140			
19	3779488325	403	Large	1417946963	36580			
20	3779488325	403	Large	1417946963	10580			
21	6901033075	90	Large		22380			
22	6103097316	78	Large	1417947011	28940			
23	1052229671	29	Medium		14660			

The provider_npi field will be recoded to indicate whether the providers have attested for meaningful use. Using Excel, an IF function will be used to generate the text "Attested" when provider_npi contains a number. If the provider_npi field is blank, this will generate the text "NotAttested." Figure 7.5 displays how this is carried out in Excel. The figure depicts the method in Excel for recoding the provider_npi variable into Attested or NotAttested using the IF function. The IF function is used to determine if the value listed in the provider_npi column is a number. If the value is a number, this will return the value Attested. If the value is blank, this will return the value NotAttested. First, create a new column in the E column in Excel and label that column MeaningfulUse. The ISNUMBER function in Excel returns a TRUE if the value is a number or FALSE if the value is anything other than a number. Therefore, the ISNUMBER function can be used in an IF statement to appropriately recode the data. Type the following IF statement in cell E2: =IF(ISNUMBER(D2)=TRUE,"Attested","NotAttested") and double-click the small square icon to fill in the remainder of the column.

The third data field that will be recoded is the cbsa. Currently, the cbsa column either contains a numeric value or is blank—CBSA is a unique number that represents a specific US geographic region. If the CBSA contains a number, this indicates that the provider is located in an urban area. If the CBSA is blank, this indicates that the provider is in a rural area. The reason that this rule holds true is because in the SQL script that was used to query the data, the zip code for each provider was mapped to the CBSA. If the provider's zip code was found to be located in a CBSA, this indicates the provider is located in an urban setting. If the zip code was not found in a CBSA, the provider is located in a rural setting.

In Excel, an IF statement can be created to recode the cbsa as either "Urban" or "Rural." Figure 7.6 depicts the method in MS Excel for recoding the cbsa variable into Urban or Rural using the IF function. The IF function is used to determine if the value listed in the cbsa is numeric. If the value is numeric, Urban will be returned. If the value is blank, Rural will be returned. In the G column enter the text, "Geography." In cell G2, type the formula to recode cbsa: =IF(ISNUMBER(F2)=TRUE,"Urban","Rural") and double-click the small square icon to fill in the remainder of the column.

After recoding the data, the data preparation phase is complete. If the table with the percentiles that you calculated from the number_of_group_practice_members is still present on the spreadsheet,

Figure 7.5. Using Microsoft Excel's IF function to recode meaningful use data

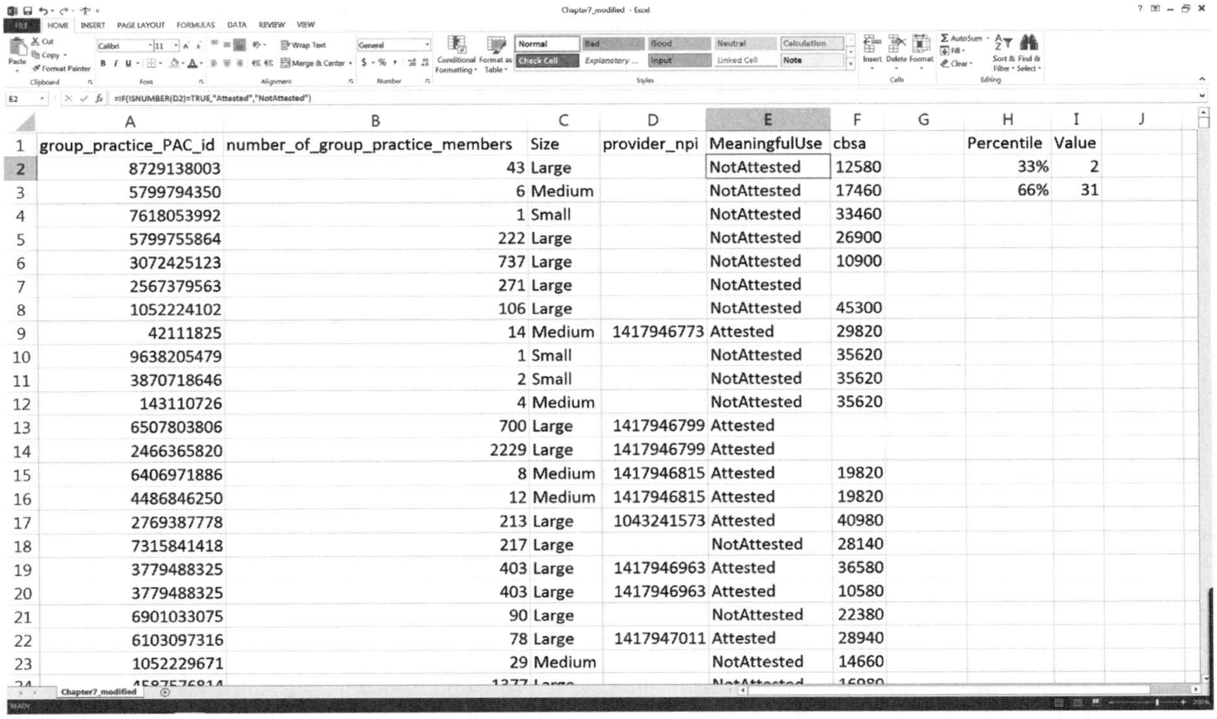

E2 =IF(ISNUMBER(D2)=TRUE,"Attested","NotAttested")

	A	B	C	D	E	F	G	H	I
1	group_practice_PAC_id	number_of_group_practice_members	Size	provider_npi	MeaningfulUse	cbsa		Percentile	Value
2	8729138003	43	Large		NotAttested	12580		33%	2
3	5799794350	6	Medium		NotAttested	17460		66%	31
4	7618053992	1	Small		NotAttested	33460			
5	5799755864	222	Large		NotAttested	26900			
6	3072425123	737	Large		NotAttested	10900			
7	2567379563	271	Large		NotAttested				
8	1052224102	106	Large		NotAttested	45300			
9	42111825	14	Medium	1417946773	Attested	29820			
10	9638205479	1	Small		NotAttested	35620			
11	3870718646	2	Small		NotAttested	35620			
12	143110726	4	Medium		NotAttested	35620			
13	6507803806	700	Large	1417946799	Attested				
14	2466365820	2229	Large	1417946799	Attested				
15	6406971886	8	Medium	1417946815	Attested	19820			
16	4486846250	12	Medium	1417946815	Attested	19820			
17	2769387778	213	Large	1043241573	Attested	40980			
18	7315841418	217	Large		NotAttested	28140			
19	3779488325	403	Large	1417946963	Attested	36580			
20	3779488325	403	Large	1417946963	Attested	10580			
21	6901033075	90	Large		NotAttested	22380			
22	6103097316	78	Large	1417947011	Attested	28940			
23	1052229671	29	Medium		NotAttested	14660			

Figure 7.6. Using Microsoft Excel's IF function to recode data as Urban or Rural

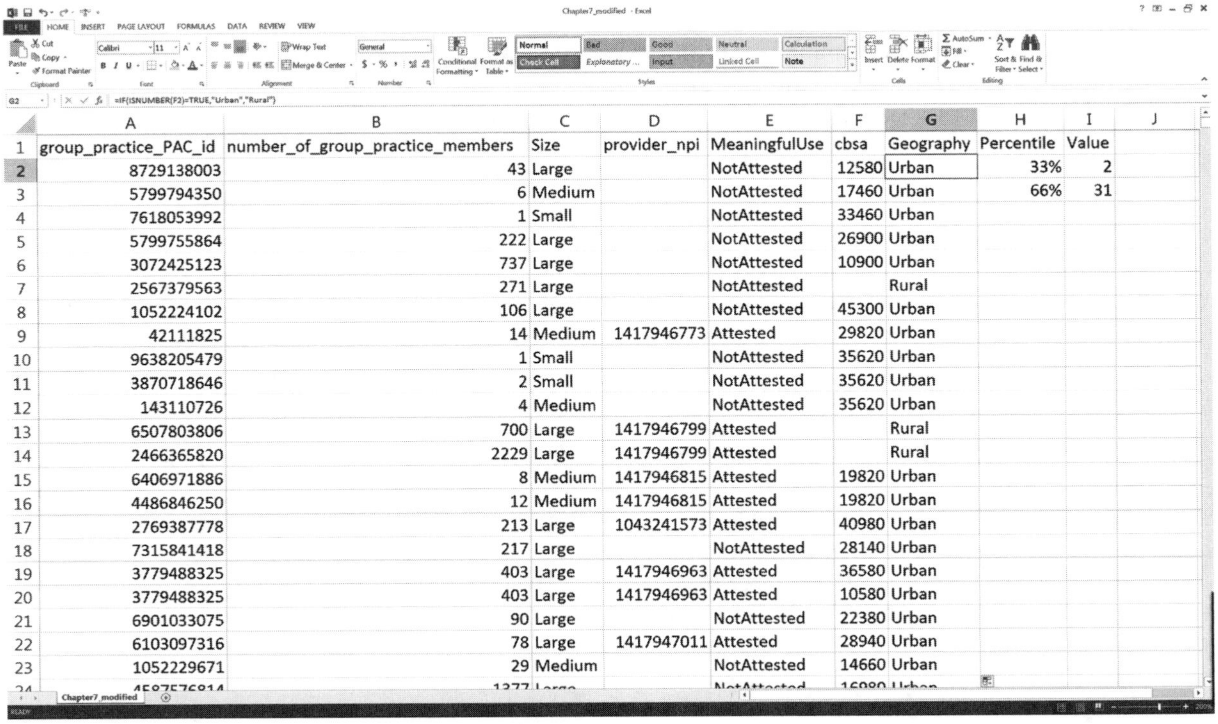

G2 =IF(ISNUMBER(F2)=TRUE,"Urban","Rural")

	A	B	C	D	E	F	G	H	I
1	group_practice_PAC_id	number_of_group_practice_members	Size	provider_npi	MeaningfulUse	cbsa	Geography	Percentile	Value
2	8729138003	43	Large		NotAttested	12580	Urban	33%	2
3	5799794350	6	Medium		NotAttested	17460	Urban	66%	31
4	7618053992	1	Small		NotAttested	33460	Urban		
5	5799755864	222	Large		NotAttested	26900	Urban		
6	3072425123	737	Large		NotAttested	10900	Urban		
7	2567379563	271	Large		NotAttested		Rural		
8	1052224102	106	Large		NotAttested	45300	Urban		
9	42111825	14	Medium	1417946773	Attested	29820	Urban		
10	9638205479	1	Small		NotAttested	35620	Urban		
11	3870718646	2	Small		NotAttested	35620	Urban		
12	143110726	4	Medium		NotAttested	35620	Urban		
13	6507803806	700	Large	1417946799	Attested		Rural		
14	2466365820	2229	Large	1417946799	Attested		Rural		
15	6406971886	8	Medium	1417946815	Attested	19820	Urban		
16	4486846250	12	Medium	1417946815	Attested	19820	Urban		
17	2769387778	213	Large	1043241573	Attested	40980	Urban		
18	7315841418	217	Large		NotAttested	28140	Urban		
19	3779488325	403	Large	1417946963	Attested	36580	Urban		
20	3779488325	403	Large	1417946963	Attested	10580	Urban		
21	6901033075	90	Large		NotAttested	22380	Urban		
22	6103097316	78	Large	1417947011	Attested	28940	Urban		
23	1052229671	29	Medium		NotAttested	14660	Urban		

remove all the contents of the table. Next, save the file as a CSV. In Excel, click File > Save As. Under the Format drop-down window, select the Comma Separated Values option. When saving the file, name the document EP_Attest and save the file to your computer's desktop. Note: When saving your file, you may receive a message:

> Some features in your workbook might be lost if you save it as CSV (Comma defined). Do you want to keep using that format?

The reason Excel provides this warning is that only the active spreadsheet in your Excel workbook will be saved. If you have additional spreadsheets included in your worksheet, those spreadsheets will be lost. Click OK.

The next step in the analysis is to import the data into RStudio for analysis.

Step 3: Import the Data

The next step in the analysis is to import the data set EP_Attest.csv into RStudio for analysis (see chapter 5 for detailed instructions for importing data into RStudio). After the data is imported into RStudio, open an R scripting window. The R scripting window is where you will enter the R code in order to analyze the data. To open a new R scripting window, go to File > New File > R Script. This will add a new tab to the upper-left quadrant of RStudio. By default, the title of the tab is Untitled1.

Within the R scripting window, you must run a line of code to attach the data set. The reason that the data set is attached is to make the column names accessible in RStudio. Without the use of the attach function, the only way to work with the data by the column names is to specify the name of the data frame followed by a dollar sign and the name of the column. For example, if a data set named AllData was imported into RStudio and there was a need to call out the column Age without attaching the data, a user would be required to use the following script: AllData$Age. If the data set is attached, a user can simply call the column by its name: Age.

To attach the data, the user should enter the following R script into the console:

```
attach(EP_Attest)
```

The attach functions save the column headers into the RStudio software for analysis. This allows us to use the column names for analysis rather than using the column names with the data set name. After running the attach function, the script will appear in the console as shown in figure 7.7.

Step 4: Descriptive Statistics

Once the data is imported and attached into RStudio, the first type of analysis that should be conducted to familiarize yourself with the data is the **descriptive statistics**. Descriptive statistics simply refer to "a set of statistical techniques used to describe data such as means, frequency distributions, and standard deviations; statistical information that describes the characteristics of a specific group or population" (White 2013).

The data used to answer our research question includes categorical data. Categorical data is frequently described by counting the frequency that different categories occur. In this case, there are three categorical data elements: MeaningfulUse, Size, and Geography. In RStudio, the table function can be used to obtain a frequency of a data element broken down into groups.

The data element MeaningfulUse has two categories, Attested and NotAttested. Using the table function in RStudio, the number of providers that attested and did not attest for meaningful use can be obtained by running the following code:

```
table(MeaningfulUse)
```

Figure 7.7. Demonstration of running the attach function

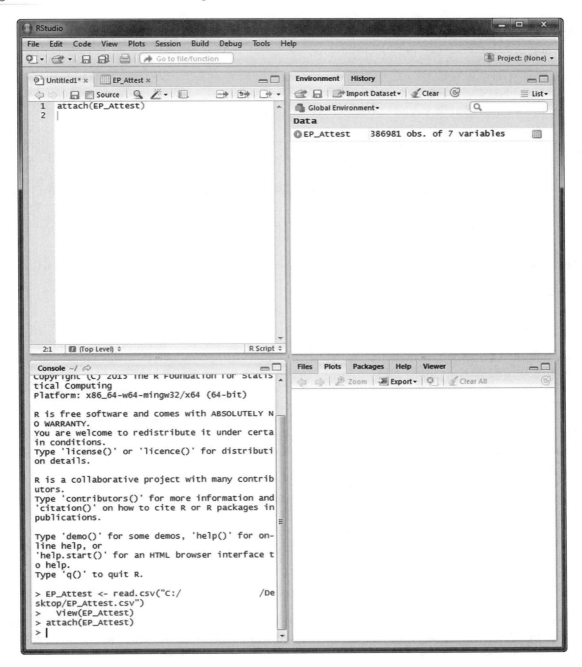

The output from this function is the following:

```
MeaningfulUse
   Attested NotAttested
     213606      173375
```

The output tells us that there were 213,606 practices with providers that attested for meaningful use and 173,375 practices that did not have providers attest. Therefore, there were more providers that did attest than there were providers that did not attest.

The same function can be used to get a frequency of each group listed under the Size data element:

```
table(Size)
```

The output from this function is the following:

```
Size
   Large   Medium    Small
  131158   108874   146949
```

This output shows that the number of large practices was equal to 131,158, medium was 108,874, and small was 146,949. Therefore, there were roughly an equal number of providers from large and small practices and fewer from medium-sized practices.

Finally, the frequency of each group for the Geography data element was determined using the following script:

```
table(Geography)
```

The output from this function is the following:

```
Geography
  Rural    Urban
  41524   345457
```

This output shows that the number of providers in urban settings (n=345,457) was far greater than that of providers in rural settings (n=41,524).

Cross-tabulations, also known as **contingency tables**, are simply a table of frequency distributions (a table that displays the number of times an observation occurs). Cross-tabulations can be beneficial for comparing the frequency of providers when defining two groups. For instance, to determine how many providers attested and did not attest for meaningful use for each of the three different-sized practices, the tapply function can be used in RStudio. The tapply function allows us to combine variables and return a table that returns the results for each level across the factors:

```
tapply(group_practice_PAC_id,list(MeaningfulUse,Size),length)
```

The output from this function is the following:

```
                Large   Medium    Small
Attested       124128    62509    26969
NotAttested      7030    46365   119980
```

The results show the largest number of providers that did not attest for meaningful use were located in small practices, while the largest number of providers that did attest for meaningful use were located in large practices. Despite these findings, we still need to conduct a statistical analysis to determine if these observed differences are significant.

Another table needs to be created to count how many providers attested and did not attest for meaningful use when the provider is located in a rural or urban setting:

```
tapply(group_practice_PAC_id,list(MeaningfulUse,Geography),length)
```

The output from this function is the following:

```
                Rural    Urban
Attested        27228   186378
NotAttested     14296   159079
```

The output shows that the greatest number of providers that did not attest were in urban settings and the greatest number of providers that did attest were in urban settings. A statistical analysis is required in order to empirically determine if the differences in the number of providers that attested in rural and urban settings is significantly different.

Step 5: Statistical Analyses

As mentioned previously, we need to conduct two statistical procedures to determine the following:

1. Is the frequency of providers that attested for meaningful use different among small, medium, and large practices?
2. Is the frequency of providers that attested for meaningful use different between rural or urban settings?

To answer these questions, a statistical procedure needs to be adopted that can handle qualitative data presented as a frequency, that is, data that are categorical and are based upon frequency of occurrence. The **chi-squared goodness of fit test** is the appropriate procedure to use in this situation. Chi-squared statistical tests are used to test for relationships between categorical variables. The assumptions for the chi-squared statistical goodness of fit test include that the data are categorical, the observations are independent (for example, the same individual is not observed multiple times), the groups are mutually exclusive (that is, for each categorical variable each individual observation can only be in one group), and there must be at leave five expected frequencies in each categorical variable (Laerd n.d.). Chi-squared is often represented by the symbol χ^2, which is the Greek symbol *chi* squared. The following code can be used to conduct a chi-squared test comparing meaningful use attestation by size of group practice.

```
chisq.table2<-
tapply(group_practice_PAC_id,list(MeaningfulUse,Size),length)

chisq.test(chisq.table2)
        Pearson's Chi-squared test

data: chisq.table2
X-squared = 163393.6, df = 2, p-value < 2.2e-16
```

The p-value is presented at <2.2e−16. This is formatted in scientific notation. Essentially, one must move the decimal place 16 places to the left. Therefore, the p-value from this test is 0.00000000000000022. Because the p-value is much less than 0.05, it suggests that there is enough evidence to reject the null hypothesis and conclude that there are significant differences in the number of providers that attested and did not attest to meaningful use when located in small, medium, or large practices.

The chi-squared goodness of fit tests whether the observed frequencies are significantly different than the expected frequencies. The expected frequencies are calculated by completing the following equation:

Expected cell frequency = (Row total) × (Column total)/(Grand total of all cells)

You can develop the expected frequencies using RStudio by using the following code. If the null hypothesis were true, the expected values would be equal to the following:

```
chisq.test(chisq.table2)$expected
             Large    Medium    Small
Attested    72396.67  60096.33  81113
NotAttested 58761.33  48777.67  65836
```

Next, we need to determine which of the observed frequencies is farthest from the expected frequencies. The observed frequencies are the frequencies that were calculated and observed regarding the number of providers that attested and did not attest for meaningful use for each of the practice sizes. We can calculate how different the observed frequencies are compared to the expected frequencies by measuring the residuals. To determine

Table 7.1.   Summary of the observed frequencies (O), expected frequencies (E), and residuals (R) when comparing the group size practice and meaningful use status

	Large Practices	Medium Practices	Small Practices
Attested	O: 124128.00	O: 62509.00	O: 26969.00
	E: 72396.67	E: 60096.33	E: 81113.00
	R: 192.26	R: 9.84	R: −190.11
Not Attested	O: 7030.00	O: 46365.00	O: 119980.00
	E: 58761.33	E: 48777.67	E: 65836.00
	R: −213.41	R: −10.92	R: 211.02

which group had the furthest deviation from the expected frequency, look at the residuals and identify the largest and smallest number.

```
chisq.test(chisq.table2)$residuals
               Large        Medium         Small
Attested      192.2624     9.841768   -190.1101
NotAttested  -213.4066   -10.924123    211.0175
```

These results suggest that providers that did not attest for meaningful use and were located in a small practice or providers that did not attest to meaningful use and were located in a large practice had the greatest deviation from what was observed compared to the expected frequency. We can easily compare the observed and expected frequencies by looking at them together in a table. Table 7.1 shows the observed frequencies, expected frequencies, and residuals for each of the groups.

Looking at the observed frequency of providers that did not attest for meaningful use and were located in a small practice, the observed value was 119,980 while the expected value was 65,836. Because the observed value was so much higher than the expected value, there was evidence that there were higher than expected providers in small practices that did not attest for meaningful use. Also, the observed number of providers in a large practice that did not attest to meaningful use was 7,030 while the expected value was 58,761.33. Since the observed value was so much lower than the expected value, there were fewer than expected providers in large practices that did not attest for meaningful use. Collectively, these results suggest providers in small practices are less likely to attest than providers in larger practices.

To investigate whether these findings also hold for providers in rural and urban settings, another chi-squared goodness of fit test is performed. For this test, we will be developing a contingency table to compare the number of providers that attested and did not attest to meaningful use for both rural and urban regions:

```
chisq.table1<-
tapply(group_practice_PAC_id,list(MeaningfulUse,Geography),length)

chisq.test(chisq.table1)
        Pearson's Chi-squared test with Yates' continuity correction
data:  chisq.table1
X-squared = 2023.659, df = 1, p-value < 2.2e-16
```

Again, the p-value is much lower than 0.05. The p-value suggests that there is enough evidence to reject the null hypothesis and conclude that there are significant differences in the number of urban and rural providers that attested and did not attest to meaningful use.

If the null hypothesis were true, the expected values would be equal to the following:

```
chisq.test(chisq.table1)$expected
              Rural      Urban
Attested     22920.44   190685.6
NotAttested  18603.56   154771.4
```

Table 7.2. Summary of the observed frequencies (O), expected frequencies (E), and residuals (R) when comparing the association between practice location and meaningful use status

	Rural	Urban
Attested	O: 27228.00	O: 186378.00
	E: 22920.44	E: 190685.60
	R: 28.45	R: −9.86
Not Attested	O: 14296.00	O: 159079.00
	E: 18603.56	E: 154771.40
	R: −31.58	R: 10.94

The goodness of fit tests whether the observed frequency are significantly different than the expected frequencies. To determine which group had the furthest deviation from the expected frequency, we can look at the residuals and identify the largest and smallest number.

```
chisq.test(chisq.table1)$residuals
                Rural       Urban
Attested     28.45245   -9.864436
NotAttested -31.58153   10.949284
```

These results suggest that providers that did not attest for meaningful use and were located in a rural area had the greatest deviation from what was observed compared to the expected frequency. Again, we can compare the observed and expected frequencies in a table (table 7.2).

Looking at the observed frequency of rural providers that did not attest for meaningful use, the value is 14,296, which is lower than the expected frequency of 18,603.56. Also, the observed value of providers that did not attest in an urban setting was 159,079, which is slightly higher than the expected value of 154,771.40. Together, these results suggest that providers in rural settings actually had a lower than expected number of providers that did not attest for meaningful use when compared to providers in urban settings.

Discussion

The results of this analysis indicate that eligible professionals in small practices are significantly less likely to attest to meaningful use and, therefore, receive financial incentive payments than eligible professionals in large practices ($p < 0.001$). The results also indicate that eligible professionals who practice in rural settings are significantly more likely to attest to meaningful use than providers in urban settings ($p < 0.001$).

These findings are inconsistent with previous research on the topic, which found that urban providers were significantly more likely to attest than rural providers, and that primary care providers were significantly less likely to attest to meaningful use than providers overall (Casey et al. 2013). One explanation for why rural providers are now attesting at a higher rate than urban providers is the impact of federal programs focused on assisting small and rural providers achieve the objectives related to meaningful use, including adopting, implementing, and using health information technology. For example, the Health Information Technology Regional Extension and Assistance Center Program that is funded by the Office of the National Coordinator for Health Information Technology provided five years of funding to 62 independent centers in the United States to work solely with small primary care practices and small hospitals. Previous research did demonstrate that providers and hospitals working with regional extension centers were more likely to attest to meaningful use than those not working with regional extension centers. In fact, the study found that rural providers were far more likely to sign up for regional extension centers than urban providers (Casey et al. 2013).

Conclusion

Using data on meaningful use attestations, data regarding healthcare providers who bill for Medicare services, and Census information to determine urban and rural location of providers, we were able to demonstrate differences in meaningful use attestation across practice size and geographic location. Health information technology and, specifically, electronic health record utilization are being promoted as a patient safety tool, so these findings are useful for understanding how healthcare providers are adopting technology and where there are gaps that need to be addressed. Future research could look at meaningful use attestation across specific provider specialties to provide further explanation of observed differences.

Review Exercises

Instructions: Answer the following questions.

1. Define a contingency table.

2. Choose the statement that is considered the null hypothesis:
   a. The average readmission rate is not equal between urban and rural hospitals.
   b. The average readmission rate is equal between urban and rural hospitals.
   c. The average readmission rate is greater in urban versus rural hospitals.
   d. The average readmission rate is lower in urban versus rural hospitals.

3. A chi-squared test was used to determine if there was an association between smoking status and heart disease. Data were collected from a hospital on the number of people who smoke and who do not smoke and how many of these people have heart disease versus does those who not have heart disease. The results of the chi-squared test revealed a p-value less than the alpha of 0.05. Therefore, there was enough evidence to reject the null hypothesis and conclude that there is a significant association between smoking status and heart disease. The following table displays the residuals from the analysis. Interpret the findings from these residuals:

```
chisq.test(chisq.table1)$residuals
             Has heart disease   Does not have heart disease
Smoker              32.3                    -22.5
Non-smoker         -26.2                     16.5
```

4. True or False: Categorical data can be summarized by calculating an average.

5. True or False: The p-value of 2.2e-16 is less than 0.05.

References

Blumenthal, D. 2009. Stimulating the adoption of health information technology. *West Virginia Medical Journal* 105(3):28–29.

Blumenthal, D. and M. Tavenner. 2010. The "meaningful use" regulation for electronic health records. *New England Journal of Medicine* 363(6):501–504.

Casey, M.M., I. Moscovice, and J. McCullough. 2013. Rural primary care practices and meaningful use of electronic health records: The role of regional extension centers. *Journal of Rural Health* 30(3):244–251.

Centers for Medicare and Medicaid Services. 2014. EP Recipients of Medicare EHR Incentive Program Payments. http://www.cms.gov/Regulations-and-Guidance/Legislation/EHRIncentivePrograms/DataAndReports.html

Centers for Medicare and Medicaid Services. 2015. Medicare.gov Hospital Compare. http://www.medicare.gov/hospitalcompare/search.html

Furukawa, M.F., J. King, V. Patel, C.J. Hsiao, J. Adler-Milstein, and A.K. Jha. 2014. Despite substantial progress In EHR adoption, health information exchange and patient engagement remain low in office settings. *Health Affairs (Millwood)* 33(9):1672–1679.

Government Accountability Office. 2012. Electronic Health Records: First Year of CMS's Incentive Programs Shows Opportunities to Improve Processes to Verify Providers Met Requirements. http://www.gao.gov/products/GAO-12-481

King, J., V. Patel, and M.F. Furukawa. 2012. Physician Adoption of Electronic Health Record Technology to Meet Meaningful Use Objectives: 2009–2012. In *ONC Data Brief*. Washington, DC: Office of the National Coordinator for Health Information Technology.

Laerd. n.d. Chi-Square Goodness-of-Fit Test in SPSS. *Laerd Statistics*. https://statistics.laerd.com/spss-tutorials/chi-square-goodness-of-fit-test-in-spss-statistics.php

McCullough, J., M. Casey, I. Moscovice, and M. Burlew. 2011. Meaningful use of health information technology by rural hospitals. *Journal of Rural Health* 27(3):329–337.

US Census Bureau. 2011. ZCTA to CBSA. https://http://www.census.gov/geo/reference/zctas.html

White, S. 2013. *A Practical Approach to Analyzing Healthcare Data*, 2nd ed. Chicago, IL: AHIMA.

Population Health: Hazardous Air Pollutants and County Level Health Measures

Valerie Watzlaf, PhD, RHIA, FAHIMA and
Dilhari DeAlmeida, PhD, RHIA

Learning Objectives

- Describe the value of open source data for examining relationships between small particulate measures of lead and infant birth weight
- Conduct statistical analysis (descriptive statistics, correlation, regression) using RStudio to determine a relationship between average small particulate lead values and infant birth rates across US counties
- Interpret population health outcomes as it relates to hazardous air pollutant indicators
- Formulate a set of educational material for indicators and measure of choice as per the results
- Interpret statistical tests, such as linear regression, to show relationships and statistical significance
- Distinguish how the results generated on air pollutants and population health compare to current literature on the subject

Key Terms

Best-fit line
Continuous variables
Correlation
Descriptive statistics
Histogram
Least squares regression line
Normally distributed
Population health
Residual
R-squared value
Simple linear regression

Open source data, although massive and sometimes ominous, can be used to examine **population health** outcomes. Most of the open source data are widely available through government resources such as the data. gov website, which houses over 138,445 data sets (Data.gov 2015). Healthdata.gov provides links to open source data sets from government agencies such as the Centers for Disease Control and Prevention (CDC), National Institutes of Health (NIH), and the Agency for Healthcare Research and Quality (AHRQ), just to name a few (HealthData.gov 2015). Although open source data from government websites contain large amounts of data, much of those data have not been examined or analyzed for population health outcomes. For example, one area that is in need of further research is the examination of air pollution data and its effect on population health. Although there has been research performed that shows a relationship between sociodemographic variables such as age, race, and education, it is still unclear why these disease disparities occur or why some vary across different geographic locations (ALA 2014; Zou et al. 2014; Tian et al. 2010; Zeka et al. 2008). Furthermore, through the Clean Air Act the US Environmental Protection Agency (EPA) has set National Ambient (Outdoor) Air Quality Standards (NAAQS) for particulate matter that are less stringent than the standards set by the World Health Organization (WHO). However, ultrafine particulates have no current national or global recommendations for daily or annual exposure limits (EPA 2013, 2008). Outdoor air pollution in both cities and rural areas was estimated to cause 3.7 million premature deaths worldwide per year in 2012 (WHO 2014). This mortality is due to exposure to small particulate matter (10 microns or less in diameter [PM10]), which causes cardiovascular disease, respiratory disease, and cancers (WHO 2014). Also, particulate matter and its effect on infants has not been researched with effective epidemiological studies solely in the United States (Data.gov 2015; Dadvand et al. 2013; Saravia et al. 2013).

Evaluation of population health outcomes is of utmost importance today as we move to a healthier nation. One of the many initiatives toward this effort is seen in the US Department of Health and Human Service's Healthy People 2020 initiative and its efforts toward moving to improved air quality indicators, which would result in better health outcomes and a healthier population overall (HHS 2011).

Therefore, this research will explore the association between air pollution particulate matter and its effect on infant health, particularly focusing on the effect of Lead PM and birth weight and premature birth. All variables will be examined using open source data that are available from the United States government, such as the EPA and CDC.

Research Question and Hypothesis

Is there a relationship between the rate of air pollution particulates (specifically Lead PM2.5 LC—Particulate Lead 2.5 microns or less in diameter, local conditions) measured in US counties and infant health (low birth weight, very low birth weight, and premature birth)?

The dependent variable for the proposed study is the rate of infant health for US counties, because the dependent variable is the variable that is being measured. In the case of the proposed research question, there is one independent variable: Lead PM2.5 LC. Lead PM2.5 LC is considered a measure of air quality by the Environmental Protection Agency.

Hypotheses

The research question will require more than one hypothesis. The hypotheses will include the following:

$H1_0$: There is not a relationship between the average concentration of Lead PM2.5 LC and the rate of infants born with low birth weight in US counties.

$H1_A$: There is a relationship between the average concentration of Lead PM2.5 LC and the rate of infants born with low birth weight in US counties.

$H2_0$: There is not a relationship between the average concentration of Lead PM2.5 LC and the rate of infants born with very low birth weight in US counties.

$H2_A$: There is a relationship between the average concentration of Lead PM2.5 LC and the rate of infants born with very low birth weight in US counties.

$H3_0$: There is not a relationship between the average concentration of Lead PM2.5 LC and the rate of infants born prematurely in US counties.

$H3_A$: There is a relationship between the average concentration of Lead PM2.5 LC and the rate of infants born prematurely birth in US counties.

Checklist

To answer our research question, a specific process of data acquisition, preparation, and discovery is required. The following steps will be explained in detail:

1. Extract data sets from MySQL
   a. Select appropriate columns of data
   b. Join columns of data using MySQL queries
2. Data preparation
   a. Review data set for erroneous values
3. Import the data into RStudio
4. Perform descriptive statistics on the variables of avg_value, lbw, vlbw, and premature
5. Conduct similar linear regressions to examine the relationship between lead levels and measures of infant health at the US county level

The Analysis

This section will provide a step-by-step description of obtaining and analyzing the data required to answer the proposed research question.

Step 1: Data Extraction

In order to carry out the analysis, the following data are needed:

- A list of all US counties with measures of average concentrations of lead PM2.5 LC
- A measure of percent of births that are considered low birth weight (<2,500 g) for each county
- A measure of percent of births that are considered very low birth weight (<1,500 g) for each county
- A measure of percent of births that are considered premature births (<37 weeks) for each county

Three data sets need to be combined to obtain the needed data to answer the proposed research question. The first data set is named daily_hazardous_air_pollutants and obtained from the US Environment Protection Agency (EPA 2014a). This data set provides air pollutant measures, including sample time and duration, for all states

Figure 8.1. SQL script and returned data for combining three data sets

```
SELECT
state_geocodes.state,
state_geocodes.county_name,
daily_hazardous_air_pollutants.parameter_name,
AVG(daily_hazardous_air_pollutants.arithmetic_mean),
measures_of_birth_and_death.lbw,
measures_of_birth_and_death.vlbw,
measures_of_birth_and_death.premature
FROM state_geocodes
        JOIN
    daily_hazardous_air_pollutants
ON daily_hazardous_air_pollutants.state_geocodes_id = state_geocodes.state_
geocodes_id
        JOIN
    measures_of_birth_and_death
ON measures_of_birth_and_death.state_geocodes_id = state_geocodes.state_
geocodes_id
WHERE
daily_hazardous_air_pollutants.parameter_name LIKE '%Lead%'
AND daily_hazardous_air_pollutants.arithmetic_mean > 0
GROUP BY state_geocodes.county_code;
```

(Continued)

Figure 8.1. SQL script and returned data for combining three data sets *(Continued)*

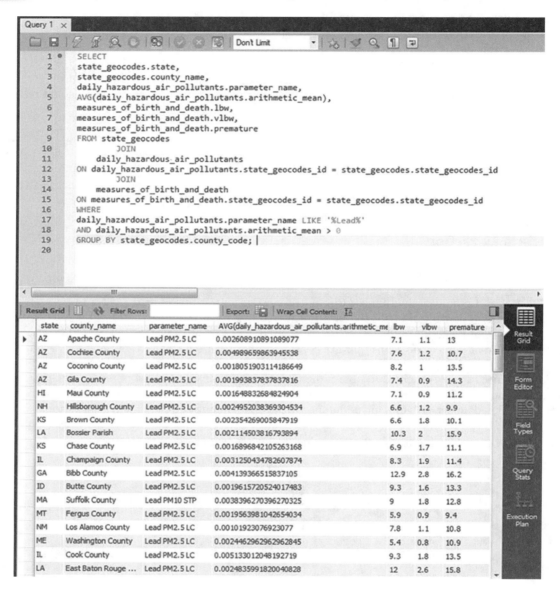

and counties in the United States. Each state and county is identified by a unique code, and the data set also includes the core-based statistical areas (CBSA) for each county to assist in determining rural and urban status.

The second data set is named measures_of_birth_and_death and is derived from the Community Health Status Indicator data set that was made available by the US Department of Health and Human Services (CDC 2015). This data set provides measures of birth and death, including low birth weight, very low birth weight, and premature births for every US county. The data set includes a variety of other measures related to birth and death, such as infant mortality rates, suicide rates, and cancer rates. Each state and county is identified by a unique code.

The third data set is state_geocodes and is derived from the US Census Bureau and includes the state and county names for each US county where a measurement of air quality has been reported.

The three data sets will be combined using MySQL scripts. The scripts will be constructed so that only the following data elements are extracted: county, average concentration of Lead PM2.5 LC, measure of low birth weight, measure of very low birth weight, measure of premature births, and the CBSA. Figure 8.1 displays the

SQL script that was used to combine the three data sets and also the first few rows of the output that were derived from the query. Note that you must alter a setting in MySQL so that the output shows all of the results rather than just showing the first 1,000 rows (see chapter 4).

Step 2: Data Preparation

Data preparation is often the most labor-intensive and, arguably, the most important step in the analytics process. The purpose of data preparation is to ensure the correct data—in the correct format—are used for the analysis. Since the SQL query that was used extracted data in a format that was ready for further analysis, there are no additional steps required for data preparation in Microsoft Excel. Therefore, we can export the data from MySQL Workbench and save the data in a CSV file and name the file HAP. After you open HAP. csv, you should see the following columns in Excel:

- state: The name of the state
- county_name: The name of the county
- parameter_name: The name of the hazardous air pollutant
- AVG(daily_hazardous_air_pollutants_arithmetic_mean): The average daily measure for the hazardous air pollutant
- lbw: Percentage of infants born with low birth weight
- vlbw: Percentage of infants born with very low birth weight
- premature: Percentage of infants born prematurely

Renaming Column Headers in Excel
When we import this data into RStudio, these column header names will become the names of different fields in a data frame. RStudio will do its best working with names that have spaces in them, but it would be better to make each of these field names shorter now while in Excel, rather than changing them in RStudio (or worse—typing long field names in RStudio each time we want to use them). Table 8.1 contains the names we will use when renaming the column headers. To rename column headers in Excel, simply click each individual cell, highlight the contents, delete the content, enter the new column name, and click return. Repeat this process for each column header.

Reviewing Data Sets for Erroneous Values
One of the first steps in data preparation is to carefully examine if the data include erroneous values or blanks. An erroneous value may be a value that was used as a filler. A filler is often used as a default value to indicate a blank field. For example, the value −1111.1 may be used to represent a blank field entry. It is best to eliminate the fillers from your data set because data often hold a numeric value. If numeric fillers are included in the data set, this can skew the results when calculating the mean or alter the results when performing inferential statistical analyses (for a detailed description of how to delete these values from the data set, see chapter 7).

Table 8.1.   Original and revised column names within Excel

Original Name	Revised Name
state	state
county_name	cnty
parameter_name	parameter
AVG(daily_hazardous_air_pollutants_arithmetic_mean)	avg_value
lbw	lbw
vlbw	vlbw
premature	premature

The CSV that was exported from MySQL does include several instances of erroneous values. For instance, when examining the lbw, vlbw, and premature, the value –1111.1 does appear for several counties. These values do need to be removed in order to obtain accurate results. The erroneous values can be removed in Excel. First, highlight columns E, F, and G. Next, in the Home tab select Find & Select. A drop down will appear where you can select Replace. A Find and Replace window will appear; you will enter text in the Find what textbox and Replace with textbox. In the Find what textbox, type –1111.1 and leave the Replace with blank. Choose the Replace All option. A window will appear saying there were nine replacements made. Click OK. The data preparation phase is now complete. Remember to save the file as a CSV. In Excel, click File > Save As. Under the Format drop-down window, select the Comma Delimited Values option. When saving the file, name the document HAP and save the file. Note: When saving your file, you may receive a message:

> Some features in your workbook might be lost if you save it as CSV (Comma defined). Do you want to keep using that format?

The reason Excel provides this warning is that only the active spreadsheet in your Excel workbook will be saved. If you have additional worksheets included in your file, those spreadsheets will be lost—in short, only the worksheet that is open when you save the filed is retained. Click OK.

The next step in the analysis is to import the data into RStudio for analysis.

Step 3: Import the Data

Importing data into RStudio is a relatively straightforward process (see chapter 5 for detailed instructions for importing data into RStudio). To import the CSV file that was prepared for the analysis under Step 2, click Import Dataset and choose the From Text File option in the drop-down window. Navigate to the HAP.csv file that was saved in the final action of Step 2, highlight the file, and click Import.

After the data is imported into RStudio, open an R scripting window. The R scripting window is where you will enter the R code in order to analyze the data. To open a new R scripting window, go to File >New File > R Script. The first step is to attach the data set. The reason that the data set is attached is to make the column names accessible in RStudio. Without the use of the attach function, the only way to work with the data by the column names is to specify the name of the data frame followed by a dollar sign and the name of the column. For example, if a data set named AllData was imported into RStudio and there was a need to call out the column Age without attaching the data, a user would be required to use the following script: AllData$Age. If the data set is attached, a user can simply call the column by its name: Age.

To attach the data, the following R script into the console:

```
attach(HAP)
```

Step 4: Descriptive Statistics

Once the data is imported and attached into RStudio, the first type of analysis that should be conducted to familiarize yourself with the data is the **descriptive statistics**. The data we are using to answer our research question includes **continuous variables**. Continuous variables are commonly described by calculating the mean, median, standard deviation, and range. In this case, there are four continuous variables: avg_value, lbw, vlbw, and premature. In RStudio, the summary function can be used to obtain basic descriptive statistics for quantitative variables (figure 8.2).

The summary function is very useful to gaining understanding about the data you are working with, and figure 8.2 demonstrates how RStudio can quickly summarize data. In four quick lines of code you have the minimum value for each quantitative variable (Min.); the value that is at the 25th percentile of the variable (1st Qu.); the value that is exactly in the middle of the variable once they are ordered from low to high (Median); the average value for the variable (Mean); the value that is at the 75th percentile of the variable (3rd Qu.); the maximum value for the variable (Max.); and a count of the number of blank entries (NAs). These data are informative to our research question. For example, the mean of the percentages of lbw is 7.9 percent and the maximum value is 13.6 percent (therefore, this means that there is a county that has about a 6 percent higher rate of infants being born with low birth weight than the average). Now look at the variable vlbw. The mean is 1.4 percent and the maximum value is 3.2 percent, thus demonstrating that there is much less variability in the measures of very low birth weight among US counties.

An important step in the data analysis process is to determine if data are **normally distributed** as certain statistical techniques have assumptions that data is **normally distributed,** which refers to the probability of measures falling within a certain range. Normal distribution is referred to as following a bell-shaped curve. One technique used to check for normal distribution is to depict that data using **histograms,** which is simply a graphical way to show the distribution of continuous data. We are looking to see if the data is normally distributed (that is, the data is approximately even on both sides of the mean). To create a histogram for each variable of interest, simply use the following R codes:

```
hist(lbw, xlab="Average Births Considered Low Birth Weight by US county")

hist(vlbw, xlab="Average Births Considered Very Low Birth Weight by US county")

hist(premature, xlab="Average Births Considered premature by US county")

hist(avg_value, xlab="Average Lead PM2.5 LC by US County")
```

The output from the first histogram code is shown in figure 8.3.

Figure 8.2. Calculating descriptive statistics using R's summary function

```
summary(avg_value)
   Min. 1st Qu.  Median    Mean 3rd Qu.    Max.
0.001000 0.001822 0.002530 0.003189 0.003690 0.016870
summary(lbw)
   Min. 1st Qu.  Median    Mean 3rd Qu.    Max.    NA's
  4.400   6.650   7.800   7.878   9.000  13.600    2
summary(vlbw)
   Min. 1st Qu.  Median    Mean 3rd Qu.    Max.    NA's
  0.300   1.100   1.400   1.461   1.800   3.200    6
summary(premature)
   Min. 1st Qu.  Median    Mean 3rd Qu.    Max.    NA's
  7.10   10.78   12.40   12.43   14.00   19.20    1
```

Figure 8.3. Histogram of average births considered low birth weight by US county

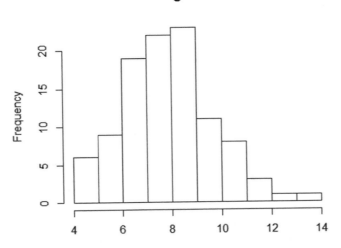

Histogram of lbw

Source: Used with permission from RStudio.

The histogram depicts a normal distribution of data, and we can feel comfortable using this variable for statistical analysis because it is symmetric around the mean. The histogram is showing us that, for example, approximately 6 counties have an average lbw rate between 4 and 5 percent; 10 counties have an average lbw rate between 5 and 6 percent, and so on. Figure 8.4 shows a histogram for very low birth weight, and you can see that it also has a normal distribution. We can also see that, for example, 45 counties have an average vlbw rate between 1 and 1.5 percent. Figure 8.5 depicts premature births by US county and also demonstrates a normal distribution.

Figure 8.4. Histogram of average births considered very low birth weight by US county

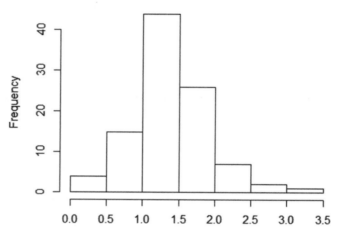

Source: Used with permission from RStudio.

Figure 8.5. Histogram of average births considered premature by US county

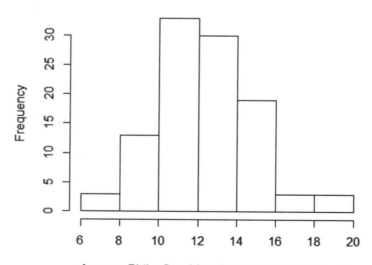

Source: Used with permission from RStudio.

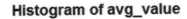

Figure 8.6. Histogram of average lead PM2.5 LC by US county

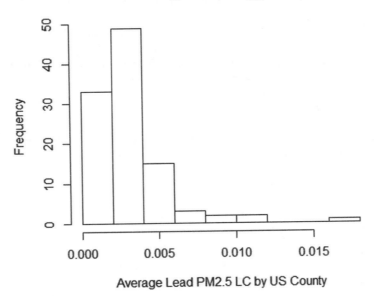

Source: Used with permission from RStudio.

Figure 8.6 is the final histogram depicting the distribution of the measurements of Lead PM2.5 LC for US counties. You can see that the data are not normally distributed, but skewed to the right. The data on this chart inform us that the vast majority of US counties have average Lead PM2.5 LC rates less than 0.005.

Step 5: Statistical Analyses

In order to determine if there is any **correlation** (a relationship of dependence) between these variables that we have summarized, we need to conduct multiple statistical procedures to determine the following:

1. Is there a relationship between the average Lead PM2.5 LC and the rate of infants born with low birth weight in US counties?
2. Is there a relationship between the average Lead PM2.5 LC and the rate of infants born with very low birth weight in US counties?
3. Is there a relationship between the average Lead PM2.5 LC and the rate of infants born prematurely in US counties?

To answer these questions, a statistical procedure needs to be adopted that can handle continuous data. The **simple linear regression** is the appropriate procedure to use in this situation. The purpose of the simple linear regression is to examine the correlation between two variables and "is used to characterize the linear relationship between a dependent variable and one independent variable" (White 2013). In short, it is creating a model by using two variables. For the purposes of this chapter, the dependent variables include the three measures of infant health (lbw, vlbw, and premature). The independent variable (or predictor variable) is avg_value (Lead PM2.5 LC). In short, we are trying to predict the outcome of, for example, low birth weight from rates of lead levels that have been measured in US counties. An equation for a regression line is y=a+bx, where a is the y-intercept and bx is the slope. A complete description of simple linear regression is beyond the scope of this text, but is critical to understand that simple linear regression is calculated by developing the slope of a line and determining if that slope is significantly different than zero. Simple linear regression fits a straight line, which is called the **least squares regression line**, through all of the data points in the analysis. This line is also understood as the **best-fit line**—it is called the best-fit line because it provides the best approximation of the trend based upon all data points included in a scatterplot. A **residual** is the distance a data point is from the least squares regression line. The least squares regression line is drawn through the best data points so that the sum of the squared residuals are as small as possible. The mathematics underlying simple linear regression has been summarized in other publications (White 2013).

Let us begin by using RStudio to conduct a simple linear regression to examine if there is a relationship between the average Lead PM2.5 LC values and low birth weights in US counties. Conducting a simple linear regression in RStudio is a process that includes five steps. The first step is to create and name a model using the R function lm (linear model). The following is the R script for developing the model:

```
lin1<- lm(lbw~avg_value)
```

The second step in the process is to use RStudio to summarize the statistics of the model using the R function summary. The following is the R script for summarizing the model:

```
summary(lin1)
```

The output from this function is the following:

```
Call:
lm(formula = lbw ~ avg_value)

Residuals:
  Min   1Q Median   3Q  Max
-4.434 -1.076 -0.306 1.069 5.535

Coefficients:
      Estimate Std. Error t value Pr(>|t|)
(Intercept) 7.0009   0.2897 24.164 < 2e-16 ***
avg_value 271.3942  72.6059  3.738 0.000308 ***
---
Signif. codes: 0 '***' 0.001 '**' 0.01 '*' 0.05 '.' 0.1 ' ' 1

Residual standard error: 1.726 on 101 degrees of freedom
 (2 observations deleted due to missingness)
Multiple R-squared: 0.1215,  Adjusted R-squared: 0.1128
F-statistic: 13.97 on 1 and 101 DF, p-value: 0.0003078
```

The output summarizes the model and the data elements included in the analysis under Call. The lm(formula = lbw ~ avg_value) formula is the formula you developed for your linear model. As shown, the linear model we created was based on evaluating the relationship between avg_value of Lead and lbw. The call summarizes the variables that we included in our model—simply confirm the variables were those you intended to include in the analysis.

The second section of the model summary (labeled "Residuals") presents the regression residuals, also known as errors. As a reminder, the least squares regression line described above is intended to minimize error, so the residuals should be small. The fact that we have very small numbers is a good sign for our model.

The next section is labeled "Coefficients," which includes information about our linear model. We can derive the equation for the best-fit line from the information listed in the Coefficients section. The y-intercept is shown as the value listed in the line item labeled as "Intercept" and under the Estimate column. The slope of the best-fit line is listed in the line item labeled as "lbw" and under the Estimate column. Therefore, the equation for the best-fit line for this linear model is $y=7+271.4x$. The equation of the best-fit line can be used to predict a y-value when we observe a specific x value. For instance, we can predict the low birth weight rates for a specific average value of small particulate lead matter. If the average value of small particulate lead matter was 0.001 micrograms per cubic meter, we can multiply this value by 271.4 (see previous equation) to get 0.2714. We then add this to 7 and obtain the y-intercept of 7.27. That is, with an average value of small particulate lead matter at 0.001 micrograms per cubic meter the predicted low birth rate is 7.27 percent. Also, the results of our linear regression will test if the slope of our best-fit line (271.4x) is significantly different from zero.

The Coefficients section also contains information about the standard error of the y-intercept and the slope of the line. The t value is the estimate divided by the standard error. The standard error is an estimate of the standard deviation of the coefficient. The amount the coefficient varies across cases. It can be thought of as a measure of the precision with which the regression coefficient is measured. If a coefficient is large compared to its standard error, then the coefficient is most likely different from 0 and a small p-value will result.

For our purposes, we want to pay special attention to the significance or p-value—Pr (>|t|)—which is listed in the line item for lbw under the Coefficients section. This p-value shows if the slope of the best-fit line is significantly different from zero. As shown, the p-value is 0.0003, which is less than 0.05 and thus the slope of the line is significantly different than zero. Therefore, we can conclude that there is a significant association between the small particulate lead matter and low birth rates. If the slope of the line is a negative number, we interpret the relationship as a negative association. If the slope is a positive number, we can interpret the relationship as a positive association. Given the fact that we have a positive number for the slope of the best-fit line, we can conclude that there is a significant positive association between small particulate lead matter and low birth rates.

The final value that is of relevance is the R-squared value. The **R-squared value** is the proportion of the observed values of y explained by the linear regression of y on x. In other words, the R-squared value explains the strength of the relationship between the two quantitative variables. The R-squared value ranges from 0 to 1. The closer the R-squared value is to 1, the stronger the association is between the two variables. A value closer to zero indicates a weak association. When looking at the multiple R-squared value in the linear regression output, we see a value of 0.1128. Since this value is closer to zero, this indicates that the strength of the relationship between small particulate lead matter and low birth rates is a weak association.

We should always interpret the p-value from our linear model and the R-squared value together when interpreting the results of our linear model. Even though we have a significant positive association between small particulate lead matter and low birth rates, the strength of that relationship is weak.

The third and fourth steps in the process are to plot the data and draw the least squares regression line to assist us interpret the results of the statistical output. The following is the R script for plotting the data and adding the line to the plot:

```
plot(lbw~avg_value)
abline(lin1, col="red")
```

The output from these R scripts are shown in figure 8.7. The average value of Lead PM2.5 LC is on the x-axis and average rate or percent of low birth weight is on the y-axis. The line shows that there is a positive correlation between average lead levels and average rates of low birth weights in US counties. In short, as lead levels rise in specific geographic locations the probability of infants being born with a lower birth weight increases.

We will now replicate this process for the other two measures of interest (vlbw and premature). See figure 8.8 for the linear regression plot.

```
lin2<- lm(vlbw~ avg_value)
summary(lin2)
Call:
lm(formula = vlbw ~ avg_value)

Residuals:
    Min      1Q  Median      3Q     Max
-1.03374 -0.30270 -0.05096 0.26024 1.68696

Coefficients:
            Estimate Std. Error t value Pr(>|t|)
(Intercept) 1.20554    0.08139   14.81  < 2e-16 ***
avg_value   78.42518   20.31847   3.86 0.000205 ***
---
Signif. codes: 0 '***' 0.001 '**' 0.01 '*' 0.05 '.' 0.1 ' ' 1

Residual standard error: 0.4728 on 97 degrees of freedom
  (6 observations deleted due to missingness)
Multiple R-squared: 0.1331,    Adjusted R-squared: 0.1242
F-statistic: 14.9 on 1 and 97 DF, p-value: 0.0002046

plot(vlbw~avg_value)
abline(lin2, col="red")
```

Figure 8.7.   Relationship between lead PM2.5 LC and low birth weight

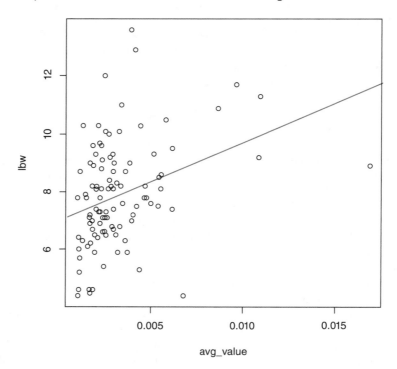

Source: Used with permission from RStudio.

Figure 8.8.   Relationship between lead PM2.5 LC and very low birth weight

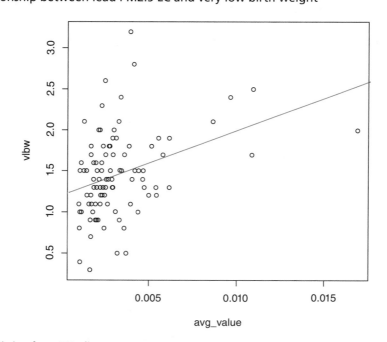

Source: Used with permission from RStudio.

Similar to the results with low birth weight, these results indicate that there is a positive correlation between lead levels and the percentage of births considered very low birth weight in US counties. See figure 8.9 for the linear regression plot.

```
lin3<- lm(premature~ avg_value)

summary(lin3)

Call:
lm(formula = premature ~ avg_value)

Residuals:
   Min   1Q Median   3Q   Max
-6.3888 -1.5665 -0.1497 1.5598 6.5407

Coefficients:
         Estimate Std. Error t value Pr(>|t|)
(Intercept)  11.373    0.381 29.848 < 2e-16 ***
avg_value   328.130   95.913  3.421 0.000898 ***
---
Signif. codes: 0 '***' 0.001 '**' 0.01 '*' 0.05 '.' 0.1 ' ' 1

Residual standard error: 2.289 on 102 degrees of freedom
  (1 observation deleted due to missingness)
Multiple R-squared: 0.1029,  Adjusted R-squared: 0.09414
F-statistic: 11.7 on 1 and 102 DF, p-value: 0.0008983

plot(premature~ avg_value)

abline(lin3, col="red")
```

Again, because the p-value is less than 0.001, the results indicate that there is a positive relationship between lead levels and the percentage of births that are considered premature in US counties.

Figure 8.9.   Relationship between lead PM2.5 LC and premature births

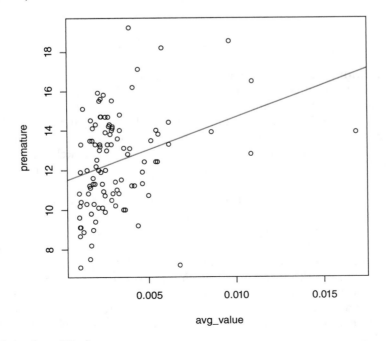

Source: Used with permission from RStudio.

Based upon these results, we can reject the null hypotheses and conclude that there is a significant relationship between average values of Lead PM2.5 LC and rates of low birth weights, very low birth weights, and premature births at the US county level.

Discussion

With the development of a multitude of healthcare delivery systems and consumer-oriented healthcare, population health management has become and will be a vital part of everyday healthcare. A great resource for utilizing effective methods for population health management is the use of publicly available open source data sets. This chapter focused on one such entity: namely the air pollutant lead in US counties. The authors specifically focused on lead particulate matter with a lead count of 2.5 (Lead PM2.5 LC). According to the EPA, lead particulate matter that are less than 2.5 micrometers in diameter are of concern since those particles have the ability to pass through the throat and nose and enter the lungs (EPA 2014b). One segment of the population that may be at risk for consuming such particles are infants. This chapter focused on the outcomes of low birth weight, very low birth weight, and premature birth of infants based upon the level of Lead PM2.5 LC in US counties.

The results of this analysis indicate that there is a significant relationship between US Lead PM2.5 LC and infant birth weight. We saw this relationship for all levels of birth weight; low birth weight (R squared=0.1128; p=0.000308), very low birth weight (R squared=0.1242, p=0.000205), and premature weight (R-squared=0.09414, p=0.000898).These findings are consistent with previous research in which all particulate matter was examined in several different counties for infant weight and specifically for respiratory effects in children (Dadvand et al. 2013; Saravia et al. 2013). However, the R-squared value is low, thereby indicating the strength of the relationship is present but weak. One potential reason for the low R-squared value is the number of US counties with the lead measure available. Only 276 of the 3,144 US counties had data available. Also, we only examined data on lead; other small particulate values in the data set could be explored and pooled for further analysis, such as nickel, arsenic, beryllium, cadmium, chromium, manganese, and mercury. Furthermore, in our analysis we did not control for other confounding factors that may play a part in the dependent variable of infant weight—maternal complications or comorbidities, maternal risk factors such as smoking, infant complications or comorbidities—which may also lead to low birth weight. Therefore, further research is needed to examine a variety of small particulate types as well as determining if additional data sets include maternal and infant risk factors as mentioned.

Conclusion

Using data on air pollution, such as lead small particulate matter, and health measures, such as infant birth weight, enabled us to see a relationship that affects population health. Using RStudio to analyze multiple data sets related to lead and infant weight helped to determine a significant relationship between these variables. These findings are useful to examine other types of relationships to see if they also exist, such as other pollutants in the United States that are at small particulate measures (<2.5 microns in diameter). Future research could examine other pollutants such as nickel, arsenic, cadmium, and such, as well as other risk factors related to maternal and infant health for further explanation of observed relationships.

The results depicted a significant association between the lead particulate matter exposures versus the three outcome measures; however, the R-squared value was low, conferring that there is a weak relationship. One potential reason for this could be the fact that the data was available for only 276 of the 3,144 counties. Thus, there are implications for future research. As we continue to collect healthcare-related data on all consumers, it would be crucial to have an established set of data governance standards and principles behind any data that would need to be analyzed. With the growing number of open source data sets and open source software tools to analyze them, today's healthcare consumers are able to review and analyze a variety of different outcomes measures in a variety of different settings. Although this chapter only highlighted an air pollutant (lead) measure in a certain population (infants), this could be further analyzed for other populations at risk.

Review Exercises

Instructions: Choose the best answer.

1. Select the correct order of steps used in this chapter to analyze the data set(s).
   a. Extract data, data preparation, import the data, and apply statistical analysis
   b. Extract data, import the data, data preparation, and apply statistical analysis
   c. Extract data, apply statistical analysis, data preparation, and import the data
   d. Data preparation, extract data, import the data, and apply statistical analysis

2. It is important to eliminate erroneous filler values from the data set because:
   a. It does not look nice
   b. They could hold a numeric value which could skew the results
   c. They are not the numbers you expected
   d. They are blank

3. After importing data to RStudio, which of the following would be the first step to follow?
   a. Specify the data import order
   b. Use the attach function to attach the data set
   c. Run the MySQL command on the data set
   d. Conduct data preparation

4. The four variables used in this study include:
   a. Three dependent variables (low birth weight, very low birth weight, and premature birth weight) and one independent variable (Lead PM2.5)
   b. Two dependent variables and two independent variables
   c. Continuous variables
   d. Both a and c

5. R-squared values range from:
   a. 0 to 100
   b. 0 to 10
   c. –1 to 1
   d. 0 to 1

References

American Lung Association. 2014. State of the Air Disparities in the Impact of Air Pollution. http://www.stateoftheair .org/2014/health-risks/health-risks-disparities.html

Centers for Disease Control and Prevention. 2015. Community Health Status Indicators. http://wwwn.cdc.gov/Community Health/homepage.aspx?j=1

Dadvand, P., J. Parker, M.L. Bell, M. Bonzini, M. Brauer, L.A. Darrow, U. Gehring, S.V. Glinianaia, N. Gouveia, and E.H. Ha. 2013. Maternal exposure to particulate air pollution and term birth weight: A multi-country evaluation of effect and heterogeneity. *Environmental Health Perspectives* 121(3):267–373.

Data.gov. 2015. The home of the US Government's Open Data. http://www.data.gov

Department of Health and Human Services. 2011. http://www.healthypeople.gov/

Environmental Protection Agency. 2013. Clean Air Act in a Nutshell. http://www.epa.gov/air/caa/pdfs/CAA_Nutshell.pdf

Environmental Protection Agency. 2008. National Ambient Air Quality Standards 2008. http://www.epa.gov/air/criteria. html

Environmental Protection Agency. 2014a. Air Quality Data for the CDC National Environmental Public Health Tracking Network. http://www.epa.gov/heasd/research/cdc.html

Environmental Protection Agency. 2014b. Fine Particle (PM2.5) Designations: Frequent Questions. http://www.epa.gov/ pmdesignations/faq.htm

HealthData.gov. 2015. HealthData.gov Home Page. http://www.healthdata.gov

Saravia, J., G.I. Lee, S. Lomnicki, B. Dellinger, and S.A. Cormier. 2013. Particulate matter containing environmentally persistent free radicals and adverse infant respiratory health effects: A review. *Journal of Biochemical and Molecular Toxicology* 27(1):56–68.

Tian, N., J.G. Wilson, and F.B. Zhan. 2010. Female breast cancer mortality clusters within racial groups in the United States. *Health & Place* 16(2):209–218.

US Census Bureau. 2011. ZCTA to CBSA. https://http://www.census.gov/geo/reference/zctas.html

White, S. 2013. *A Practical Approach to Analyzing Healthcare Data,* 2nd ed. Chicago, IL: AHIMA.

World Health Organization. 2014. 2014 Ambient (Outdoor) Air Quality and Health. http://www.who.int/mediacentre/factsheets/fs313/en/

Zeka, A., S.J. Melly, and J. Schwartz. 2008. The effects of socioeconomic status and indices of physical environment on reduced birth weight and preterm births in Eastern Massachusetts. *Environmental Health* 7:60.

Zou, B., F. Peng, N. Wan, K. Mamady, and G.J. Wilson. 2014. Spatial cluster detection of air pollution exposure inequities across the United States. *PloS One* 9(3):e91917.

Comparative Effectiveness Research: Case Study of Hospital Readmissions

Shauna M. Overgaard, MHI

Learning Objectives

- Compare outcomes across hospitals by a variety of organizational characteristics
- Demonstrate the use of logistic regression to identify predictors of cardiovascular disease within hospitals
- Demonstrate the use of logistic regression to determine the effect of emergency services in the likelihood of a hospital scoring above or below the national average for heart failure 30-day readmission rate

Key Terms

Dichotomous
Logistic regression
Odds ratio
Simple logistic regression (SLR)

Heart failure is marked by frequent exacerbations where the heart is unable to pump enough blood and oxygen to support other organs. These exacerbations often result in hospitalization and death, where nearly half of individuals die within five years of diagnosis (Heidenreich et al. 2011). The cost of heart failure care in the United States in 2009 was reported by the American Heart Association (AHA) to be an estimated $37.2 billion, a major contributor being high rates of hospitalization (Heidenreich et al. 2011). Treatment guidelines have worked to reduce the risk for emergency care and hospitalization by increasing patient education, working to improve adherence to treatment and thus preventing clinical deterioration (Hunt 2005). As hospitals seek to identify improvement methods for heart-failure outcomes, the rate of readmission is utilized as a valuable measure of performance. The AHA is leading national efforts in reducing the rate of heart failure readmission through programs such as Get With The Guidelines® Heart Failure, an in-hospital program for care improvement through the promotion of stable adherence to the latest scientific treatment guidelines (AHA 2015). It has been shown that improved adherence to heart failure guidelines translates to improved clinical outcomes in patients (Fonarow et al. 2011). The AHA uses the rate of 30-day readmission as a measure of quality performance in the assessment of successful adherence to guidelines (Hernandez et al. 2011). Within the literature, there are other factors to consider that may be influencing a hospital's rate of readmission. For example, the possible threshold effect due to the number of beds a hospital has available to admit patients (Fisher et al. 1994). In this chapter, logistic regression is employed to assess the effect, if any, of emergency services in determining the odds of a hospital's performance by measure of readmission rate. The odds of performing better or worse than the US national average rate of 30-day readmission will be computed using the coefficients derived from a logistic regression model.

Research Question and Hypothesis

Is there a relationship between accessibility to emergency services and heart failure 30-day readmission rate?

A **simple logistic regression (SLR)** analysis can be used to determine whether and to what degree emergency services affect a hospital's rate of readmission. A SLR is a statistical procedure that is used when you have one categorical variable with two values and one quantitative variable, and you want to know whether variation in the quantitative variable causes variation in the categorical variable. The dependent variable will be **dichotomous**, that is, the outcome will always be one of two factors. In the case of the proposed analysis, the values for the dichotomous dependent variable include better than the national average or worse than the national average readmission rate.

Hypotheses

H_0: There is not a relationship between accessibility to emergency services and heart failure 30-day readmission rate.

H_A: There is a relationship between accessibility to emergency services and heart failure 30-day readmission rate.

Checklist

To answer our research question, a specific process of data acquisition, preparation, and discovery is required. The following steps will be explained in detail:

1. Extract data sets from MySQL
   a. Select the appropriate columns of data
2. Data preparation with Microsoft Excel
   a. Rename the column headers
3. Descriptive statistics in Excel
   a. Generate a pivot table
4. Conduct statistical procedures: logistic regression, calculation of odds ratio

The Analysis

Now that the research question and hypotheses are written, the variables necessary to answer the research question are identified, and the appropriate statistical procedures for the project are selected, the process for analyzing the data may commence.

Step 1: Data Extraction

In order to carry out the analysis, the following data elements are needed: provider id, 30-day readmission rate, and emergency services. After generating the data frame using the SQL script, export and save the data in an Excel workbook. Note: All data required for answering the research question are included in the database associated with this textbook. Figure 9.1 displays the SQL script that was used to query the data and also the first few rows of the output that was derived from the query. Keep in mind that you must alter a setting in MySQL so that the output shows all of the results rather than just showing the first 1,000 rows (see chapter 4). After executing each query, export the data to a CSV file and save the file as HF. For detailed instructions regarding exporting data from MySQL Workbench to CSV format, see chapter 4.

Figure 9.1.   SQL script and returned data for combining three data sets

```
SELECT
    hospital_general_information.provider_id,
    readmissions_complications_deaths.measure_name,
    readmissions_complications_deaths.compared_to_national,
    hospital_general_information.emergency_services
FROM
    hospital_general_information
        JOIN
    readmissions_complications_deaths ON hospital_general_information.
    provider_id = readmissions_complications_deaths.provider_id
WHERE
    measure_id = 'READM_30_HF'
        AND
    (readmissions_complications_deaths.compared_to_national='Better than
    U.S. National Rate' OR
    readmissions_complications_deaths.compared_to_national='Worse than
    U.S. National Rate');
```

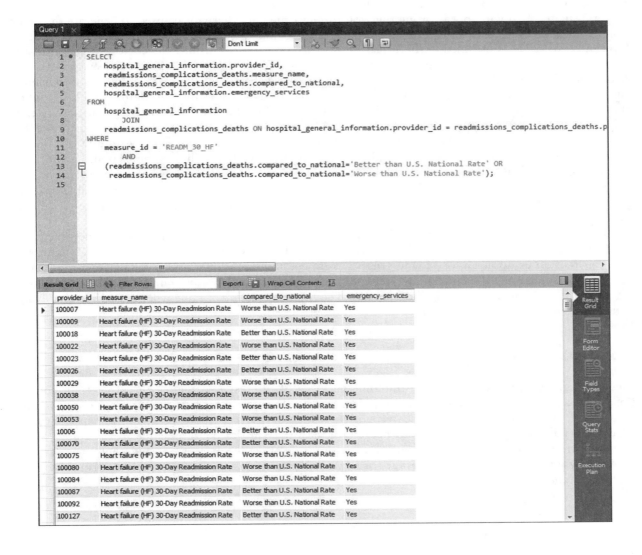

Step 2: Data Preparation

The data used within this analysis are from the Hospital Compare website, which are official data from the Centers for Medicare and Medicaid Services (CMS 2015). Open the HF.csv file that was exported from MySQL Workbench with Excel. You should see the following four columns of data (each observation represents a single US hospital):

- provider_id: A unique identification number given to each care provider (namely, hospital).
- measure_name: Has one level, heart failure (HF) 30-day readmission rate. 30-day readmission rate is the rate of readmission within 30 days following hospital discharge for heart failure. If a readmission occurs beyond 30 days, it is then an independent event. Within the model we use the corresponding fields within the compared_to_national variable to determine if the heart failure readmission rate for a single hospital is different than the national average.
- compared_to_national: Has two levels—better than US national rate and worse than US national rate.
- emergency_services: Presence of an emergency department at the hospital.

Step 3: Descriptive Statistics

An efficient way to summarize the data that are in Excel is through the use of pivot tables. A pivot table can be generated to count the number of providers within our selection criteria. To create a pivot table, click into any cell that has data. Select PivotTable listed under the Insert tab (see figure 9.2a). Next, the window shown in figure 9.2b will appear prompting you to select the data that will be used to generate the pivot table. Typically, Excel will select the appropriate range of data, but you should confirm that the text "HF!$A$1:$D$277" is included in the Table/Range textbox. After confirming the correct range of data is entered, click OK. Figure 9.2c displays the resulting pivot table. The right side of the screen includes the PivotTable Fields, which are the columns of data in the spreadsheet. Listed under the fields are four bins: filters, columns, rows, and values. The fields listed in the PivotTable Fields (or PivotTable Field List) will be dragged into the respective bins to summarize the data. The filters bin will add criteria to the data so that only specific data are displayed. The columns bin will summarize each value of a field and display the discrete name of the values in columns. The rows bin will summarize each value of a field and display the discrete name of the values in rows. The values bin is the variable that will be summarized. Quantitative variables can be summarized using various descriptive statistics such as mean or standard deviation. Qualitative variables can be summarized using counts. We can display the results of our pivot table by dragging the "emergency" field into the rows bin, "compare" column into the columns bin, and the "pid" column into the values bin.

The resulting pivot table is shown in figure 9.2d. As displayed, the discrete values for the emergency field are listed as row labels and those for the compare field are listed as column labels. To count the number of hospitals that do or do not have an emergency department and have a HF 30-day readmission rate that is better or worse than the US national rate, the pid field is included in the values bin. By default, the count of pid in each condition is included in the summary. The results of the pivot table will be used for calculating odds ratios and the logistic regression.

Step 4: Statistical Analyses

Logistic regression is used when the outcome variable of interest is categorical, rather than continuous. Just as with linear regression, logistic regression allows us to look at the effect of multiple predictors on an outcome. In this case we will investigate whether there is a relationship between accessibility to emergency services and heart failure 30-day mortality rate using SLR. Table 9.1 displays the frequency of US hospitals with and without emergency services and whether they perform better or worse than the national average for heart failure readmission rates, as derived from the pivot table (see table 9.1).

Figure 9.2.   Creating a Microsoft Excel pivot table

a.
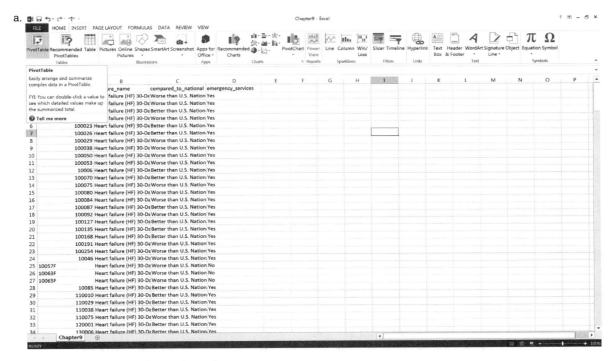

Source: Used with permission from Microsoft.

b.
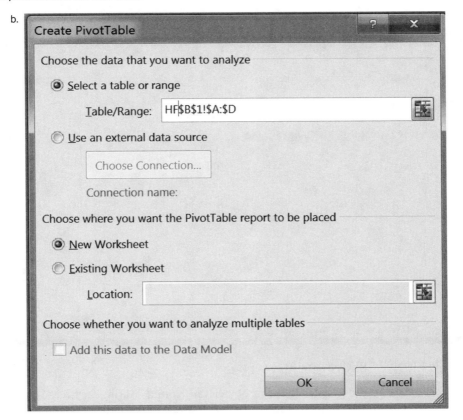

Source: Used with permission from Microsoft.

(Continued)

Figure 9.2.   Creating a Microsoft Excel pivot table *(Continued)*

c.

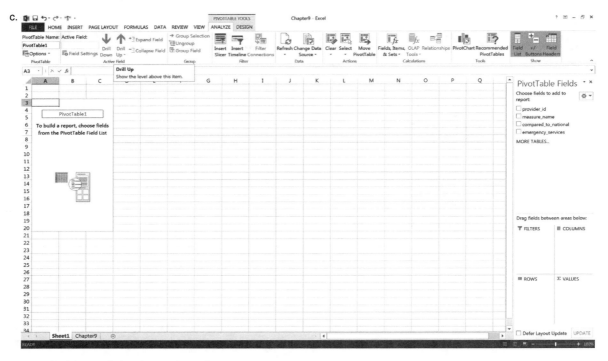

Source: Used with permission from Microsoft.

d.

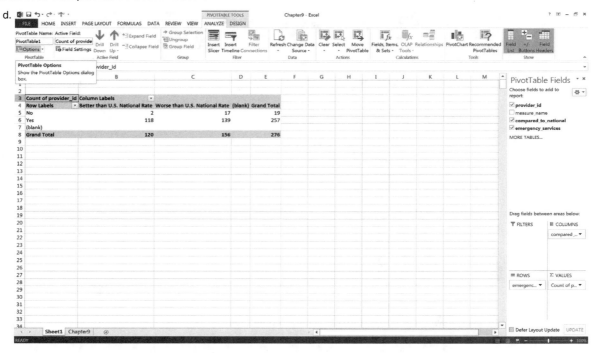

Source: Used with permission from Microsoft.

An **odds ratio** is a descriptive statistic that can be derived from a contingency table or the coefficients of a logistic regression, for example. It is a measure of effect size and provides an index for the strength of association (or nonindependence) between two values. The formula for the odds ratio (OR) is Oddsgroup1/Oddsgroup2. Using the data from the previous table, we can calculate the odds of being better than the US national rate for hospitals with emergency services versus without emergency services using the formula:

$$OR = (118/139)/(2/17) = 7.22$$

Table 9.1. Heart failure readmission rates for US hospitals by availability of emergency services

Emergency Services	Heart Failure (HF) 30-day Readmission Rate		Grand Total
	Better Than US National Rate	Worse Than US National Rate	
Yes	118	139	257
No	2	17	19
Grand total	120	156	276

Thus, we say that hospitals with emergency services have a 7.22 times greater odds of performing better than the US national rate than hospitals without emergency services.

The odds of being worse than the US national rate for hospitals with emergency services versus without emergency services is:

OR = (139/118)/(17/2) = 0.14

Here we can say that hospitals with emergency services have an 86 percent (1 – 0.14) lower odds of being worse than the US national rate than hospitals without emergency services. Note that 0.14 was subtracted from 1 in order to convert the odds ratio to percentage form. If the odds ratio is less than 1, the conversion subtracts the odds ratio from 1 and multiplies by 100. If the odds ratio is greater than 1, the conversion subtracts 1 from the odds ratio and multiplies by 100.

When calculating the odds ratio, we have the odds of the event in the group of interest divided by the odds of the event in the comparison group. To ensure the logistic regression is generated appropriately, we need to simplify our data set so that our group of interest, hospitals with a readmission rate better than the US national rate, is coded as 1 and the comparison group, hospitals with a readmission rate worse than the US national rate, is coded as 0. In other words, the event itself will be coded as 1 and the nonevent as 0. This is done in order to weight the variables so that they accurately reflect the presence or lack of a factor (namely, better = 1, or worse = 0). We now apply logistic regression to our example. To begin this process, open RStudio. Rather than importing data into RStudio, we will be manually entering the information that is needed for further analysis.

Analyzing the Data in RStudio

After you have accessed RStudio, open an R scripting window. The R scripting window is where you will enter the R code in order to analyze the data. To open a new R scripting window, go to File > New File > R Script. In RStudio, we begin by creating three variables that represent different components of the table we created in figure 9.2—a variable to identify 30-day readmission rate, a variable for emergency services, and a variable containing counts for each readmission rate–emergency services combination. Recall that within the contingency table, the counts within the cells depict the frequency with which hospitals do or do not have emergency services, and whether hospitals within those categories have readmission ratings that are better or worse than the national average. Rather than importing the contingency table, we can generate three variables for later use in modeling and attribute this set to a data frame named readmission.id using the following RStudio command:

```
readmission.id <- data.frame(readmission=factor(c("1","1","0","0")),
eservices=factor(c("1","0","1","0")), count=c(118,2,139,17))
```

Next, we verify our variables were assigned appropriately using the structure function in R, str():

```
str(readmission.id)
```

Using this command we view the following output. Note that the $ indicates that a column name follows.

```
> str(readmission.id)
'data.frame':       4 obs. of 3 variables:
$readmission:       Factor w/2 levels "0","1": 2 2 1 1
$eservices:         Factor w/2 levels "0","1": 2 1 2 1
$count:             num 118 2 139 17
```

This output shows that we created a data frame of four observations and three variables. That is, we have four rows and three columns of data. One column is named readmission and has two levels, 0 and 1. The series of numbers at the end of the $ readmission line signifies that the second variable (1) appears in the first two observations and the first variable (0) appears twice in the last two observations. The next column is eservices and again has two levels, 0 and 1. The last column of data is count and is numeric, with four different values.

The glm() function is used to fit a logistic regression model. The glm stands for generalized linear model. The word *general* refers to the dependence on potentially more than one independent variable. Also, a generalized linear model can accommodate a dependent variable that is binary or count and does not depend on calculating a mean.

In R, the first attributes we need to supply to the glm function are the columns we want to compare. Since we want to compare the count of hospitals with readmission rates greater than or worse than the national rate based on whether the hospital has emergency services or not, the first variable we must supply to our glm function is readmission. Next, we enter a tilde (~). Since we want to compare readmissions by emergency services, we include eservices as our next variable. Here, our example data set already contains the counts for each combination of factor levels so we need to include the "weights=" attribute. If we omit the weights attribute, R will attempt to count the variables automatically, but since we are basing our linear model on a table of data this would cause an error. Additionally, because we intend to fit a logistic model we are requesting a binary outcome; therefore, we must specify the "family='binomial'" attribute. Finally, we will be naming our logistic model readmission.logit. Naming the model.logit is a reminder that the computation of the log-odds (the coefficients within the logistic regression model) is contained in the solution; however, this is not necessary—users may name their model anything they like. The following command will generate our logistic regression model:

```
readmission.logit <-glm(readmission ~ eservices, weights=count,
data=readmission.id, family="binomial")
```

We then use the summary() function to view the results of our fitted logistic regression model in order to view the coefficients and their respective p-values:

```
summary(readmission.logit)
```

We view our output:

```
> summary(readmission.logit)

Call:
glm(formula = readmission ~ eservices, family = "binomial", data =
readmission.id, weights = count)

Deviance Residuals:
  1 2 3 4
  13.554 3.001 -13.071 -1.945

Coefficients:
            Estimate   Std. Error   z value   Pr(>|z|)
(Intercept) -2.1401     0.7474      -2.863    0.00419 **
eservices1   1.9763     0.7578       2.608    0.00911 **

- - -
```

```
Signif. codes: 0 '***' 0.001 '**' 0.01 '*' 0.05 '.' 0.1 ' ' 1

(Dispersion parameter for binomial family taken to be 1)

Null deviance: 377.91 on 3 degrees of freedom
Residual deviance: 367.35 on 2 degrees of freedom
AIC: 371.35

Number of Fisher Scoring iterations: 4
```

This output provides the log-odds, which is the logarithm of the odds $p/(1 - p)$, where p = probability of success. The log-odds is later used to compute the odds ratio. We can derive an equation for our log-odds using the output from our logistic regression that is shown in red. The equation begins with the log odds, which is equal to 0.0 when the probability in question is equal to 0.50, smaller than 0.0 when the probability is less than 0.50, and greater than 0.0 when the probability is greater than 0.50. The method for deriving the equation for a logistic regression is similar to the method used for deriving the equation for our best-fit line for a linear regression. In the case of a logistic regression, the equation is $\beta 0 + \beta 1x$, where $\beta 0$ = the intercept, and $\beta 1x$ = the slope:

$$\text{log-odds} = \beta 0 + \beta 1x$$

The intercept is the log odds when x is equal to zero. The slope is the rate at which the predicted log odds increases (or, in some cases, decreases) with each successive unit of x. When the slope is exponentiated, this describes the proportionate rate at which the predicted odds changes with each successive unit of x.

The y-intercept of the logistic regression equation is derived from the output of the logistic regression model. In the output, the y-intercept is listed under the Estimate column in the row labeled (Intercept). The value for the y-intercept is –2.1401. The slope is also listed under the Estimate column, but in the row labeled eservices1. With the values of the coefficients inserted, the equation becomes log-odds = –2.1401 + 1.9763x, where x = 1 if the hospital has emergency services and x = 0, if it does not. We can also verify by the second line of the red output as 1 in eservices indicates that this variable is modeled for x = 1.

Next, we will use the output from the logistic regression model fit in R to calculate the odds ratio and construct its 95 percent confidence interval. We need to calculate the odds ratio of being better than the US national rate for hospitals with emergency services versus without emergency services. To determine the odds of being better than the US national rate for hospitals with emergency services compared to those without, calculate the OR by taking the log(odds) for hospitals with eservices minus the log(odds) for hospitals without eservices. This is the same OR value we calculated earlier directly from the contingency table. It is important to note that the value of using RStudio to compute the OR is the fact that this information is easily gained. Specifically, using the coefficients (log-odds in this example) and their respective standard errors, the confidence intervals can be computed, which describe the range expected to contain the parameter of interest at a certain percentage of the time over the course of many separate replications of the analysis.

We can use RStudio and the logistic regression model we generated earlier to do the calculations for the odds ratio. Since the OR is simply the slope exponentiated, which is a coefficient from our model (readmission. logit), we can extract this value from the model and exponentiate in one step using the exp() and coef() functions in R:

```
exp(coef(readmission.logit))
```

The output will be the following:

```
(Intercept) eservices1
0.1176471 7.2158262
```

The value in the column labeled eservices1 (7.2158262) is our odds ratio. This means that hospitals with emergency services are 7.22 times more likely to have a HF 30-day readmission rate better than the US national rate.

Using the natural log scale, we can now construct the 95 percent confidence interval of the odds ratio of being better than the US national rate for hospitals with emergency services versus without emergency services.

95% C.I. for $\beta 1$:

$\beta 1 +/- 1.96 * se(\beta 1)$

Each of these values can be obtained from the output of the logistic regression model labeled readmission. logit. The value for $\beta 1$, which is our slope is shown under the Estimate column in the row labeled eservices1. Listed under the Std.Error column in the row labeled eservices1 is the value for $se(\beta 1)$:

$1.9763 +/- 1.96 * (0.7578) = (0.49, 3.46)$

This is the confidence interval (CI) for the log(odds). Notice that this interval does not contain 0. To construct the CI of the OR rather than the log(odds), exponentiate each value of the confidence interval for the previous log(odds):

$(\exp(0.49), \exp(3.46)) = (1.63, 31.82)$

This is the confidence interval for the OR. Notice that this interval does not contain 1.

We can also derive these confidence intervals using the function confint.default() in R for the log(odds) and for the OR, respectively:

```
confint.default(readmission.logit)

              2.5 %        97.5 %
Intercept)   -3.6048652   -0.6752668
eservices1    0.4910738    3.4614796

exp(confint.default(readmission.logit))
              2.5 %        97.5 %
Intercept)    0.02719111   0.5090206
eservices1    1.63406989  31.8640888
```

We can test the significance of the parameter estimate with the Wald test of the confidence intervals, which means if the CI for an estimate (or log(odds)) contains 0, the variable is not significantly associated with the outcome. Equivalently, if the CI for an OR contains 1, the variable is not significantly associated with the outcome. We already know that the CI for the log(odds) does not contain 0 and the CI for the OR does not contain 1. The statistical hypotheses tested are:

H_0: $\beta 1 = 0$ versus H_A: $\beta 1 \neq 0$

We can obtain the Wald test statistic (specifically the Wald z-statistic) and p-value from the coefficients section in the coefficients. These coefficients are shown in the output after executing the command summary (readmission. logit). In the output, the Wald z-statistic is listed under the Estimate in the row that is labeled eservices1. The p-value is shown is listed under Pr(>|z|) in the row labeled eservices1. The Wald z-statistic for the eservices coefficient is 1.9763 with p-value <0.05. As the p-value is less than an alpha of 0.05, we reject the null hypothesis and conclude that emergency services is significantly related to heart failure 30-day readmission rate. When we constructed the confidence interval of the log(OR), we took notice that the CI did not contain 0. Similarly, the CI of the OR did not contain 1. Both of these observations lead to the same conclusion as the Wald test: We reject the null hypothesis.

Discussion

Given these results, it appears that hospitals with emergency services are more likely to perform above the national average on the rate of heart failure 30-day readmission. It is possible, as shown in the work of others, that there may be a threshold effect at play (Fisher et al. 1994). Individuals in systems without emergency services might be referred directly for admission to the hospital, thereby increasing the rate of readmission in hospitals without emergency services.

Interestingly, if we apply the same logistic regression methodology, but replace the rate of hospitalization with the rate of mortality (refer to the question prompts at the end of the chapter), we see opposing trends. In fact, hospitals without emergency services have a 5.31 times greater odds of performing better than the national rate of mortality than hospitals with emergency services.

Conclusion

In summary, we have discovered that the presence of emergency services in a hospital is significantly related to heart failure 30-day readmission rate. In fact, by employing logistic regression we have shown that hospitals with emergency services have a 7.22 times greater odds of performing better than the US national rate than do hospitals without emergency services. Further, hospitals with emergency services have an 86 percent (1 – 0.14) lower odds of being worse than the US national rate than do hospitals without emergency services.

Review Exercises

Instructions: Answer the following questions.

1. Using the following table, compute each step of the logistic regression analysis but replace HF 30-readmission rate with HF 30-day mortality rate.

Emergency Services	Heart Failure (HF) 30-day Readmission Rate		Grand Total
	Better Than US National Rate	Worse Than US National Rate	
No	13	2	15
Yes	164	134	298
Grand total	177	136	313

2. What is an odds ratio and how can it be computed?

References

American Heart Association. 2015. Get With The Guidelines®-Heart Failure. http://www.heart.org/HEARTORG/HealthcareResearch/GetWithTheGuidelines/GetWithTheGuidelines-HF/Get-With-The-Guidelines-Heart-Failure-Home-Page_UCM_306087_SubHomePage.jsp

Centers for Medicare and Medicaid Services. 2015. Medicare.gov Hospital Compare. http://www.medicare.gov/hospitalcompare/search.html

Fisher E., J. Wennberg, and T. Stukel. 1994. Hospital readmission rates for cohorts of Medicare beneficiaries in Boston and New Haven. *New England Journal of Medicine* 331(15).

Fonarow G.C., N.M. Albert, A.B. Curtis, M. Gheorghiade, J.T. Heywood, Y. Liu, et al. 2011. Associations between outpatient heart failure process-of-care measures and mortality. *Circulation* 123(15):1601–1610.

Heidenreich P.A., J.G. Trogdon, O.A. Khavjou, J. Butler, K. Dracup, M.D. Ezekowitz, et al. 2011. Forecasting the future of cardiovascular disease in the United States: A policy statement from the American Heart Association. *Circulation* 123(8):933–944.

Hernandez A.F., G.C. Fonarow, L. Liang, P.A. Heidenreich, C. Yancy, and E.D. Peterson. 2011. The need for multiple measures of hospital quality: Results from the Get With The Guidelines®-Heart Failure registry of the American Heart Association. *Circulation* 124(6):712–719.

Hunt S.A. 2005. ACC/AHA 2005 guideline update for the diagnosis and management of chronic heart failure in the adult: A report of the American College of Cardiology/American Heart Association Task Force on Practice Guidelines (Writing committee to update the 2001 guidelines for the evaluation and management of heart failure). *Journal of the American College of Cardiology* 46:e1–e82.

Comparing Medicare Spending per Patient and Patient Satisfaction Scores

Ryan Sandefer, MA, CPHIT and David Marc, MBS, CHDA

Learning Objectives

- Define patient satisfaction and value-based purchasing
- Demonstrate the relationship between patient experience of care and Medicare spending in US hospitals
- Conduct a simple linear regression and one-way ANOVA to determine association between variables

Key Terms

Association
Continuous variable
Hospital Value-Based Purchasing Program
Normally distributed
One-way ANOVA
Patient satisfaction
R-squared value
Simple linear regression
Tukey HSD

Patient satisfaction is a critical component of the US healthcare delivery system. According to one researcher, "patient satisfaction is increasingly used as a measure of health system performance through public reporting and pay-for-performance schemes" (Farley et al. 2014).

The Institute of Medicine has put patient-centered outcomes as one of six key dimensions of a high-quality healthcare system (Rozenblum et al. 2013). There is no agreed upon definition of patient satisfaction. Two definitions of **patient satisfaction** are an "individual's evaluation of his or her healthcare experience" (Shirley and Sanders 2013) and "the degree to which the individual regards the healthcare service or product or the manner in which it is delivered by the provider as useful, effective, or beneficial" (NLM 2015).

Research has indicated that patient satisfaction is correlated with improved hospital care (Jha et al. 2008). Higher patient satisfaction is associated with reduced hospital readmissions, lower inpatient mortality, and improved clinical guideline adherence (Boulding et al. 2011; Glickman et al. 2010). Other research has shown that among hospitals that perform major surgical procedures, hospitals with higher patient satisfaction have higher quality and more efficiency (Tsai et al. 2014). Also, larger hospitals were shown to have lower patient satisfaction scores (Young et al. 2000).

Due to the importance of patient satisfaction on the impact of clinical outcomes, patient satisfaction has become a top priority for the Centers for Medicare and Medicaid Services (CMS). CMS recently updated its **Hospital Value-Based Purchasing Program**, which rewards acute-care hospitals with incentive payments for providing quality care. Payments are provided based upon a hospital's total performance score, which includes a clinical process of care domain and a patient experience of care domain. The patient experience of care domain accounts for 30 percent of the total performance score and is measured by scores on eight dimensions of patient experience:

- nurse and doctor communication
- cleanliness and quietness
- responsiveness of hospital staff
- pain management
- communication about medications
- discharge information
- overall rating (CMS 2012)

The purpose of this chapter is to evaluate the relationship between patient satisfaction and Medicare spending per patient among US acute-care hospitals participating in the Hospital Value-Based Purchasing Program.

Research Question and Hypothesis

Is there a difference in average Medicare spending per patient when comparing hospitals by patient experience of care domain score?

The dependent variable for the proposed study is the average patient experience of care domain score for hospitals, because the dependent variable is the variable we are measuring. In the case of the proposed research question, there is one independent variable: Medicare spending per beneficiary. Medicare spending per beneficiary is an average dollar amount for each hospital in the data set—it is an average Medicare payment per Medicare patient for each hospital. The analysis for answering the proposed research question will include

1. A comparison of the average Medicare spending per beneficiary dollar amount and patient experience of care domain score groups
2. An association between the patient experience of care domain score and Medicare spending per beneficiary dollar amount

Hypotheses

Given that the research question is measuring patient experience of care scores by Medicare spending and by Medicare spending by groups, there is more than one set of hypotheses.

$H1_0$: There is not a relationship between the patient experience of care domain score and hospital Medicare spending by patient.
$H1_A$: There is a relationship between the patient experience of care domain score and hospital Medicare spending by patient.

$H2_0$: There is no difference in the patient experience of care domain score by spending group.
$H2_A$: At least one spending group has a different patient experience of care domain score when compared to at least one other spending group.

Checklist

To answer the research question, a specific process of data acquisition, preparation, and discovery is required. The following steps will be explained in detail:

1. Extract data sets from MySQL
   a. Select required columns of data from database
   b. Join columns of data using MySQL queries
2. Data preparation
   a. Review data set for erroneous values

3. Import the data into RStudio
4. Perform descriptive statistics on the variables of mspb and uw.pt.ex.sc
5. Conduct simple linear regressions to examine the relationship between spending and patient experience of care

The Analysis

This section will provide a step-by-step description of obtaining and analyzing the data required to answer the proposed research question.

Step 1: Data Extraction

In order to carry out the analysis, the following data are needed:

- A list of all hospitals in the United States participating in the CMS Value-Based Purchasing Program
- A patient experience of care domain score for each hospital
- A Medicare spending per beneficiary score amount for each hospital

Two data sets need to be combined to obtain the needed data to answer the proposed research question. The first data set is named hospital_value_based_purchasing and obtained from the Centers for Medicare and Medicaid Services (CMS 2015). This data set includes measures related to the Hospital Value-Based Purchasing Program, including weighted and unweighted scores for clinical processes, outcomes, and patient experience of care for all hospitals that are participating in this Medicare program. The data set also includes each hospital's unique Medicare identification number, hospital name, address, and other geographic-related information.

The second data set is named medicare_hospital_spending_per_patient and is also obtained from the Centers for Medicare and Medicaid Services (CMS 2015). This data set provides measures of average spending per patient for hospital inpatient services, including cost of care for a variety of DRGs and MS-DRGs. The data set also provides a measure of the average hospital spending per patient for each US hospital. A variety of other data elements are also included that allow us to refine our analysis, including measure start and end date, measure name, hospital name, county name, and other elements.

The two data sets will be combined using MySQL scripts. The scripts will be constructed so that only the following data elements are extracted: unique hospital ID, Medicare spending per patient score, and hospital value-based purchasing patient experience of care domain score. Figure 10.1 displays the SQL script that is used to combine the two data sets and also the first few rows of the output that was derived from the query. Note that

Figure 10.1. SQL script and returned data for combining three data sets

```
SELECT hospital_general_information.provider_id,
medicare_hospital_spending_per_patient.measure_id,
medicare_hospital_spending_per_patient.score,
hospital_value_based_purchasing.unweighed_patient_experience_of_care_
domain_score

FROM hospital_general_information

JOIN medicare_hospital_spending_per_patient

ON hospital_general_information.provider_id=medicare_hospital_spending_per_
patient.provider_id

JOIN hospital_value_based_purchasing

ON hospital_general_information.provider_id=hospital_value_based_purchasing.
provider_id;
```

(Continued)

Figure 10.1.   SQL script and returned data for combining three data sets *(Continued)*

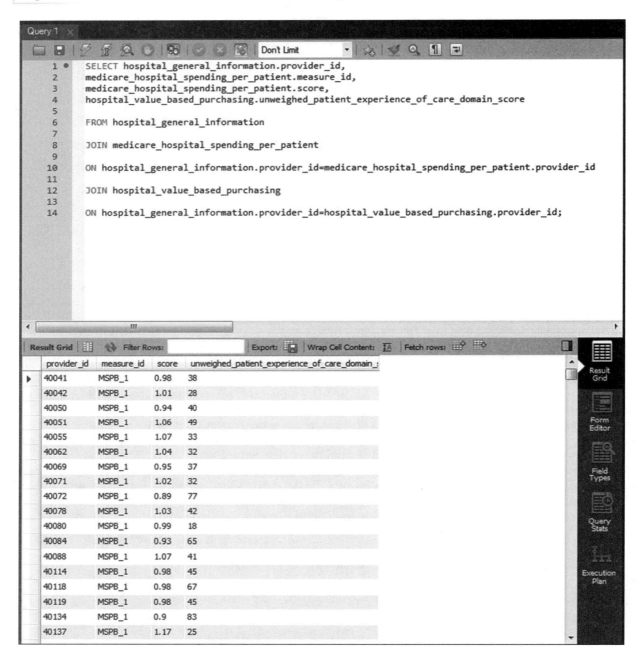

you must alter a setting in MySQL so that the output shows all of the results rather than just showing the first 1,000 rows (see chapter 4). After executing each query, export the data to a CSV file and save the file as pt_sat. For detailed instructions regarding exporting data from MySQL Workbench to CSV format, see chapter 4.

Step 2: Data Preparation

Data preparation is critical for the analysis process. To make this data set easier to work with and meaningful for our analysis, we are going to prepare the data in Excel prior to importing it into RStudio. Open the pt_sat.csv file that was exported from MySQL Workbench with Excel. You should see the following four columns of data (each observation represents a single US hospital):

- provider_id: The code number assigned to an individual inpatient hospital.
- measure_id: The name of the specific measure from the Hospital Value-Based Purchasing Program. For our purposes, we are focused on MSPB_1, which is defined as "a claims-based measure that includes risk-adjusted and price-standardized payments for all Part A and Part B services provided from 3 days prior to a hospital admission (index admission) through 30 days after the hospital discharge" (CMS 2015).
- score: The measure that represents the average Medicare spending per patient across each hospital. The score is represented as a ratio. The number is either greater than or less than one. If it is greater than one, the hopsital's Medicare spending is greater than the national average; if the number is less than 1, the hospital's Medicare spending is lower than the national average.
- unweighed_patient_experience_of_care_domain_score: The measure for the unweighted patient experience of care domain score. This score is calculated by summing the hospital's HCAHPS (Hospital Consumer Assessment of Healthcare Providers and Systems) base score (0 to 80) and the HCAHPS consistency score (0 to 20). These two measures are based upon the individual scores for each hospital across all dimensions of the HCAHPS survey, which includes 27 to 32 questions (there is a standard and expanded version of the survey that affects the number of questions included).

Renaming Column Headers in Excel

When we import these data into RStudio, these column header names will become the names of R objects after we attach the data set. Although RStudio is able to work with names that have spaces in them, it is best practice to change the field names in Excel, rather than changing them in RStudio or typing long field names in RStudio each time. Table 10.1 contains the names we will use when renaming the column headers. To rename column headers in Excel, simply click on each individual cell, highlight the contents, delete the content, enter the new column name, and hit return. Repeat this process for each column header.

Reviewing Data Sets for Erroneous Values

One of the first steps in data preparation is to carefully examine if the data include erroneous values or blanks. Although the CSV that was exported from MySQL does not include any erroneous values or blanks, it is still important to review the data set for errors and issues.

Recoding a Variable in Excel

After you have reviewed the data for accuracy and completeness, you need to create a new column of data. For the purpose of this chapter we want to compare four different groups of hospitals. We will group the hospitals by their average patient experience of care score—we will group them into quartiles (that is, the lowest

Table 10.1. Original and revised column names within Excel

Original Name	Revised Name
provider id	pid
measure_id	mid
score	mspb
unweighed_patient_experience_of_care_domain_score	uw.pt.ex.sc
Column E	pt.ex.group

Source: Used with permission from RStudio.

25 percent of hospitals will be one group, 26 to 50 percent will be the second group, 51 to 75 percent the third group, and 76 percent and greater the highest group).

The first step in this process is to identify the percentiles. Click into any open cell, input the following formula, and hit enter:

= PERCENTILE(D : D,0.25)

This function should return the value of 26. This means that 25 percent of all numbers in this column fall below the number 26. We need to repeat this same function to identify the remaining quartiles by using these formulas:

= PERCENTILE(D : D,0.50)

= PERCENTILE(D : D,0.75)

These two functions should return the values 39 and 52, respectfully. Because we know that 75 percent of all values in this column fall below the number 52, we know anything higher than that is in the top 25th percentile. Based on this information, our quartiles are defined as the following:

- Group 1 (lowest average patient experience of care score): scores less than or equal to 26
- Group 2 (lower-middle average patient experience of care score): scores between 27 and 39
- Group 3 (upper-middle average patient experience of care score): scores between 40 and 52
- Group 4 (highest average patient experience of care score): scores greater than or equal to 53

The next step in the process is to group these hospitals based upon these values. This can be done using Excel's IF function. Click into cell E2 and input the following formula:

= IF(D2 < 26,1,IF(AND(D2 >= 26,D2 < 39),2,IF(AND(D2 >= 39,D2 < 52),3,4)))

After you enter this formula, press the return key to run it. This function is forcing Excel to enter the number 1 in the cell E2 if the number in the cell D2 is in Group 1, if the number is between 26 and 39 the formula is forcing Excel to populate the cell with a number 2, and so on all the way to 4. The number 3 should be returned in cell E2. To populate the entire column, click into cell E2 and double-click the fill handle (square in the bottom right-hand corner of the cell that holds the formula). This will auto fill the formula for all cells in the column. The entire column should now be populated, and each cell should include a number between 1 and 4. Quickly review the column to test that numbers are binned appropriately; for example, numbers less than 26 in column D are equal to 1 in column E. Important note: please click into cell E1 and name the column pt.ex.group.

The last step in the process is to remove the formula that we just created to avoid potential issues with future analyses. Highlight column E by clicking on the E above the column header. The entire column should be highlighted. On the Excel Menu bar (Mac) or Home tab (Windows), select Edit and then Copy. After you have chosen Copy, go back to the Menu bar or Home tab and select Edit and then Paste Special. A menu will appear with multiple options. Choose the option that says paste Values. This pastes the numbers into the column and removes the formula.

After reviewing the data, the data preparation phase is complete. Remember to save the file as a CSV. In Excel, select File > Save As. Under the "Format" or "Save as type" drop-down window, select the Comma Separated Values option. When saving the file, name the document pt_sat and save the file to your computer's desktop. When saving your file, you may receive a message:

Some features in your workbook might be lost if you save it as CSV (Comma defined). Do you want to keep using that format?

The reason Excel provides this warning is that only the active spreadsheet in your Excel workbook will be saved. If you have additional worksheets included in your file, those spreadsheets will be lost—in short, only the worksheet that is open when you save the file is retained. Click OK or Yes.

Step 3: Import the Data

The next step in the analysis is to import the data set pt_sat.csv into RStudio for analysis (see chapter 5 for detailed instructions for importing data into RStudio).

After the data are imported into RStudio, open an R scripting window. The R scripting window is where you will enter the R code in order to analyze the data. To open a new R scripting window, go to File > New File > R Script. The first step is to attach the data set. The reason that the data set is attached is to make the column names accessible in RStudio—for a detailed description of the attach function, see chapter 5.

To attach the data, the following R script into the console:

```
attach(pt_sat)
```

Step 4: Descriptive Statistics

Once the data are imported and attached into RStudio, the first type of analysis that should be conducted to familiarize yourself with the data is the descriptive statistics. The data we are using to answer our research question include a **continuous variable**. Continuous data are commonly described by calculating the mean, median, standard deviation, and range. In this case, there is one continuous variable: mspb (Medicare spending per beneficiary). In RStudio, the summary function can be used to obtain basic descriptive statistics for quantitative variables. The following code can be entered to obtain these variables:

```
summary(mspb)
```

The following is the output from the summary function, which provides the minimum value, the value at the 25th percentile, the median, the mean, the value that is at the 75th percentile, and the maximum value:

Min.	1st Qu.	Median	Mean	3rd Qu.	Max.
0.7100	0.9500	0.9900	0.9914	1.0300	1.3600

We see that the mean of the data is 0.9914, the minimum value is 0.71 and the maximum value is 1.36.

While the summary output is informative, we can also create a histogram to visualize the distribution of the data. To create a histogram, use the following code:

```
hist(mspb)
```

The histogram that is created in RStudio is illustrated in figure 10.2. An important step in the data analysis process is to determine if data are **normally distributed,** that is, that the data are approximately equal on both sides of the mean, which is commonly referred to as following a bell-shaped curve. Certain statistical techniques have assumptions that data are normally distributed; if this assumption is not satisfied the results of the statistical procedure may be compromised. We see that the data are normally distributed. The shape of the data tells us that there is nearly an equal number of hospitals with Medicare spending per patient on each side of the mean and, therefore, the data are not skewed.

The next step is to create a second histogram that depicts the unweighted patient experience of care domain score. Again, it is important to check the distribution of each variable we plan to use in our analysis. Use the following script to create the histogram:

```
hist(uw.pt.ex.sc)
```

The histogram that we created is shown in figure 10.3. Similar to the histogram we created previously, the data appears to be normally distributed because they resemble a bell-shaped curve. The shape of the data tells us that there is nearly an equal number of hospitals with patient experience of care scores on each side of the mean and, therefore, the data are not skewed.

Now that we have a sense of the distribution of the data, the next step is to gain a better understanding of the data by the patient experience of care groups we created using Excel earlier. We created four groups based upon the values at each of the data's quartiles—the first group represents all data at and below the 25th

Figure 10.2.   Histogram of Medicare spending per patient

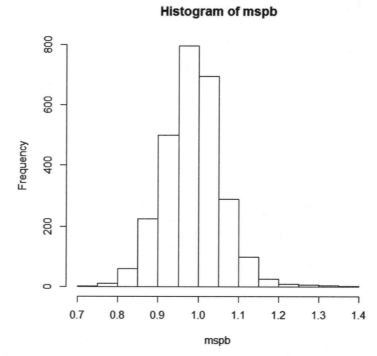

Source: Used with permission from RStudio.

Figure 10.3.   Histogram of unweighted patient experience of care score

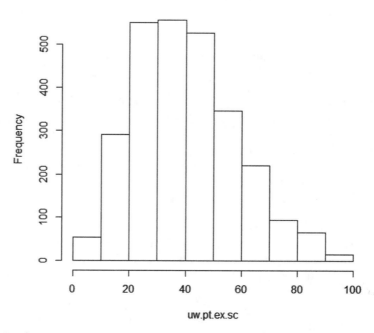

Source: Used with permission from RStudio.

percentile, the second group is the data between the 26th and 50th percentile, the third group is the data between the 51st and 75th percentile, and the fourth group is all data above the 76th percentile.

To obtain the average Medicare spending per beneficiary for each of these groups, we will need to use R's tapply function. This function allows us to combine multiple columns of data (much like a contingency table) and perform a variety of analyses on the data. To calculate the mean score for each group, use the following script:

```
tapply(mspb,pt.ex.group,mean)
```

This script combined the columns mspb and pt.ex.group and calculated the mean for each group. The output from this script is the following:

```
        1           2           3           4
1.0104147   0.9997167   0.9875036   0.9697118
```

This output shows that the average Medicare spending per patient is 1.01 for hospitals in the lowest quartile for patient experience of care, while the average Medicare spending per patient is 0.97 for hospitals in the highest quartile for patient experience of care. The Medicare spending per patient measure represents the average Medicare spending per patient compared to the national average—if below 1.0, the hospital spends less per patient than the national average; if above 1.0, the hospital spends more per patient than the national average. In short, these findings indicate that patients with higher patient satisfaction also have lower overall Medicare spending. We will need to use a statistical procedure to test if this finding is significant. However, before we delve into the statistical procedure, we need to use R's tapply function to calculate some additional descriptive statistics.

We will use tapply to calculate the standard deviation (useful for understanding the variation in our data) for the same two variables of mspb and pt.ex.group using the following script:

```
tapply(mspb,pt.ex.group,sd)
```

This script combined the columns mspb and pt.ex.group and calculated the standard deviation for each group. The output from this script is the following:

```
         1            2            3            4
0.07348135   0.07400348   0.06619272   0.06504458
```

The output from the standard deviation shows that the standard deviation for Medicare spending per patient is higher for hospitals in the first quartile (0.073) than hospitals in the fourth quartile (0.065). The standard deviation provides a measure of the variation in the data and is often an indicator if there are extreme values in the data set. If the standard deviation is low, it means that the data are close to the mean. If it is high, it means that the data are spread further from the mean.

One way to visualize all of these descriptive statistics is through the use of a boxplot (also known as a box and whiskerplot). The boxplot graphically illustrates the 25th percentile, the mean, the 75th percentile, the minimum value, the maximum value, and the minimum and maximum values within 1.5*interquartile (1.5 IQR) range (1.5 times the difference between the 25th and 75th percentile). In short, boxplots are very powerful for visualizing quantitative information.

We will now create a boxplot for Medicare spending per patient for each of our patient experience of care groups using this script:

```
boxplot(mspb~pt.ex.group, ylab="MSPB Rate", xlab="Patient Experience of
Care Domain Score Groups")
```

The resulting boxplot is shown in figure 10.4. Medicare spending is plotted on the y-axis, and the patient groups are listed on the x-axis. From this chart, we can see that the average Medicare spending per patient is highest in group 1 and lowest in group 4. The median is indicated by the bold black line within the box. The upper bounds of the box represent the 75th percentile for the data, and the lower bounds of the box represent the 25th percentile. The whiskers (the dotted lines with the bar extending from the top and bottom

Figure 10.4.   Box and whiskerplot of Medicare spending by patient experience of care groups

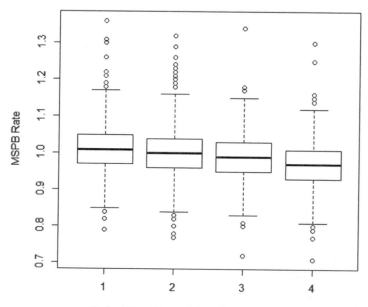

Source: Used with permission from RStudio.

on the box) represent 1.5 IQR. Anything above and below those whiskers (represented as circles) may be considered an outlier, so this chart helps identify potential issues with your data.

Now that we have used RStudio to explore the distribution of the data and calculate some descriptive statistics, we can use it to test if there is any statistical significance in Medicare spending by patient experience of care domain score groups.

Step 5: Statistical Analyses

In order to determine if there is an **association** (a relationship between two measured variables) between these variables that have been summarized, we need to conduct multiple statistical procedures to determine the following:

1. Is there a difference in the average Medicare spending per patient for US acute-care hospitals across groups of US hospitals based upon their patient experience of care domain scores?
2. Is there a relationship between the average Medicare spending per patient for US acute-care hospitals and the average patient experience of care domain score for US acute-care hospitals?

To answer these questions, we will use two different statistical procedures—a one-way ANOVA and a simple linear regression.

A **one-way ANOVA** will be used to compare the average Medicare spending of hospitals based upon the groupings of hospitals by their patient experience of care domain score. For detailed instruction regarding conducting one-way ANOVAs see chapter 8. A one-way ANOVA is used to compare a mean across more than two groups—we are comparing a mean across four groups. The dependent variable for this statistical procedure is mspb (Medicare spending per patient), and the independent variable is pt.ex.group (the average patient experience of care domain score by group). We will use RStudio to conduct the one-way ANOVA by using the following script:

```
anova1<-aov(mspb~as.factor(pt.ex.group))
```

We have named our model anova1. When writing R scripts it is important to realize that you will be assigning meaning to different variables by a naming them and storing the values in R's memory for later use. That is what is happening in this example. By naming our model anova1, we can store the model in memory and run additional statistics on that model or return to the model in the future. When we create a model in R, such as the one in this example, we need to separate the name from the function by including a less than sign (<) followed by a hyphen (-). The next element of the script is to use R's aov function (which stands for "analysis of variance"), followed by an open parentheses. We then enter the dependent variable (the variable that is stored as the mean). For our purposes this is the variable mspb. We separate the dependent variable by a tilde (~), and then insert the independent variable (the grouping variable). For our example, this is the pt.ex.group variable. However, because the data for this variable are stored as integers, RStudio needs to be told not to interpret the variable as numbers but as factors (that is, categories). Thus, we must include "as.factor()" to force R to use the data as categorical versus continuous data. Categorical data are data that represent a nonnumeric data, such as categories of hospitals by some patient satisfaction scores (think of them as groups). On the other hand, continuous data are numeric data that do not represent a group, but are measured on a continuous scale, such as hospital spending. The last step is to ensure our parentheses are closed.

Now that we have the ANOVA stored in RStudio, the next step is to summarize the model using R's summary function. The following script should be used to summarize the model:

```
summary(anova1)
```

The output from this script is the following:

```
                        Df Sum Sq Mean Sq F value Pr(>F)
as.factor(pt.ex.group)    3  0.612 0.20416   41.99 <2e-16 ***
Residuals              2716 13.205 0.00486
---
Signif. codes: 0 '***' 0.001 '**' 0.01 '*' 0.05 '.' 0.1 ' ' 1
```

The output provides several statistics, including the degrees of freedom (Df), Sum of Squares (Sum Sq), the Sum of Squares divided by the degrees of freedom (Mean Sq), the F statistic, and the p-value for the F statistic (Pr(>F)). For our purposes, we see in the last column labeled Pr(>F) that the p-value is less than 0.05, which means the F statistic is greater than the F critical value. Therefore, we conclude that there is a significant difference in Medicare spending between one group and at least one other group. The issue is that we do not know for sure which groups are significantly different. Determining differences between groups requires an additional statistic, a post-hoc test.

A common post-hoc test that is performed with an ANOVA is the Tukey honest significant difference (HSD) test. The **Tukey HSD** performs a significance test using single pairwise comparisons of the dependent variable across pairs of the independent variable. Therefore, the MSPB variable will be compared across each pairing of the patient experience of care domain groups. To perform a TukeyHSD post-hoc test in R, you must use the following script:

```
TukeyHSD(anova1)
```

Here is the output:

```
        Tukey multiple comparisons of means
        95% family-wise confidence level

Fit: aov(formula = mspb ~ as.factor(pt.ex.group))

$`as.factor(pt.ex.group)`
          diff           lwr            upr        p adj
2-1 -0.01069796 -0.02053401  -0.0008619042 0.0267610
3-1 -0.02291107 -0.03279042  -0.0130317110 0.0000000
4-1 -0.04070286 -0.05057883  -0.0308268845 0.0000000
3-2 -0.01221311 -0.02179788  -0.0026283323 0.0058813
4-2 -0.03000490 -0.03958619  -0.0204236097 0.0000000
4-3 -0.01779179 -0.02741753  -0.0081660576 0.0000126
```

The output provides several critical pieces of information for our analysis. First, it provides the Fit, which summarizes what data were analyzed (mspb ~as.factor(pt.ex.group)). The remainder of the analysis consists of pairwise comparisons for each group of hospitals. For example, the first line of output under "$'as. factor(pt.ex.group)'" provides the statistics when comparing the average Medicare spending per patient between hospitals that fall within the first group of patient experience of care and hospitals that fall within the second group of patient experience of care. The statistics include Diff (the difference in means between the two groups), lwr (the lower value of the confidence interval), upr (the upper value of the confidence interval), and p adj (the p-value for the pairwise comparison). These comparisons are done between each group in the model.

The results indicate that there is a significant difference between each group because the p adj (p-value) is less than 0.05 for each pairwise comparison. If you recall from our boxplot in figure 10.4, Medicare spending per beneficiary was highest for group one and lowest for group four. The key takeaway from this analysis is that there is a clear relationship between cost of care and patient experience of care.

The second analysis we will conduct is a **simple linear regression** (for a detailed discussion of simple linear regression, see chapter 13) to examine the correlation between the variables of average Medicare spending per patient and average patient experience of care domain score per hospital. Simple linear regression "is used to characterize the linear relationship between a dependent variable and one independent variable" (White 2013). For the purposes of this chapter, and similar to the analysis we conducted with the one-way ANOVA, the dependent variable is the variable mspb. The independent variable (or predictor variable) is pt.ex.group. In general with this analysis, we are attempting to predict the Medicare spending per beneficiary among US hospitals from hospital average patient experience of care domain scores.

We will now use RStudio to conduct a simple linear regression to examine if there is a relationship between the average Medicare spending per beneficiary and the patient experience of care domain score for hospitals. Conducting a simple linear regression in RStudio is a process that includes five steps. The first step is to create and name a model using the R function lm (which stands for linear model). The following is the R script for developing the model:

```
lin1<- lm(mspb~uw.pt.ex.sc)
```

The second step in the processes is to use RStudio to summarize the statistics of the model using the R function summary. The following is the R script for summarizing the model:

```
summary(lin1)
```

The output from this function is the following:

```
Call:
lm(formula = mspb ~ uw.pt.ex.sc)

Residuals:
     Min       1Q    Median       3Q       Max
 -0.26383  -0.04204  -0.00070  0.04158  0.35706

Coefficients:
              Estimate Std. Error t value Pr(>|t|)
 (Intercept)  1.028e+00  3.279e-03  313.44  <2e-16 ***
 uw.pt.ex.sc -8.953e-04  7.392e-05  -12.11  <2e-16 ***
 ---
 Signif. codes:  0 '***' 0.001 '**' 0.01 '*' 0.05 '.' 0.1 ' ' 1

 Residual standard error: 0.06945 on 2718 degrees of freedom
 Multiple R-squared:  0.05121,  Adjusted R-squared:  0.05086
 F-statistic: 146.7 on 1 and 2718 DF,  p-value: < 2.2e-16
```

The output summarizes the model and the data elements included in the analysis under Call. The formula lm(formula = mspb ~ uw.pt.ex.sc) is the formula developed for the linear model. As shown, the linear model we created was based on evaluating the relationship between mspb and uw.pt.ex.sc. The best way to use this information is to confirm that we used the correct variables when constructing our model.

The second section of the model summary (labeled Residuals) presents the regression residuals, also known as errors. As a reminder, the least squares regression line described previously is intended to minimize error, so the residuals should be small. The fact that we have very small numbers is a good sign for our model.

The next section is labeled Coefficients, which includes information about our linear model. We can derive the equation for the best-fit line from the information listed in the Coefficients section (see chapter 13 for a detailed discussion). In short, the best-fit line provides a description of the direction of a line and thus illustrates the correlation between two variables. The y-intercept is shown to be 1.028, and the slope is –0.00089. The estimate for uw.pt.ex.sc included e-04, which is scientific notation for how we should interpret the number. It means we must move the decimal four places to the left). Given this information, we can construct the equation of the best-fit line as y = 1.028 – 0.00089x. As shown, the slope is negative indicating that the relationship between the Medicare spending per patient and patient experience of care domain score is negative.

The Coefficients section also contains information about the standard error of the y-intercept and the slope of the line. The t value is the estimate divided by the standard error. The standard error is an estimate of the standard deviation of the coefficient. That is, the amount the coefficient varies across cases. It can be thought of as a measure of the precision with which the regression coefficient is measured. If a coefficient is large compared to its standard error, then the coefficient is probably different from 0 and a small p-value will result.

For our purposes, we want to pay special attention to the significance or p-value Pr (>|t|), which is listed in the line item for lbw under the Coefficients section. This p-value shows if the slope of the best-fit line is significantly different from zero. As shown, the p-value less than 0.0001, which is less than 0.05 and thus the slope of the line is significantly different than zero. Therefore, we can conclude that there is a significant association between the hospital Medicare spending per beneficiary and hospital patient experience of care domain scores. If the slope of the line is a negative number, we interpret the relationship as a negative association. If the slope is a positive number, we can interpret the relationship as a positive association. Given the fact that we have a negative number for the slope of the best-fit line, we can conclude that there is a significant negative association between Medicare spending and patient experience of care domain scores.

The final value that is of relevance is the r-squared value. The **r-squared value** is the proportion of the observed values of y explained by the linear regression of y on x. In other words, the r-squared value explains the strength of the relationship between the two quantitative variables. The r-squared value ranges from 0 to 1. The closer the r-squared value is to 1, the stronger the association is between the two variables. A value closer to zero indicates a weak association; a value closer to 1 indicates a strong association. When looking at the multiple r-squared value in the linear regression output, we see a value of 0.05121. Since this value is close to zero, this indicates that the strength of the relationship between Medicare spending per beneficiary and patient experience of care domain scores is a weak association. If you recall, because the slope of our line is negative, together the r-squared value and the slope indicate that we have weak negative association.

We should always interpret the p-value from our linear model and the r-squared valued together when interpreting the results of our linear model. Even though we have a significant negative association between these two variables, the strength of that relationship is weak.

The third and fourth steps in the process are to plot the data and draw the least squares regression line to help us interpret the results of the statistical output. The following is the R script for plotting the relationship between mspb and uw.pt.ex.sc:

```
plot(mspb~uw.pt.ex.sc, xlab="Patient Experience of Care Domain Score",
ylab="MSPB Rate")
```

To add the best-fit line to the plot, run the abline function after creating the plot:

```
abline(lin1, col="red")
```

The output from these R scripts are shown in figure 10.5. The average value of MSPB for US hospitals is on the y-axis and average percentage of patient experience of care domain score is on the x-axis. The line shows

Figure 10.5.   Relationship between MSPB and patient experience of care domain score

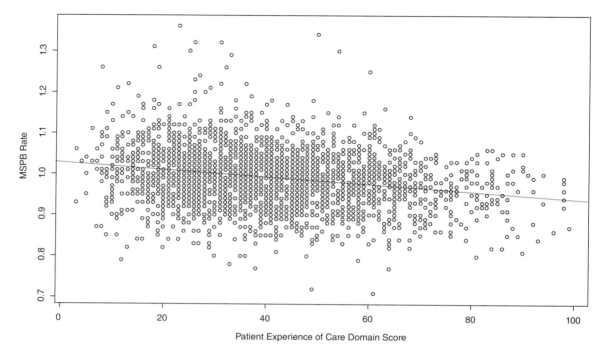

Source: Used with permission from RStudio.

that there is a weak negative correlation between Medicare spending per beneficiary and patient experience of care domain scores in US hospitals. In short, although the relationship is weak, there is a trend to suggest that as Medicare spending per patients decreases, patient experience of care domain scores increases in US hospitals.

Discussion

The results of this study reveal that hospitals with lower patient experience of care domain scores tend to have higher Medicare spending per beneficiary. These findings confirm results from previous studies that found that patients receiving more care do not have better outcomes or higher satisfaction (Fisher et al. 2003; Fowler et al. 2008).

Healthcare costs continue to be a major problem in the United States, and this research further confirms that there is not a clear association between the amount of care as measured by cost per patient and the satisfaction with care as measured by the patient experience of care. There are implications of this research. First, there needs to be a greater focus on healthcare quality outcomes among US hospitals, including a great emphasis on utilizing patient satisfaction as a key measure of performance. Second, because patient experience of care accounts for 30 percent of the Hospital Value-Based Purchasing Program overall score, and is therefore intimately tied to hospital reimbursement, it is extremely important for hospitals to continuously monitor and improve their scores in order to avoid hospital payment penalties.

Conclusion

This research revealed a negative relationship between hospital spending and patient satisfaction. Future research using the same data sets could explore the association between hospital spending per patient and individual HCAHPS survey responses. For example, is there a relationship between patient satisfaction with nurse communication and Medicare spending per beneficiary? Additional analyses could also explore identifying which HCAHPS survey question best predicts Medicare spending per patient.

Review Exercises

Instructions: Answer the following questions.

1. True or False: Patient experience of care accounts for 70 percent of the total performance score under the requirements of the Hospital Value-Based Purchasing Program.

2. When interpreting the results of a simple linear regression, how would you interpret an r-squared value of 0.99?

3. A Tukey post-hoc test would be used for which of the following statistical procedures?
   a. Simple linear regression
   b. Two-sample t-test
   c. One-way ANOVA
   d. All of the above

4. Using the as.factor function in RStudio forces which of the following on data in a vector?
   a. Numeric data to be categorical data
   b. Categorical data to be numeric data
   c. A vector to be a data frame
   d. None of the above

5. True or False: When interpreting R output related to simple linear regression, a positive slope and a r-squared value that is close to 1.0 would indicate that there is a strong positive association between two numeric variables.

References

Boulding, W., S.W. Glickman, M.P. Manary, K.A. Schulman, and R. Staelin. 2011. Relationship between patient satisfaction with inpatient care and hospital readmission within 30 days. *American Journal of Managed Care* 17(1):41–48.

Centers for Medicare and Medicaid Services. 2012. Hospital Value-Based Purchasing Program. http://www.cms.gov/Medicare/Quality-Initiatives-Patient-Assessment-Instruments/hospital-value-based-purchasing/Downloads/FY-2013-Program-Frequently-Asked-Questions-about-Hospital-VBP-3-9-12.pdf

Centers for Medicare and Medicaid Services. 2015. Medicare.gov Hospital Compare. http://www.medicare.gov/hospital-compare/search.html

Farley, H., E.R. Enguidanos, C.M. Coletti, L. Honigman, A. Mazzeo, T.B. Pinson, K. Reed, and J.L. Wiler. 2014. Patient satisfaction surveys and quality of care: An information paper. *Annals of Emergency Medicine* 64(4):351–357.

Fisher, E.S., D.E. Wennberg, T.A. Stukel, D.J. Gottlieb, F.L. Lucas, and E.L. Pinder. 2003. The implications of regional variations in Medicare spending. Part 2: Health outcomes and satisfaction with care. *Annals of Internal Medicine* 138(4):288–298.

Fowler, F.J., P.M. Gallagher, D.L. Anthony, K. Larsen, and J.S. Skinner. 2008. Relationship between regional per capita Medicare expenditures and patient perceptions of quality of care. *Journal of the American Medical Association* 299(20):2406–2412.

Glickman, S.W., W. Boulding, M. Manary, R. Staelin, M.T. Roe, R.J Wolosin, E.M. Ohman, E.D. Peterson, and K.A. Schulman. 2010. Patient satisfaction and its relationship with clinical quality and inpatient mortality in acute myocardial infarction. *Circulation: Cardiovascular Quality and Outcomes* 3(2):188–195.

Jha, A.K., E.J. Orav, J. Zheng, and A.M. Epstein. 2008. Patients' perception of hospital care in the United States. *New England Journal of Medicine* 359(18):1921–1931.

National Library of Medicine. 2015. Patient Satisfaction. http://www.ncbi.nlm.nih.gov/mesh/68017060

Rozenblum, R., J. Donzé, P.M. Hockey, E. Guzdar, M.A. Labuzetta, E. Zimlichman, and D.W. Bates. 2013. The impact of medical informatics on patient satisfaction: A USA-based literature review. *International Journal of Medical Informatics* 82(3):141–158.

Shirley, E.D. and J.O. Sanders. 2013. Patient satisfaction: Implications and predictors of success. *Journal of Bone & Joint Surgery* 95(10):e69, 1–4.

Tsai, T.C., E.J. Orav, and A.K. Jha. 2015. Patient satisfaction and quality of surgical care in US hospitals. *Annals of Surgery* 261(1):2–8.

White, S. 2013. *A Practical Approach to Analyzing Healthcare Data*, 2nd ed. Chicago, IL: AHIMA.

Young, G.J, M. Meterko, and K.R. Desai. 2000. Patient satisfaction with hospital care: Effects of demographic and institutional characteristics. *Medical Care* 38(3):325–334.

Chapter 11

Evaluating Excessive Hospital Readmissions: The Geographic Impact

Susan H. Fenton, PhD, RHIA, FAHIMA

Learning Objectives

- Define the Hospital Readmission Reduction Program
- Discuss whether unnecessary hospital readmissions should be considered a sign of poor care quality
- Identify a minimum of three factors that can contribute to hospital readmissions
- Combine three disparate data sets needed to answer a research question
- Assess data types and descriptive statistics to select an appropriate statistical test
- Evaluate the impact of geographic region on hospital readmissions for selected conditions using a one-way ANOVA

Key Terms

Analysis of variance
Hospital Readmissions Reduction Program
Normal distribution
Pairwise comparisons

Qualifying for payment incentives or preventing payment penalties from being enacted are important and becoming more important with each passing year. This is true for most healthcare providers, including hospitals and physicians. However, as with all elements used for healthcare reimbursement, once measures such as hospital readmissions begin to be used, there can be unexpected consequences and surprising findings. This chapter will focus on the economic impact of hospital readmissions using a variety of statistical tests. It is important to remember that this type or similar analyses can be conducted for all quality and performance measures.

The Patient Protection and Affordable Care Act, signed into law on March 23, 2010, included a section titled **Hospital Readmissions Reduction Program** (US Congress 2010). This program requires payment penalties for hospitals with excess readmissions for specified conditions beginning with discharges on or after October 1, 2012 (US Congress 2010). Because the list of conditions changes yearly, this chapter will not review those conditions, but will only state that readmission rates can be calculated for most conditions. The most current data and information can be found on the Readmissions Reduction page of the CMS website (2014).

The issue of hospital readmissions as a concern and potential indicator of quality of care has been examined for decades. An analysis of Medicare hospital readmissions was first published in 1985 (Anderson and Steinberg 1985). They used a 60-day time frame for readmissions, as opposed to the Centers for Medicare and Medicaid Services (CMS) standard 30-day time frame. Of the 20 variables examined, 10 were found to be statistically significant as a predictor of hospital readmission within 60 days. The five predictive demographic variables were patient age, gender, race, coverage of the stay by Medicare, and whether the patient qualified for supplemental Medicaid coverage. Clinical predictors included the number of discharges in the 60 days before the admission, classification of the principal diagnosis as chronic or nonchronic, and whether or not surgery was performed. The predictive hospital variables included whether the hospital was urban or rural and bed size. Interestingly, as early as 1985 researchers were urging hospitals to try and reduce readmissions in an effort to reduce Medicare costs (Anderson and Steinberg 1985).

In 2000, other researchers explored the question of whether hospital readmission rates were even a useful measure of quality of care. Their findings that many of the causes of readmission are unmodifiable by hospitals (Benbassat and Taragin 2000) continued to be echoed by a new team of researchers in 2012 (Joynt and Jha 2012). The 2012 research team listed three reasons why the readmission reduction program may not result in necessarily improved quality of care:

1. Many of the factors that contribute to readmissions are outside of a hospital's control.
2. The payment reduction policies may not be the best for achieving the goals of discharge planning and care coordination.
3. The focus on readmission reduction may cause facilities with limited resources to forego other quality initiatives (Joynt and Jha 2012).

This is at odds with a study that maintained hospital readmissions were "the avoidable byproduct of fragmented and ill-incentivized healthcare delivery" that could be effectively addressed with payment incentives and penalties (Kocher and Adashi 2011). It is reasonable to conclude that consensus regarding the hospital readmission reduction program does not exist.

One of the challenges encountered in regard to hospital readmissions is geographic differences. In 2002, the results of a research study examining hospital readmission rates from three European countries (Finland, Scotland, and the Netherlands) and three states in the United States (New York, California, and Washington) found geographical differences (Westert et al. 2002). The analysis for this study focused on the conditions of chronic obstructive pulmonary disease (COPD), congestive heart failure (CHF), asthma, diabetes, stroke, and the total hip replacement procedure. The overall takeaway from this study is that hospital readmission rates do vary geographically and the explanatory causes of hospital readmission also vary (Westert et al. 2002). The European countries with the longest initial hospital stays had the lowest readmission rates; however, this was not found in the United States. In the United States, the patients with the longer initial stays had the highest rates of readmission (Westert et al. 2002). This study provides additional evidence that excessive hospital readmissions is a multifactorial problem that likely includes environmental factors such as the structure of the country and state healthcare system, after-care systems, and the availability of long-term care, among other factors.

Examining all of the data, including geographic location, surrounding hospital readmissions is necessary to determine which factors contribute to their causation, as well as their prevention. The remainder of this chapter will provide the guidance for health information management (HIM) professionals and others to study hospital readmission factors from a wide variety of perspectives, including geographical variation.

Research Question and Hypothesis

Is there a difference in the average number of prospective payment system (PPS) hospital readmissions related to the measures of heart failure, acute myocardial infarction, or pneumonia based upon geographic location?

The dependent variable (the measured variable) for this research question is the average rate of hospital readmissions for three different clinical measures: heart failure (HF), acute myocardial infarction (AMI), or pneumonia (PN). The independent variable (the comparison variable) will be geographic location as measured by the US region where the hospital is located. To answer this research question, the analysis will compare the average rate of readmissions for each measure across each geographic region. There are four geographic regions that will be compared: Midwest, Northeast, South, and West.

Hypotheses

The research question will require more than one hypothesis. The hypotheses will include the following:

$H1_0$: There is no statistically significant difference in the average number of readmissions related to acute myocardial infarction in PPS hospitals located in the Midwest, Northeast, South, and West regions.

$H1_A$: There is a statistically significant difference in the average number of readmissions related to acute myocardial infarction in PPS hospitals in at least one of the following regions: Midwest, Northeast, South, and West.

$H2_0$: There is no statistically significant difference in the average number of readmissions related to heart failure in PPS hospitals located in the Midwest, Northeast, South, and West Regions.

$H2_A$: There is a statistically significant difference in the average number of readmissions related to heart failure in PPS hospitals in at least one of the following regions: Midwest, Northeast, South, and West.

$H3_0$: There is no statistically significant difference in the average number of readmissions related to pneumonia in PPS hospitals located in the Midwest, Northeast, South, and West Regions.

$H3_A$: There is a statistically significant difference in the average number of readmissions related to pneumonia in PPS hospitals in at least one of the following regions: Midwest, Northeast, South, and West.

Checklist

To answer the research question, a specific process of data acquisition, preparation, and discovery is required. The following steps will be explained in detail:

1. Extract data sets from MySQL
   a. Select required columns of data from database
   b. Join columns of data using MySQL queries
2. Data preparation with Microsoft Excel
   a. Assess the data to ensure there are no inaccuracies, null values, or other data quality issues that could impact the validity of the results
3. Import the data into RStudio
4. Conduct descriptive statistics on the data set
   a. Develop histograms for the average readmissions rate for each of the clinical measures of heart failure, acute myocardial infarction, or pneumonia
5. Conduct a one-way ANOVA comparing the readmission rates for heart failure, acute myocardial infarction, or pneumonia in hospitals across disparate geographic regions
   a. If significance is found in one-way ANOVA, conduct a Tukey post-hoc test to identify where significant differences are present

The Analysis

Given our research question and the identified data elements needed to address the identified problem for this study, we can now begin the process of analyzing the data.

Step 1: Data Extraction

In order to carry out the analysis, the following data elements are needed. All data required for answering the research question are included in the database associated with this textbook:

- A list of all PPS hospitals in the United States
- An indicator as to whether the PPS hospital is located in the Midwest, Northeast, South, or West region
- A measure for each PPS hospital's readmission rate related to acute myocardial infarction
- A measure for each PPS hospital's readmission rate related to heart failure
- A measure for each PPS hospital's readmission rate related to pneumonia

Three data sets need to be combined to obtain the needed data to answer the proposed research question. The first data set is named hospital_general_information and was made available by CMS (2015). The data set lists all of the hospitals located in the United States, including a variety of characteristics about the organization such as address, NPI number, hospital type, ownership type, and hospital name.

The second data set is titled readmission_reduction and was also made available by CMS as a component of the Hospital Readmissions Reduction Program (CMS 2014). The data set includes the hospital name and NPI number, but also includes three variables of particular interest for this study: measure_name, number_of_discharges, and number_of_readmissions. For the purposes of the analyses, the measures for each measure are labeled as the following: acute myocardial infarction (READM-30-AMI-HRRP), heart failure (READM-30-HF-HRRP), and pneumonia (READM-30-PN-HRRP).

The third data set we will be using from the database is titled regions and is a data set made available from the US Census Bureau (Census 2011). This data set includes a variety of geographic variables. For our purposes it includes two key variables: state name and region name.

The three data sets will be combined using MySQL scripts (as illustrated in figure 11.1). The scripts will be constructed so that only the following data elements are extracted: hospital_name, state, measure_name, number_of_discharges, number_of_readmissions, excess_readmission_ratio, and region_name (see figure 11.1).

Note that you must alter a setting in MySQL so that the output shows all of the results rather than just showing the first 1,000 rows (see chapter 4).

Figure 11.1 includes the SQL script that combines the three required data sets and extracts only the relevant data elements. The hospital_general_information data set was mapped to the readmission_reduction data set using the hospitals unique provider number (NPA). These two data sets were joined with the regions data set by mapping the regions variable state variable to the state variable in the hospital_general_information. The top section of the figure depicts the MySQL script that was used to obtain the data. The bottom section of the figure depicts the first few rows of the output that was derived from the query. The final step of this process is to export the data as a CSV file. Name the file Readmissions and save the file. For detailed instruction on saving CSV files from MySQL Workbench see chapter 4.

Step 2: Data Preparation

Data preparation is a critical step in every analytics project. To begin the process, open the CSV file in Excel created in step one (the file is named Readmissions). The data set should include six columns of data with column headers named as the following:

Figure 11.1. SQL script and returned data for combining three data sets

```
SELECT
      hospital_general_information.hospital_name,
      hospital_general_information.state,
      readmisson_reduction.measure_name,
      number_of_discharges,
      number_of_readmissions,
      excess_readmission_ratio,
      regions.region_name

FROM hospital_general_information

JOIN readmission_reduction

ON
hospital_general_information.provider_id=readmission_reduction.provider_id

JOIN regions

ON hospital_general_information.state_code=regions.state_code

WHERE readmission_reduction.number_of_discharges>0 AND
readmission_reduction.number_of_readmissions>0;
```

(Continued)

Figure 11.1. SQL script and returned data for combining three data sets *(Continued)*

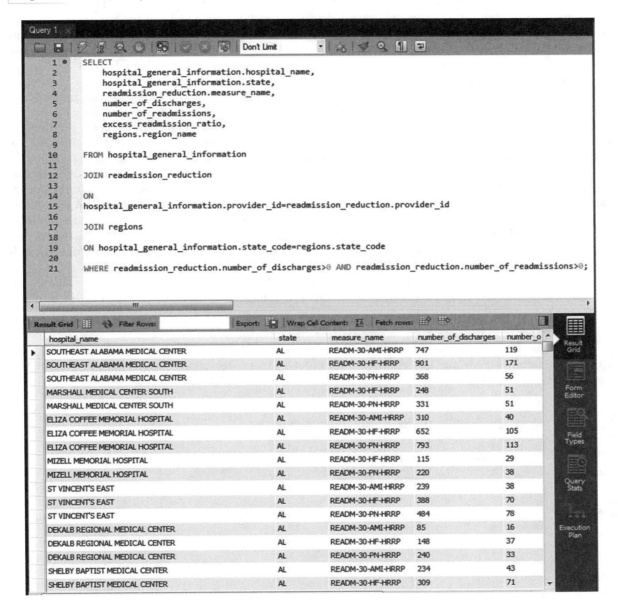

- hospital_name: This column includes the hospital name for PPS hospitals in the United States; each hospital may be listed multiple separate times, depending upon the specific quality measures the organization opts to submit.
- state: This column includes the state abbreviation for the location of every hospital in the United States.
- measure_name: This column includes the following three 30-day readmission measures: acute myocardial infarction (READM-30-AMI-HRRP), heart failure (READM-30-HF-HRRP), and pneumonia (READM-30-PN-HRRP).
- number_of_discharges: This column provides the total number of discharges for each hospital associated with each readmission measure.
- number_of_readmissions: This column provides the total number of readmissions for each hospital associated with each readmission measure.
- excess_readmission_ratio: This column provides the CMS-generated ratio of excess readmissions based upon a comparison to the national average and based upon the number of patients with the condition. The ratio is calculated using the National Quality Forum's risk adjustment methodology (CMS 2014).
- region_name: The final column provides the region where each hospital is located and consists of four different values (Midwest, Northeast, South, and West).

Removal of Erroneous Values

One of the common issues with data analysis projects is missing or incorrect data within the data set. Carefully examine the data to ensure that there are not missing or erroneous value. Because the data set consists of 7,458 rows of observations, we will use Excel's sorting and filtering feature to search for null or erroneous values. To do this, first select the Sort and Filter option listed under the Home tab (Windows) or main menu bar (Mac) (see figure 11.2 for the Windows option).

Next, select the Filter option from the drop-down menu (see figure 11.3).

By adding a filter, a drop-down arrow has been added to each of the column header cells (see figure 11.4).

When the arrow next to each column header is selected you have the ability to sort and filter the data in many different ways. First, you will notice that each individual value that is included in the column is listed in this window. This tool is very useful for determining if there are unexpected values in columns with very few options. For example, if you click in drop-down arrow in the measure_name cell, only the three readmission measures we are interested in for this study are displayed. This tells us that there are no missing or erroneous values in the column. You can also test this for the state and region_name columns, and you will find there are no missing or erroneous states or regions included in these columns. This feature of Excel also provides some useful filtering features, including limiting by specific words (for example, contains "west"). You will notice when you open the filter for the number_of_readmissions column, the lowest value for any hospital is 11 and the highest is 907. There are no hospitals with zeros. You can replicate this for each of the other numeric columns to ensure the data are clean.

The last step is to use Excel's ISBLANK function to search for blank values in any of the columns. To conduct this, click into cell H2 in the Readmissions data set. Enter the following Excel function:

```
=IF(OR(ISBLANK(A2),ISBLANK(B2),ISBLANK(C2),ISBLANK(D2),ISBLANK(E2),
ISBLANK(F2), ISBLANK(G2)), "Blank", "Complete")
```

This function combines the IF and ISBLANK functions to tell Excel to search for blanks in any of the columns related to each observation and if there are any cells blank to return "Blank" in H2.

Figure 11.2. Using Microsoft Excel's sorting and filtering feature

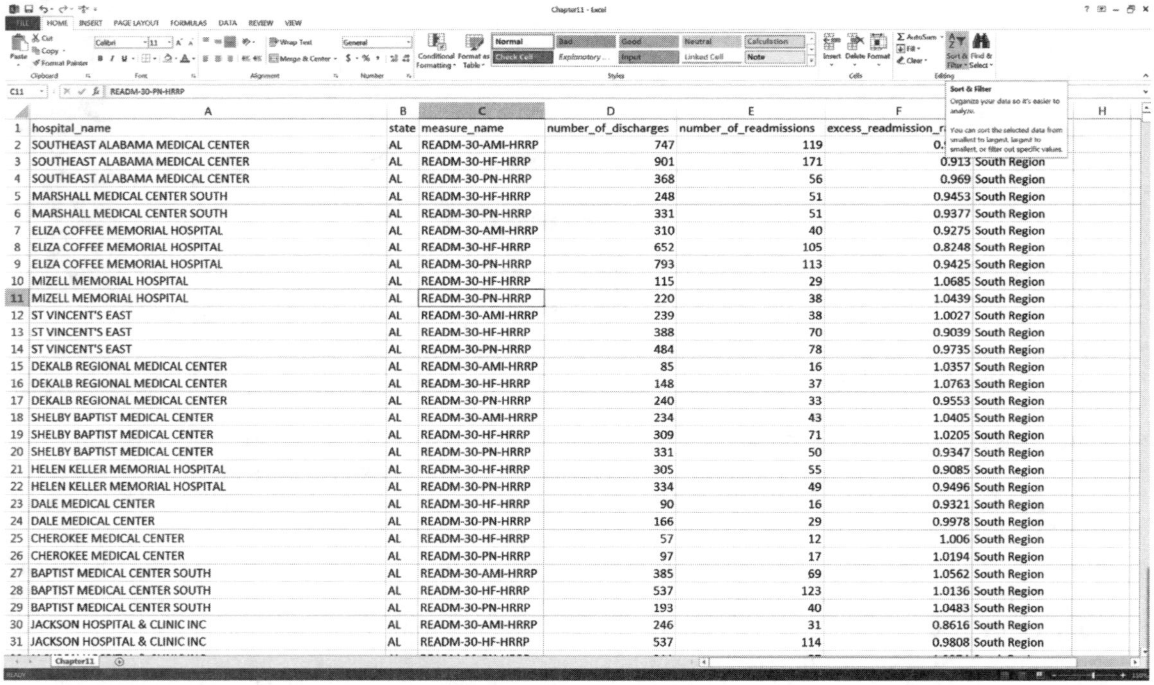

	A	B	C	D	E	F	G
1	hospital_name	state	measure_name	number_of_discharges	number_of_readmissions	excess_readmission_r	
2	SOUTHEAST ALABAMA MEDICAL CENTER	AL	READM-30-AMI-HRRP	747	119	0.	
3	SOUTHEAST ALABAMA MEDICAL CENTER	AL	READM-30-HF-HRRP	901	171	0.913	South Region
4	SOUTHEAST ALABAMA MEDICAL CENTER	AL	READM-30-PN-HRRP	368	56	0.969	South Region
5	MARSHALL MEDICAL CENTER SOUTH	AL	READM-30-HF-HRRP	248	51	0.9453	South Region
6	MARSHALL MEDICAL CENTER SOUTH	AL	READM-30-PN-HRRP	331	51	0.9377	South Region
7	ELIZA COFFEE MEMORIAL HOSPITAL	AL	READM-30-AMI-HRRP	310	40	0.9275	South Region
8	ELIZA COFFEE MEMORIAL HOSPITAL	AL	READM-30-HF-HRRP	652	105	0.8248	South Region
9	ELIZA COFFEE MEMORIAL HOSPITAL	AL	READM-30-PN-HRRP	793	113	0.9425	South Region
10	MIZELL MEMORIAL HOSPITAL	AL	READM-30-HF-HRRP	115	29	1.0685	South Region
11	MIZELL MEMORIAL HOSPITAL	AL	READM-30-PN-HRRP	220	38	1.0439	South Region
12	ST VINCENT'S EAST	AL	READM-30-AMI-HRRP	239	38	1.0027	South Region
13	ST VINCENT'S EAST	AL	READM-30-HF-HRRP	388	70	0.9039	South Region
14	ST VINCENT'S EAST	AL	READM-30-PN-HRRP	484	78	0.9735	South Region
15	DEKALB REGIONAL MEDICAL CENTER	AL	READM-30-AMI-HRRP	85	16	1.0357	South Region
16	DEKALB REGIONAL MEDICAL CENTER	AL	READM-30-HF-HRRP	148	37	1.0763	South Region
17	DEKALB REGIONAL MEDICAL CENTER	AL	READM-30-PN-HRRP	240	33	0.9553	South Region
18	SHELBY BAPTIST MEDICAL CENTER	AL	READM-30-AMI-HRRP	234	43	1.0405	South Region
19	SHELBY BAPTIST MEDICAL CENTER	AL	READM-30-HF-HRRP	309	71	1.0205	South Region
20	SHELBY BAPTIST MEDICAL CENTER	AL	READM-30-PN-HRRP	331	50	0.9347	South Region
21	HELEN KELLER MEMORIAL HOSPITAL	AL	READM-30-HF-HRRP	305	55	0.9085	South Region
22	HELEN KELLER MEMORIAL HOSPITAL	AL	READM-30-PN-HRRP	334	49	0.9496	South Region
23	DALE MEDICAL CENTER	AL	READM-30-HF-HRRP	90	16	0.9321	South Region
24	DALE MEDICAL CENTER	AL	READM-30-PN-HRRP	166	29	0.9978	South Region
25	CHEROKEE MEDICAL CENTER	AL	READM-30-HF-HRRP	57	12	1.006	South Region
26	CHEROKEE MEDICAL CENTER	AL	READM-30-PN-HRRP	97	17	1.0194	South Region
27	BAPTIST MEDICAL CENTER SOUTH	AL	READM-30-AMI-HRRP	385	69	1.0562	South Region
28	BAPTIST MEDICAL CENTER SOUTH	AL	READM-30-HF-HRRP	537	123	1.0136	South Region
29	BAPTIST MEDICAL CENTER SOUTH	AL	READM-30-PN-HRRP	193	40	1.0483	South Region
30	JACKSON HOSPITAL & CLINIC INC	AL	READM-30-AMI-HRRP	246	31	0.8616	South Region
31	JACKSON HOSPITAL & CLINIC INC	AL	READM-30-HF-HRRP	537	114	0.9808	South Region

Source: Used with permission from Microsoft.

Figure 11.3. Microsoft Excel's sorting and filtering option

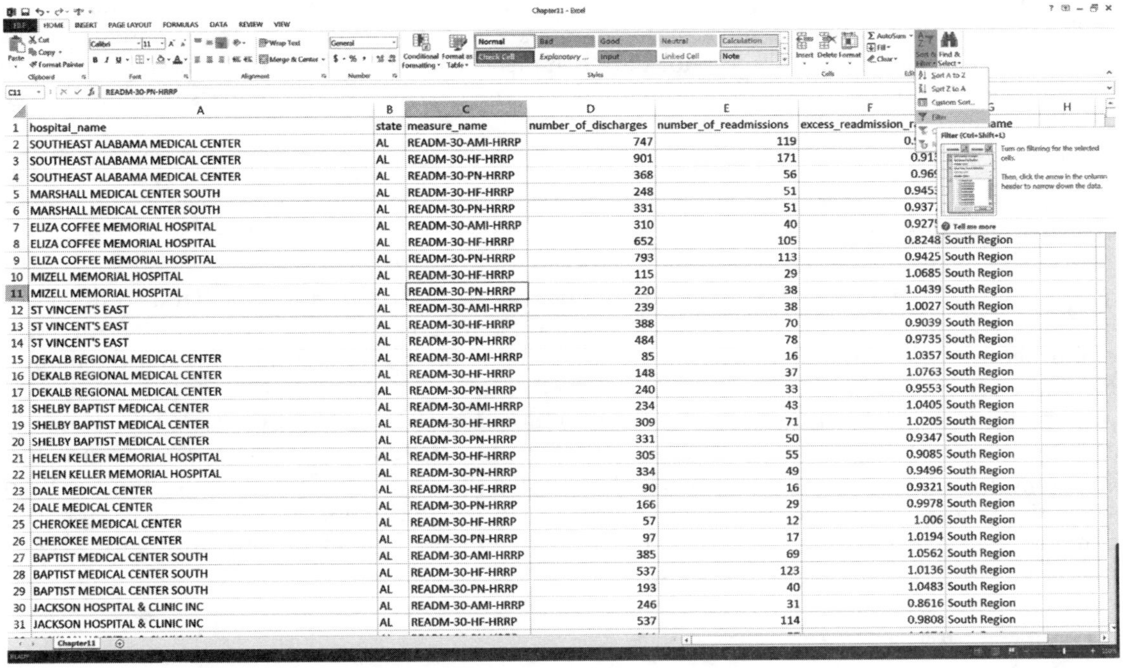

Source: Used with permission from Microsoft.

Figure 11.4. Microsoft Excel's sorting and filtering drop-down arrow

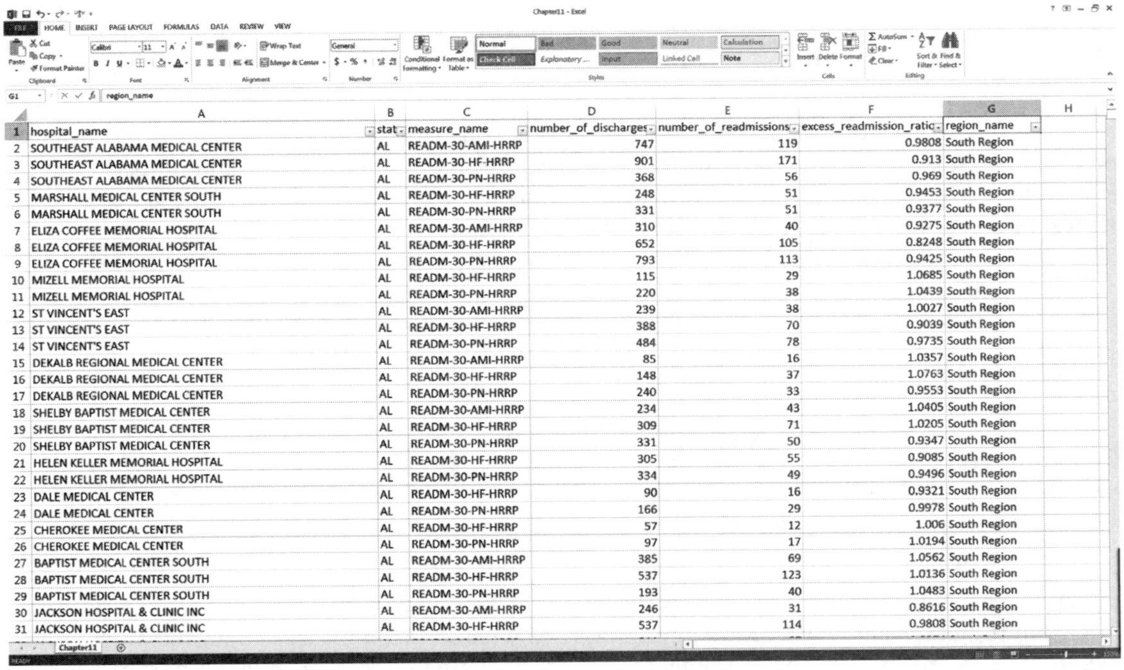

Source: Used with permission from Microsoft.

If all cells are populated with data, the function is telling Excel to return "Complete" in H2. After adding the formula to cell H2, double-click the small square icon on the bottom-right of cell H2. This will fill in the rest of the cells with the above formula. Once this is done you can replicate the filtering steps above to determine the number of Blanks and Complete observations in this data set. After completing this process, we now understand that all observations are complete. There are no zeros or missing values, and we can feel confident that our data set is ready for analysis. The next step in the analysis is to import the data into RStudio for analysis.

Step 3: Import the Data

Be sure to save the file as a CSV file and then import the file into RStudio (for a detailed description of how to import data into RStudio, see chapter 5). After importing the data successfully into RStudio, output will be returned in the console to display the path where the file was imported from and the name of the file. This output confirms that the data were successfully imported into RStudio and that you can view all of the observations in the RStudio environment. RStudio adopts the name of the CSV file as the name of the data frame in the RStudio environment (that is, it is named Readmissions). After the data are imported into RStudio, open an R scripting window. The R scripting window is where you will enter the R code in order to analyze the data. To open a new R scripting window, go to File > New File > R Script. The next step in the importing process is to attach the data to make the variables easier to work with. Use the following script:

```
attach(Readmissions)
```

As a reminder, the attach function allows you to simply use the column names for all analyses in RStudio. To confirm that the data have been imported and attached properly, use the following script to return only the first six rows of data across all columns in the data set:

```
head(Readmissions)
```

The output in the RStudio accurately reflects our data set; thus we can move on to the next step in the analysis.

Step 4: Descriptive Statistics

Our first analysis involves conducting descriptive statistics on the data (for a more in-depth discussion of descriptive statistics, see chapter 7). The first thing we want to understand is the total number of hospitals in each geographic region that are included for each readmission measure condition. This is done because we cannot presume that all hospitals report all measures and the differences may affect our results. To execute this in RStudio, we will use the tapply function and the following script:

```
tapply(hospital_name, list(region_name, measure_name), length)
```

The output from this function is the following:

	READM-30-AMI-HRRP	READM-30-HF-HRRP	READM-30-PN-HRRP
Midwest Region	434	677	662
Northeast Region	353	482	481
South Region	680	1225	1206
West Region	292	488	478

The output is rather informative for our study. First, we see that across all geographic regions far fewer hospitals are submitting the acute myocardial infarction (AMI) readmission measure than the heart failure (HF) and pneumonia (PN) measures. For example, the South region had 1,225 hospitals report HF readmission measures, but only 680 reported the AMI readmission measures. Second, this analysis informs us that there are far more hospitals reporting readmission measures in the South region than the other three regions—the South has 1,225 hospitals reporting on HF readmissions but the second highest number of hospitals reporting is 677 in the Midwest region.

Before moving on with additional descriptive statistics, we will create a variable for readmission rate. Given the differences in the raw number of hospitals reporting the measures across the geographical regions, a rate must be used to compare the results across geographical regions. The rate is created in RStudio by using the following script:

```
ReadmRate<-number_of_readmissions/number_of_discharges
```

With this script we have told RStudio to create a new variable called ReadmRate by dividing the number of readmissions by the number of discharges for each hospital in the entire data set. This allows us to simply use the variable name ReadmRate for all future analyses.

Now that we know the number of hospitals reporting measures regarding readmissions in each region, the next step is to compare the average readmission rates across each region for each condition using the following script:

```
tapply(ReadmRate, list(region_name, measure_name), mean)
```

The output from this function is the following:

	READM-30-AMI-HRRP	READM-30-HF-HRRP	READM-30-PN-HRRP
Midwest Region	0.1817637	0.2202626	0.1756788
Northeast Region	0.2186870	0.2404059	0.1845952
South Region	0.1941361	0.2345106	0.1777274
West Region	0.1722749	0.2152746	0.1636302

The output provides us the average readmission rate in each region and for each measure. While the output shows us that the readmission rate for AMI is nearly 22 percent in the Northeast region and 17 percent in the West region, we will need to conduct statistical analyses to determine if these differences are significant.

Prior to conducting analysis, it is very important to understand the distribution of your data. Creating histograms is a useful way to visualize your data and illustrate the distribution. Because we are running multiple analyses, each distribution will be created separately. We will create a histogram that plots the average readmission rates for each of the three conditions (AMI, HF, and PN) using the following scripts:

```
hist(ReadmRate[measure_name=="READM-30-AMI-HRRP"], main="Histogram of AMI
Readmissions", xlab="Readmission Rate")

hist(ReadmRate[measure_name=="READM-30-HF-HRRP"], main="Histogram of HF
Readmissions", xlab="Readmission Rate")

hist(ReadmRate[measure_name=="READM-30-PN-HRRP"], main="Histogram of PN
Readmissions", xlab="Readmission Rate")
```

These scripts are using the R hist function to plot the readmission rate when the measure is only limited to a particular value (for example, we have limited to AMI by using the following code: measure_name=="READM-30-AMI-HRRP"). We have also customized the chart labels by using the main (main heading) and xlab (x-axis label) functions. The output for these three scripts are illustrated in figures 11.5 through 11.7 that follow.

Based upon these histograms, we can conclude that the readmission rates for HF and PN are **normally distributed**, while readmission rates for AMI are skewed slightly to the right. It is very important to identify whether the data are normally distributed, as that determines which type of statistical tests can be conducted. The data are normally distributed when they are evenly spread out on either side of the mean, creating a bell curve. When comparing means between groups when the data are normally distributed, you can use **analysis of variance** (also known as ANOVA). If the data were not normally distributed, you would use the Kruskal Wallis Test, a nonparametric statistical test.

Figure 11.5.   Histogram of average readmissions for acute myocardial infarction

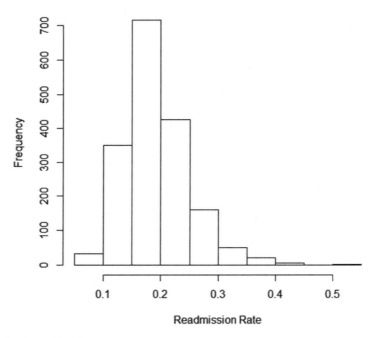

Source: Used with permission from RStudio.

Figure 11.6.   Histogram of average readmissions for heart failure

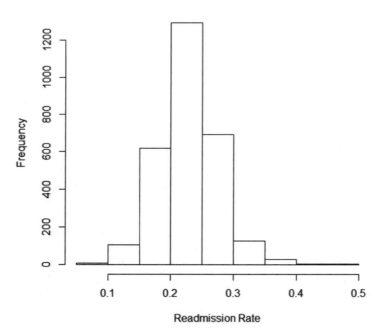

Source: Used with permission from RStudio.

Figure 11.7. Histogram of average readmissions for pneumonia

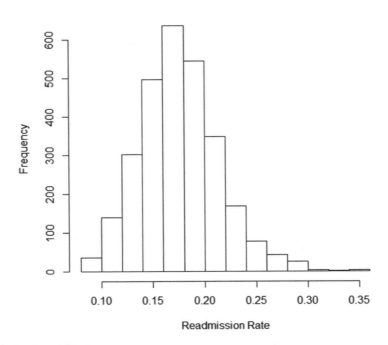

Source: Used with permission from RStudio.

Step 5: Statistical Analyses

As mentioned previously, we need to conduct a statistical procedure to determine the following:

1. Is the average hospital readmission rate for AMI different among US geographic regions?
2. Is the average hospital readmission rate for HF different among US geographic regions?
3. Is the average hospital readmission rate for PN different among US geographic regions?

To answer these questions, a statistical procedure needs to be adopted that can handle continuous data. The one-way ANOVA can be used to test if more than two groups are different from each other. For the purpose of this project, the one-way ANOVA can be used to test whether the average readmission rate for each condition (AMI, HF, and PN) for one geographic region is significantly different from at least one other geographic region. For example, the Midwest region's average readmission for the AMI condition may or may not be significantly different from at least one of the following: Northeast, South, and West). For a more in-depth discussion regarding the assumptions for the one-way ANOVA, see chapter 8.

We will now use RStudio to conduct a one-way ANOVA to test for significant differences in hospital readmission rates for specific conditions (AMI, HF, and PN) by geographic region. There are multiple steps associated with conducting a one-way ANOVA using RStudio. The first step is to name the ANOVA. For example, in the script that follows we name the first ANOVA "anova1." When you use RStudio to name this type of analysis, it is required to enter the name followed by the less than sign (<), followed by a hyphen (-). This is a naming convention particular to RStudio. The second step is to write the function for returning the ANOVA given specific data parameters. The R function for ANOVA is aov, and the data elements we are analyzing in this analysis include ReadmRate and region_name. However, because we only want to calculate the readmission rate for one specific condition for each one-way ANOVA that we conduct, we need to tell RStudio to only include a specific result. To specify a result for a given variable, add a bracket after the variable name, followed by two equal signs and the exact name in double quotation marks, and you need to close the bracket. Thus, the first of the three ANOVA analyses would be developed by writing the following script:

```
anova1<-aov(ReadmRate[measure_name=="READM-30-AMI-HRRP"]~
region_name[measure_name=="READM-30-AMI-HRRP"])
```

The script is telling RStudio to perform a one-way ANOVA to compare readmission rates (only when readmission rates are equal to AMI) by region (but only include the region data when the measure is equal to AMI).

The third step is to use RStudio to summarize the results of the ANOVA you have just conducted. The summary would be returned by simply entering the following RStudio script:

```
summary(anova1)
```

The output from this function is as follows:

```
                                             Df   SumSq   Mean   SqFvalue Pr(>F)
region_name[measure_name=="READM-30-AMI-     3    0.413  0.13778   48.85  <2e-16 ***
HRRP"]
Residuals                                    1755  4.950  0.00282
---
Signif. codes: 0 '***' 0.001 '**' 0.01 '*' 0.05 '.' 0.1 ' ' 1
```

The ANOVA output includes the degrees of freedom (DF) for the independent variable we are analyzing, the sum of squares (Sum Sq), the mean of squares (Mean Sq), the test statistic (F value), and the p-value (Pr(>F)). For our purposes, we will primarily focus on the p-value for determining statistical significance. Using the output shown as an example, we see a significant finding related to geographic region because the p-value is less than 0.05. However, this output does not tell us precisely where the significant differences are, only that there are significant differences.

The fourth step is to use RStudio to conduct a post-hoc test to determine significant differences between means for each specific group (for example, RStudio will compare the Midwest region to the other three regions). The post-hoc test will be returned by simply entering the following RStudio script:

```
TukeyHSD(anova1, ordered=T)
```

The output from this function is the following:

```
Tukey multiple comparisons of means
95% family-wise confidence level
factor levels have been ordered

Fit: aov(formula = ReadmRate[measure_name == "READM-30-AMI-HRRP"] ~ region_
name[measure_name == "READM-30-AMI-HRRP"])

$'region_name[measure_name == "READM-30-AMI-HRRP"]'
```

	diff	lwr	upr	p adj
Midwest Region-West Region	0.009488795	-0.0008475269	0.01982512	0.0852001
South Region-West Region	0.021861181	0.0123063890	0.03141597	0.0000000
Northeast Region-West Region	0.046412066	0.0356092978	0.05721483	0.0000000
South Region-Midwest Region	0.012372386	0.0039820907	0.02076268	0.0008886
Northeast Region-Midwest Region	0.036923272	0.0271353802	0.04671116	0.0000000
Northeast Region-South Region	0.024550885	0.0155922398	0.03350953	0.0000000

The Tukey HSD post-hoc test returns a substantial amount of information. First, it provides a summary of the post hoc test and summarizes the original ANOVA. It then conducts **pairwise comparisons** of differences in means for each of the independent variables (that is, each region). Pairwise comparisons provide statistical differences for each group against each other group. For example, the software compares the results from the Midwest region versus West region, Midwest region versus South region, Midwest versus Northeast region, and so on through all of the possible permutations. It also provides the difference in observed means for each comparison (diff), the lower end point of the interval (lwr), the upper end of the interval (upr), and the adjusted p-value after each comparison (p adj).

The results indicate that there are significant differences between geographic regions regarding average hospital readmissions for AMI. The differences are significant between every region except the Midwest and the West. If you recall from the descriptive statistics section, the average AMI readmission rate for the Northeast region was 22 percent. These findings indicate that average hospital AMI readmission rates in the Northeast are significantly higher than hospitals in the Midwest, South, and West.

Let us now conduct a one-way ANOVA to test for significant differences in hospital HF readmission rates by geographic region using these same four steps outlined. The following is the RStudio script:

```
anova2<-aov(ReadmRate[measure_name=="READM-30-HF-HRRP"] ~
region_name[measure_name=="READM-30-HF-HRRP"])

summary(anova2)
```

The following is the RStudio output

```
                            Df     SumSq     Mean       SqFvalue  Pr(>F)
region_name[measure_name ==  3     0.243     0.08116    41.6      <2e-16 ***
"READM-30-HF-HRRP"]
Residuals                   2868   5.595     0.00195
---
Signif. codes: 0 '***' 0.001 '**' 0.01 '*' 0.05 '.' 0.1 ' ' 1
```

The post-hoc test will be returned by entering this RStudio script:

```
TukeyHSD(anova2, ordered=T)
```

The output from this function is

```
Tukey multiple comparisons of means
95% family-wise confidence level
factor levels have been ordered

Fit: aov(formula = ReadmRate[measure_name == "READM-30-HF-HRRP"] ~
region_name[measure_name == "READM-30-HF-HRRP"])

$'region_name[measure_name == "READM-30-HF-HRRP"]'

                                 diff          lwr           upr        p adj
Midwest Region-West Region       0.004987935  -0.0017543001 0.01173017 0.2274903
South Region-West Region         0.019235980   0.0131581870 0.02531377 0.0000000
Northeast Region-West Region     0.025131234   0.0178400568 0.03242241 0.0000000
South Region-Midwest Region      0.014248045   0.0088106850 0.01968540 0.0000000
Northeast Region-Midwest Region  0.020143298   0.0133767207 0.02690988 0.0000000
Northeast Region-South Region    0.005895253   0.0002095319 0.01200004 0.0628917
```

The results from this analysis indicate there is a significant statistical difference in hospital HF readmission rates by geographic location. Similar to the first ANOVA results, there is not a statistical difference in readmission rates related to HF between the Midwest and the West regions, nor is there a difference between the Northeast and the South. This means that the Northeast and the South have significantly higher HF readmission rates than do the Midwest and the West regions. We know this because when you compare the average readmission rate for the Northeast and South regions, the value is larger than the Midwest region.

The final one-way ANOVA will test for significant differences in hospital PN readmission rates by geographic region using the same four steps. The following are the scripts and the output:

```
anova3<-aov(ReadmRate[measure_name=="READM-30-PN-HRRP"] ~
region_name[measure_name=="READM-30-PN-HRRP"])

summary(anova3)
```

	Df	SumSq	Mean	SqFvalue	Pr(>F)
region_name[measure_name == "READM-30-PN-HRRP"]	3	0.112	0.03745	26.5	<2e-16 ***
Residuals	2823	3.989	0.00141		

```
---
Signif. codes: 0 '***' 0.001 '**' 0.01 '*' 0.05 '.' 0.1 ' ' 1

TukeyHSD(anova3, ordered=T)

Tukey multiple comparisons of means
95% family-wise confidence level
factor levels have been ordered

Fit: aov(formula = ReadmRate[measure_name == "READM-30-PN-HRRP"] ~ region_
name[measure_name == "READM-30-PN-HRRP"])

$'region_name[measure_name == "READM-30-PN-HRRP"]'
```

	diff	lwr	upr	p adj
Midwest Region-West Region	0.012048592	0.006248907	0.017848277	0.0000006
South Region-West Region	0.014097191	0.008874692	0.019319690	0.0000000
Northeast Region-West Region	0.020965027	0.014724550	0.027205503	0.0000000
South Region-Midwest Region	0.002048599	-0.002625315	0.006722513	0.6730433
Northeast Region-Midwest Region	0.008916435	0.003127262	0.014705607	0.0004475
Northeast Region-South Region	0.006867836	0.001657013	0.012078658	0.0039778

These results indicate that there are significant differences between geographic regions regarding hospitals readmission related to pneumonia. We conclude this because the Tukey post-hoc analysis has a p-value less than 0.05 for all pairwise comparisons except for the comparison between the South and the Midwest. These results also lead to the conclusion that the West has the lowest readmission rate for pneumonia and it is significantly lower than all three other regions.

Overall, we reject all three null hypotheses and conclude that there are significant differences in hospital readmissions for AMI, HF, and PN by geographic region. Across all three measures, the West region has significantly lower rates of hospital readmission and the Northeast region has significantly higher rates of readmission.

Discussion

This analysis reveals that there are significant differences in hospital readmission rates for AMI, HF, and PN by geographical region. However, this is not the entire story. These findings appear to be consistent with earlier findings described in the previous studies. For example, the Northeast region has the highest rates of readmission for all of the conditions. Yet, when the descriptive statistics are examined, we see that the Northeast region has a much lower gross rate of readmissions than does the South region for all conditions—meaning that the Northeast also had the fewest discharges overall, but more of the patients were readmitted. Consequently, this leads to other questions including whether the Northeast patients initially admitted for these conditions have a greater severity of illness, with more comorbidities and a longer initial length of stay, that would cause them to be readmitted at higher rates (Westert et al. 2002); or whether the healthcare environment in the Northeast is structured so that patients with these conditions do not have access to adequate nonhospital care to prevent their readmission (Joynt and Jha 2012).

One of the things this study does not do is identify the cause of the geographical differences in hospital readmission rates for AMI, HF, and PN. Future studies on these hospital readmissions could perhaps begin to identify these by exploring patient demographics such as gender, race, ethnicity and severity of illness, as well as other variables such as hospital ownership and the availability of nonhospital supportive care, or even the time-lag between hospital discharge and follow-up appointment. Other statistical techniques such as factor analysis or logistic regression or even more complex methods such as predictive modeling could be utilized to try to identify, with some reliability, the causes contributing to hospital readmission for AMI, HF, and PN.

As with all research studies, this one does have limitations that need to be mentioned. First, this study only identifies readmissions for patient stays paid for by Medicare; thus, any findings are not generalizable to the entire population in hospitals. Another limitation is the analysis of the geographical data at the level of four distinct regions. While this makes differences easier to detect, in reality it would be very difficult to detect causal differences at this level since there are significant differences between healthcare environments in urban and rural areas within the four geographic regions, as well as patient demographics such as age or race and ethnicity, all of which are likely to have an impact on the final results.

Conclusion

The problem of hospital readmissions is complex and requires thoughtful, careful analysis of all available data. The geographical analyses performed demonstrated differences in hospital readmission rates; however, these are just the beginning as the data available via CMS do not include sufficient detail to reveal the causes for the differences. More detailed data might be utilized from electronic health record (EHR) systems. Other additional external data include data not normally considered, such as the healthcare environment and the support accessible for care transitions. Health information professionals can utilize analyses such as these to understand the impact of reimbursement and payment regulations on their operations. They can benchmark their operations against the operations of other facilities to explore whether their reported quality is higher than or lower than comparable organizations. These results can also motivate organizations to collect more data and extend their analyses to more fully understand how they can continue to improve care. It is only with this type of use of data that the US healthcare industry can improve care while controlling spending.

Review Exercises

Instructions: Choose the best answer.

1. The CMS Hospital Readmission Reduction Program:
   a. Is a simple quality measurement program to provide consumers with readmission information
   b. Is a program that clearly indicates the quality of care delivered by a hospital
   c. Reduces hospital payments when a patient with certain diagnoses is readmitted to any hospital within 30 days of discharge
   d. Obtains results that are totally dependent upon patient characteristics

2. True or False: When an ANOVA statistical test is run, the initial ANOVA results will convey the differences between the groups being compared.

3. The type of statistical test to be run is usually determined by a combination of:
   a. Data type and distribution
   b. Results desired and data type
   c. Data type and statistical package
   d. None of the above

4. True or False: Demonstrating differences in readmission rates for different conditions across the four geographical regions is not the same as determining the cause of the differences.

Instructions: Answer the following question.

5. As described in the background for this chapter, hospital readmissions can have many contributory causes. As a result, the analysis of hospital readmissions often requires data from multiple sources. Provide an example of three different types of data sources or databases that might be used and the types of data that would be found in each data source or database.

References

Anderson, G.F. and E.P. Steinberg. 1985. Predicting hospital readmissions in the Medicare population. *Inquiry* 22(3):251–258.

Benbassat, J. and M. Taragin. 2000. Hospital readmissions as a measure of quality of health care: Advantages and limitations. *Archives of Internal Medicine* 160(8):1074–1081.

Census. 2011. ZCTA to CBSA. US Census Bureau. Accessed January 12. https://www.census.gov/geo/reference/zctas.html.

CMS. 2014. Readmissions Reduction Program. http://www.cms.gov/Medicare/Medicare-Fee-for-Service-Payment/AcuteInpatientPPS/Readmissions-Reduction-Program.html

CMS. 2015. Official Hospital Compare Data. Centers for Medicaid and Medicare Services. Accessed January 12. http://www.medicare.gov/hospitalcompare/search.html

Joynt, K.E. and A.K. Jha. 2012. Thirty-day readmissions—truth and consequences. *New England Journal of Medicine* 366(15):1366–1369.

Kocher, R.P. and E.Y. Adashi. 2011. Hospital readmissions and the Affordable Care Act: Paying for coordinated quality care. *Journal of the American Medical Association* 306(16):1794–1795.

US Congress. 2010. The Patient Protection and Affordable Care Act. http://www.gpo.gov/fdsys/pkg/BILLS-111hr3590enr/pdf/BILLS-111hr3590enr.pdf

Westert, G.P., R.J. Lagoe, I. Keskimäki, A. Leyland, and M. Murphy. 2002. An international study of hospital readmissions and related utilization in Europe and the USA. *Health Policy* 61(3):269–278.

Nursing Home Quality Acquired Conditions: The Impact of Quality Measures, Staffing, Ownership, and Health Inspections on Overall Quality

Shauna M. Overgaard, MHI

Learning Objectives

- Perform a causal analysis using logistic regression to determine which independent variables affect the dependent variable
- Use Akaike Information Criterion (AIC) to measure the quality of a regression model
- Interpret adjusted R-squared value and the odds ratio for evaluating the strength of a logistic regression model
- Apply backward elimination techniques to improve a regression model
- Develop the logistic regression equation using the values of the coefficients provided from performing a logistic regression

Key Terms

Adjusted R-squared
Backward elimination
Logistic regression
Odds ratio
Parsimonious

The demand for nursing home services will likely increase as the US population ages. By the year 2050, the US population age 65 and older is expected to double from 40 million to nearly 89 million. Unfortunately, as the US population increases in age, this aging population will also decline in health. It has been estimated that the percentage of Americans 65 years and older who report having one or more chronic diseases increased from 86.9 percent in 1998 to 92.2 percent in 2008 (Dall et al. 2013).

As the US population continues to age, more and more responsibility may be placed on nursing homes and other long-term care facilities to support these citizens. With the health concerns that come with aging, it will be critical to monitor the quality of services provided in these organizations. Already, concerns surrounding the quality of care delivered in US nursing homes have prompted the development and implementation of targeted interventions (Luo et al. 2014). Research has shown that poor nursing home care is associated with insufficient staffing (Castle 2008; Mueller et al. 2006) and that for-profit nursing homes provide lower quality of care than do nonprofit nursing homes (Anic et al. 2014). Many of these reports are derived from satisfaction surveys, and although there are reported differences between the perspectives of the resident, family, and caregiver, four factors are described to be of high importance across all three perspectives:

1. Care and support
2. Food
3. Autonomy
4. Activities (Godin et al. 2015)

Although these reports are published, other research demonstrates the difficulties for patients and families associated with identifying information regarding the quality of nursing homes in their communities. Medicare.gov hosts Nursing Home Compare, a website for such quality rating comparisons of each nursing home participating in Medicare or Medicaid (2015). The site works to distinguish between high and low performing nursing homes by employing a five-star rating system built from an algorithm containing three measure types:

1. Health inspections, based on characteristics of deficiencies and complaints identified during state health inspection
2. Staffing, which contains two measures—one based on the ratio of registered nurse (RN) hours per patient, and the other based on total staffing (not including clerical or housekeeping staff)
3. Quality measures (QMs) based on a minimum data set (MDS), which include 11 QMs derived from 8 long-stay measures and 3 short-stay measures

More than 200,000 records from the health inspection data alone inform the algorithm, where weights for varying types of deficiencies are added to reflect the severity of infraction. For example, 75 points for an isolated incident, as compared to a widespread problem that is rated 175, weight a deficiency that causes immediate jeopardy to resident health or safety (CMS 2012). For more detailed information on the five-star rating computation, consult the *Design for Nursing Home Compare Five-Start Quality Rating System Technical User's Guide* (CMS 2012). The purpose of analysis within this chapter is to use information from Nursing Home Compare to predict the factors most associated with one-star quality rankings on the Medicare.gov Nursing Home Compare website.

Research Question and Hypothesis

What nursing home factors are most associated with the lowest ranking (one-star) on the Nursing Home Compare website?

The dependent variable for a logistic regression is dichotomous. That is, the dependent variable can only take on two possible outcomes. In the proposed study, the outcome (dependent) variable is the ranking of one star on the Nursing Home Compare website (namely, a hospital either has a one-star ranking or does not have a one-star ranking). The independent variables for a logistic regression are those factors that you expect to influence the dependent variable. In the case of the proposed research question, there are five independent variables within our data set that support the literature as described previously; we will examine QM rating, staffing rating, nurse staffing rating, health inspection rating, and ownership type. Four of the independent variables are quantitative and have numeric values between one and five. Ownership type is an independent variable that can be broken down into three distinct groups: government, for profit, and nonprofit. The analysis for answering the proposed research question will evaluate factors that are associated with the lowest nursing home ranking. We will employ diagnostic tests to determine which factors appear to be most predictive of a one-star rating, and from these tests we will use the coefficients, standard errors, odds ratios, confidence intervals, and p-values as our guide to compare the logistic regression models in order to select the best fit for our data.

Hypotheses

Given the research question, one central hypothesis should be proposed and tested. The hypotheses should be stated as a null (H_0) and alternative (H_A). Given the fact that the research question relates to an overall nursing home ranking of one across multiple independent variables, there typically would be more than one hypothesis. However, for this research question, we will be using **logistic regression**, which compares multiple independent variables simultaneously against one dependent variable. Since there are five independent variables, the null and alternative hypotheses can be written as follows:

H_0: *1...5 = 0*

H_A: *1...5 ≠ 0*

The null hypothesis states that we will observe the same measured outcome of our dependent variable for each level of our independent variable. The alternative hypothesis states that we will observe different measured outcomes of our dependent variable for each level of our independent variable. When there is not enough evidence to reject the null hypothesis, the conclusion is made that knowing the independent variables has no increased effects (that is, they make no difference) in predicting the dependent variable.

Checklist

To answer the research question, a specific process of data acquisition, preparation, and discovery is required. The following steps will be explained in detail:

1. Extract data sets from MySQL
   a. Select the appropriate columns
2. Data preparation with Microsoft Excel
   a. Rename column headers to maker analysis easier
   b. Recode a variable
3. Import the data into RStudio
   a. Manipulate R data frames using dplyr package
4. Conduct statistical procedures
   a. Explore data visually
   b. Develop research hypotheses based upon results

The Analysis

In this chapter, we examine the data contained in Nursing Home Compare, a component of the Medicare.gov website (CMS 2014). This data set provides nursing home–specific data for all US nursing homes that are Medicare and Medicaid certified (over 15,000 nursing homes nationwide). As previously described, the data set includes measures related to workforce staffing, clinical quality outcomes, ownership, and overall facility quality. Now that the research question and hypotheses are stated, the data elements are identified, and the appropriate statistical procedures have been determined, the data analysis process can begin.

Step 1: Data Extraction

In order to carry out the analysis, the following data elements are needed. Note: all data required for answering the research question are included in the database associated with this textbook.

- A list of all active nursing homes in the United States
- An overall rating for each nursing home
- A health inspection rating for each nursing home
- A staffing rating for each nursing home
- An RN staffing rating for each nursing home
- A QM rating for each nursing home
- An indicator for if the nursing home is a special focus facility
- The number of occupied beds for each nursing home
- The ownership type for each nursing home

The data will be selected from one table in MySQL Workbench. The nursing_home_provider_info table will be queried for the provider number, overall five-star rating, health inspection rating, staffing rating, RN staffing rating, QM rating, and ownership type. The table will be queried and combined using the MySQL scripts as shown in figure 12.1, along with the first few rows of the output that were derived from the query. Note that you must alter a setting in MySQL so that the output shows all of the results rather than just showing the first

1,000 rows (see chapter 4). After executing each query, export the data to a CSV file and save the file as fivestar. For detailed instructions regarding exporting data from MySQL Workbench to CSV format, see chapter 4.

Step 2: Data Preparation

In this chapter, we will do much of our work from within RStudio, but a few preliminary steps will be easier in Excel. Start by loading the files into Excel and examining them. The general structure for each is the same; a listing where each row is an individual nursing home. You should see the following columns:

- provnum: A unique identifier for each nursing home in the data set.
- overall_rating: The rating system features an overall five-star rating based on facility performance for three types of performance measures, each of which has its own five-star rating. The three areas included in the rating are health inspection, staffing, and QM ratings. The rating ranges from 0 to 5.
- survey_rating: Health inspection rating based on points that are assigned to individual health deficiencies according to their scope and severity. The top 10 percent (lowest 10 percent in terms of health inspection deficiency score) in each state receives a rating of 5; the middle 70 percent of facilities receives a rating of 2, 3, or 4; the bottom 20 percent receives a rating of 1.
- staffing_rating: The rating for staffing is based on case-mix adjusted measures for the total nursing hours per resident day (RN + LPN + nurse aide hours). For the staffing rating, a 1 to 5 rating is assigned based on a percentile-based method (where percentiles are based on the distribution for freestanding facilities).
- RN_staffing_rating: The rating for staffing is based on case-mix adjusted measures for the total RN nursing hours per resident day. For the RN staffing rating, a 1 to 5 rating is assigned based on a percentile-based method (where percentiles are based on the distribution for freestanding facilities).
- quality_rating: Facility ratings for QM are based on performance of nine QMs.
- ssf: An indicator if the nursing home is a special focus facility. Can take on the values of Y or N (Y = yes; N = no).
- restot: The total number of beds that are occupied by residents.
- ownership: The ownership type for the organization. There are 13 unique ownership types including: For-profit—Corporation; Nonprofit—Corporation; For-profit—Individual; For-profit—Partnership; Nonprofit—Other; Government—County; Nonprofit—Church-related; Government—City; Government—City/county; Government—State; For-profit—Limited Liability company; Government—Hospital district; Government—Federal.

Renaming Column Headers in Excel
When we import this data into RStudio, these column header names will become the names of different fields in a data frame. RStudio will do the best job it can of working with names that have spaces in them, but it

Figure 12.1.   SQL script and returned data

```
SELECT DISTINCT
    provnum,
    overall_rating,
    survey_rating,
    staffing_rating,
    RN_staffing_rating,
    quality_rating,
    ssf,
    restot,
    ownership
FROM
    nursing_home_provider_info;
```

(Continued)

Figure 12.1.   SQL script and returned data *(Continued)*

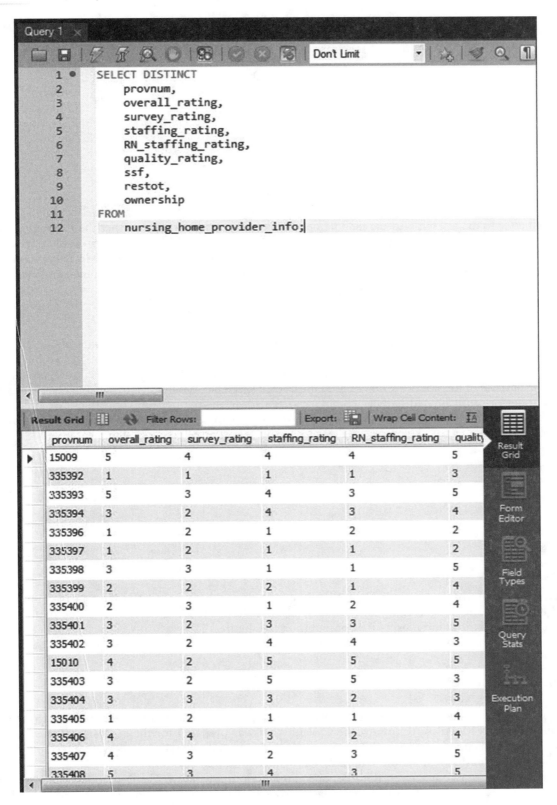

Table 12.1.   Original and revised column names within Excel

Original Name	Revised Name
provnum	provnum
overall_rating	overall
survey_rating	health_insp
staffing_rating	staff_rate
RN_staffing_rating	rn_rate
quality_rating	qual_rate
ssf	ssf
restot	restot
ownership	owner

would be better to make each of these field names shorter now, while in Excel, rather than changing them in RStudio (or worse, typing long field names in RStudio each time we want to use them). Table 12.1 contains the names we will use when renaming the column headers. To rename column headers in Excel, simply click each individual cell, highlight the contents, delete the content, enter the new column name, and click return. Repeat this process for each column header.

Recoding Data in Excel

To make analyses more powerful and understandable, it is often important to recode variables to have fewer values. For this analysis, we will create a new variable related to nursing home ownership in Excel using the IF function and recode our 13-level variable to reflect only 3 levels: for-profit = 1; government = 2; and nonprofit = 3. For the purpose of this study, we do not need the level of specificity within each ownership type; for example, differentiating for-profit limited liability companies from for-profit partnership companies. We only need to know whether a nursing home is for profit. To recode the ownership type, in J1 enter the title owner_group for the recoded column of data. We can recode this variable by using the following IF statement in cell J2:

```
=IF(I2="For profit - Corporation",1,IF(I2="For profit -
Individual",1,IF(I2="For profit - Limited Liability company",1,IF(I2="For
profit - Partnership",1,IF(I2="Government - City",2,IF(I2="Government -
City/county",2,IF(I2="Government - County",2,IF(I2="Government -
Federal",2,IF(I2="Government - Hospital district",2,IF(I2="Government -
State",2,IF(I2="Non profit - Church related",3,IF(I2="Non profit -
Corporation", 3,IF(I2="Non profit - Other", 3)))))))))))))
```

After inputting the formula, hit enter. Next, fill in the formula for the remainder of the cells in column J, click on and hover over the bottom right corner of cell J2 until the white cross turns black, then double-click to populate the rest of the column using the computation (see figure 12.2).

Once these changes have been made, save the file as a CSV file and name it fivestar.

Step 3: Import the Data

Importing data into RStudio is a relatively straightforward process (see chapter 5 for detailed instructions for importing data into RStudio). To import the CSV file that was prepared for the analysis under Step 2, click Import Dataset and choose the From Text File option in the drop-down window. Navigate to the fivestar.csv file that was saved in the final action of Step 2, highlight the file, and click Open.

After the data are imported into RStudio, open an R scripting window. The R scripting window is where you will enter the R code in order to analyze the data. To open a new R scripting window, go to File >New File > R Script. The first step is to attach the data set. An effect called "masking" may occur if a variable name is already

Figure 12.2. Recoding variables from 13 levels to 3 levels using the IF function

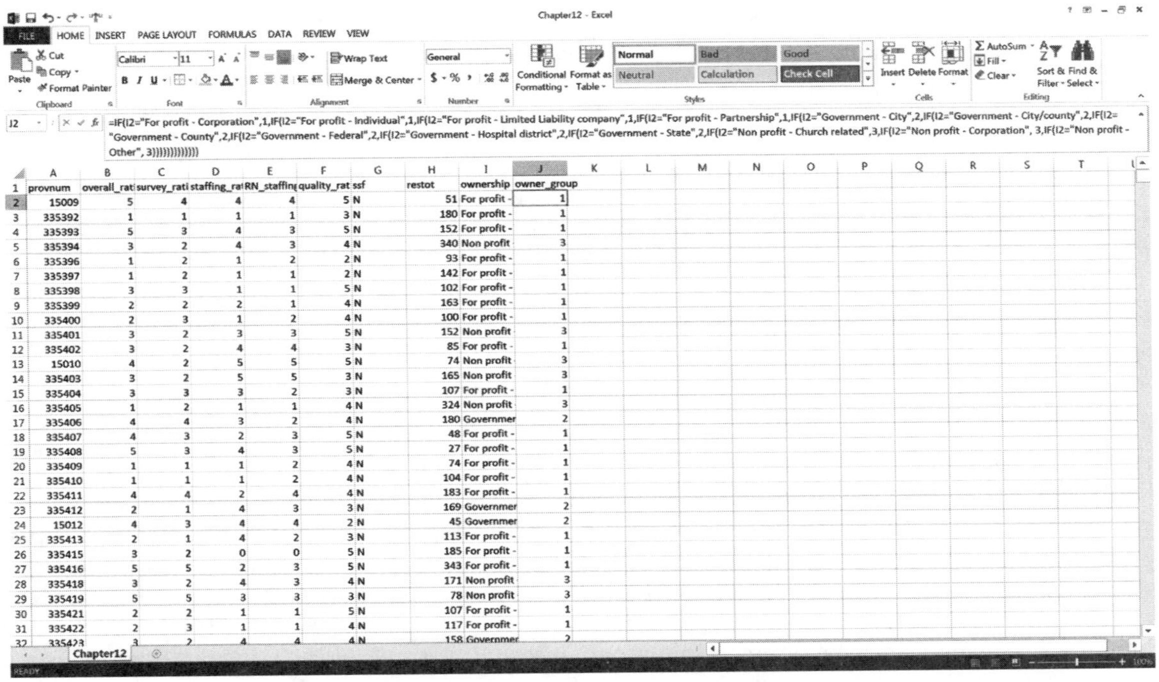

	A	B	C	D	E	F	G	H	I	J
1	provnum	overall_rati	survey_rati	staffing_ra	RN_staffing	quality_rat	ssf	restot	ownership	owner_group
2	15009	5	4	4	4	5	N	51	For profit -	1
3	335392	1	1	1	1	3	N	180	For profit -	1
4	335393	5	3	4	3	5	N	152	For profit -	1
5	335394	3	2	4	3	4	N	340	Non profit	3
6	335396	1	2	1	2	2	N	93	For profit -	1
7	335397	1	2	1	1	2	N	142	For profit -	1
8	335398	3	3	1	1	5	N	102	For profit -	1
9	335399	2	2	2	1	4	N	163	For profit -	1
10	335400	2	3	1	2	4	N	100	For profit -	1
11	335401	3	2	3	3	5	N	152	Non profit	3
12	335402	3	2	4	4	3	N	85	For profit -	1
13	15010	4	2	5	5	5	N	74	Non profit	3
14	335403	3	2	5	5	3	N	165	Non profit	3
15	335404	3	3	3	2	3	N	107	For profit -	1
16	335405	1	2	1	1	4	N	324	Non profit	3
17	335406	4	4	3	2	4	N	180	Governmer	2
18	335407	4	3	2	3	5	N	48	For profit -	1
19	335408	5	3	4	3	5	N	27	For profit -	1
20	335409	1	1	1	2	4	N	74	For profit -	1
21	335410	1	1	1	2	4	N	104	For profit -	1
22	335411	4	4	2	4	4	N	183	For profit -	1
23	335412	2	1	4	3	3	N	169	Governmer	2
24	15012	4	3	4	4	2	N	45	Governmer	2
25	335413	2	1	4	2	3	N	113	For profit -	1
26	335415	3	2	0	0	5	N	185	For profit -	1
27	335416	5	5	2	3	5	N	343	For profit -	1
28	335418	3	2	4	3	4	N	171	Non profit	3
29	335419	5	5	3	3	3	N	78	Non profit	3
30	335421	2	2	1	1	5	N	107	For profit -	1
31	335422	2	3	1	1	4	N	117	For profit -	1
32	335423	3	2	4	4	4	N	158	Governmer	2

an object in RStudio. Masking occurs when objects (such as data sets or functions) are identically named. You may choose to call the object in order to determine whether it exists in your workspace prior to attaching. This can be done by requesting the structure of an object name, using the str() function (for example, str(fivestar)). It is also good practice to detach the data set after use using the function detach() (for example, detach(fivestar)).

To attach the data, type the following R code into the console:

```
attach(fivestar)
```

Step 4: Descriptive Statistics

Prior to launching into the statistical modeling and analysis of our data set, we ought to perform some simple summary and graphical characterizations of the data. One of the first things we want to understand are the dimensions of the entire data set by using R's dim() function. The following is the code for acquiring these dimensions:

```
dim(fivestar)
```

Output from this function is as follows:

```
[1] 15632  10
```

This output indicates that there are 15,632 rows and 10 columns in the data set.

We may also be interested in knowing the mean of all numeric variables. Using the sapply() function, we can acquire the means for all variables within the fivestar data frame, while removing NA (not available) values. The sapply function differs from tapply. The sapply will apply a function to each element of a dataframe, and return a vector of results (for example, returning the mean for each column in the data frame named fivestar). The tapply function will apply a function to subsets of one vector based on the subsets of another vector, usually a factor (for example, returning mean quality rating for each ownership type for nursing homes). The sapply can be generated as follows:

```
sapply(fivestar, mean, na.rm=TRUE)
```

The following output will be displayed:

```
provnum  overall health_insp  staff_rate  rn_rate qual_rate
  NA  3.409289  2.800345  3.212193  3.266633  4.086745

  ssf   restot   owner owner_group
  NA  87.561029  NA 1.542861

Warning messages:
1: In mean.default(X[[1L]],…):
  argument is not numeric or logical: returning NA
2: In mean.default(X[[7L]],…):
  argument is not numeric or logical: returning NA
3: In mean.default(X[[9L]],…):
  argument is not numeric or logical: returning NA
```

By the three warning messages within the output, we are reminded that three of our variables are nonnumeric and are therefore returned as NA. Also, the averages for each of the quantitative variables are provided. For example, the average for the overall measure is 3.41. A mean is calculated for the variable owner_group, which is not meaningful. Since owner_group is a categorical variable that is coded with a number (for-profit = 1; government = 2; and nonprofit = 3), it is possible to calculate a mean of the number. However, the interpretation of that mean is meaningless. The average owner_group of 1.54 does not provide a better understanding of the typical or most frequent type of ownership group. Instead, the count of each ownership group is a better analysis. These summaries do offer you a better understanding of the typical values for each variable. However, to determine if there is a relationship between these variables and to test their ability to predict a five-star rating, a statistical analysis is required.

Step 5: Statistical Analyses

For the purpose of this chapter, we will conduct **backward elimination** using stepwise regression. Backward elimination is a variable selection procedure that begins with all predictors in the model, removes the predictor with the highest p-value that is greater than the prespecified critical alpha value, and refits the model. This process is repeated until all variables in the model are less than the critical alpha value. After we identify our highest predictors through backward elimination, we will convert our outcome measure to a binary variable in order to investigate what contributes to a one-star rating versus a rating greater than one star. We will then employ multiple logistic regression to determine the odds of receiving a one-star rating, given different scenarios.

Backward Elimination

Our outcome variable for this study is the nursing home overall rating. The process of backward elimination is used to identify the most robust and resourceful model that fits the data. In other words, we will be generating a model of the data that minimizes the number of variables in order to increase the stability and generalizability of the model. If we have too many variables, our model becomes dependent on the data in our sample (the observed data) because the more variables we have the greater our estimated standard errors become, which is a prediction of how far off our model is from the true fit. To take account of what variables are eligible for removal, backward elimination can be run manually; this is particularly helpful in the case of a complex hierarchy.

We begin our analysis in RStudio by viewing and creating an index of the column names we would like to use within our analysis:

```
colnames(fivestar)
```

The function will reveal the following output:

```
[1] "provnum"      "overall" "health_insp"
[4] "staff_rate" "rn_rate" "qual_rate"
[7] "ssf"          "restot"  "owner"
[10] "owner_group"
```

We can create a vector of the columns that we will be retaining for inclusion in the analysis:

```
NHcolumns <- c("overall","qual_rate", "staff_rate",
"rn_rate", "owner_group", "health_insp", "restot", "ssf" )
```

Next, we create a subset of data representing only our variables of interest (which were specified in the NH columns variables created in the prior step), and we name this data frame "NH":

```
NH<- fivestar[NHcolumns]

View(NH)

attach(NH)
```

After attaching the NH data frame, you may receive a warning stating the following: "The following objects are masked from fivestar...." As introduced earlier in this chapter, the warning notifies you of masking—that there are already objects stored in memory with the names of the columns. Again, this is occurring because the fivestar data set was previously attached. When we attach the NH data frame, this is over-writing the objects from fivestar that have the same names (for example, overall, qual_rate). Generally, masking will not be a problem; however, as you begin to increase the number of packages used, the likelihood of coming across two identically named functions from different packages—or perhaps worse, naming a data set the name of a function—will increase. For this reason, it is not always advised to attach a data set.

The next step in the process is to create our linear regression model. We set-up our model formula and view our results using the functions lm() and summary():

```
NH.lm<-lm(overall ~ qual_rate + health_insp + staff_rate +
rn_rate + as.factor(owner_group) + restot +
as.factor(ssf))
```

Calling our model (NH.lm) by running the following script will generate the coefficient:

```
NH.lm
```

The output is the following:

```
Call:
lm(formula = overall ~ qual_rate + health_insp + staff_rate +
rn_rate + as.factor(owner_group) + restot + as.factor(ssf))

Coefficients:
              (Intercept)      qual_rate      health_insp
               -0.9870177     0.3173671      0.7804446
              staff_rate       rn_rate       as.factor(owner_group)2
               0.2986339     -0.0078981      0.0827170
as.factor(owner_group)3    restot         as.factor(ssf)Y
               0.0578998     -0.0004284      -0.2092096
```

Using the summary() function applied to the stored linear model (that is, NH.lm), we can identify significant predictors within our model where the values of the coefficients have associated p-values that are less than our alpha, 0.05. Take special note of the Pr(>|t|) column while keeping in mind a critical value of 0.05. That is, anything lower than 0.05 can remain in the model:

```
summary(NH.lm)
```

The output is the following:

```
Call:
lm(formula = overall ~ qual_rate + health_insp + staff_rate +
    rn_rate + as.factor(owner_group) + restot + as.factor(ssf))

Residuals:
     Min                    1Q      Median          3Q        Max
-1.19476               -0.37301     0.00857     0.33010    2.08779

Coefficients:
                              Estimate   Std. Error  t value     Pr(>|t|)
(Intercept)                 -9.870e-01   1.953e-02   -50.547     < 2e-16 ***
qual_rate                    3.174e-01   3.911e-03    81.157     < 2e-16 ***
health_insp                  7.804e-01   3.201e-03   243.780     < 2e-16 ***
staff_rate                   2.986e-01   5.337e-03    55.956     < 2e-16 ***
rn_rate                     -7.898e-03   5.049e-03    -1.564     0.117799
as.factor(owner_group)2      8.272e-02   1.719e-02     4.812   1.51e-06 ***
as.factor(owner_group)3      5.790e-02   9.811e-03     5.901   3.68e-09 ***
restot                      -4.284e-04   7.488e-05    -5.721   1.08e-08 ***
as.factor(ssf)Y             -2.092e-01   5.416e-02    -3.863   0.000113 ***
---
Signif. codes: 0 '***' 0.001 '**' 0.01 '*' 0.05 '.' 0.1 ' ' 1

Residual standard error: 0.5015 on 15623 degrees of freedom
Multiple R-squared: 0.8623,      Adjusted R-squared: 0.8623
F-statistic: 1.223e+04 on 8 and 15623 DF, p-value: < 2.2e-16
```

Through the use of the unclass() function, we can view the information types located within our model. We may therefore locate the coefficients and the **adjusted R-squared** value within our summary() function:

```
summary(unclass(summary(NH.lm)))
```

The output is the following:

```
               Length   Class     Mode
call               2   -none-    call
terms              3   terms     call
residuals      15632   -none-    numeric
coefficients      36   -none-    numeric
aliased            9   -none-    logical
sigma              1   -none-    numeric
df                 3   -none-    numeric
r.squared          1   -none-    numeric
adj.r.squared      1   -none-    numeric
fstatistic         3   -none-    numeric
cov.unscaled      81   -none-    numeric
```

The output tells us the length, class, and mode of the information types. Note that each of these information types can be isolated. For example, just as in a call for a variable name within a data set, we can call the adjusted r-squared value from the unclass() list of options, specific to the linear model.

```
summary(NH.lm)$adj.r.squared

0.8622718
```

The adjusted R-squared value indicates that about 86 percent of our outcome variable is explained by our current model.

As discussed, we are interested in iteratively eliminating our least significant predictors to improve our adjusted R-squared value, and this can be done using backward elimination. In order to unveil the column information contained within the coefficients term, we may again use the summary() function. As you will see, the final column of the coefficients term is Pr(>|t|).

```
colnames(summary(NH.lm)$coefficients)
"Estimate" "Std. Error" "t value" "Pr(>|t|)"
```

We would like to sort our p-values in decreasing order to identify our least significant predictors, as we will eliminate the least significant predictors until only those predictors that are less than our critical alpha value remain. We can therefore extract our p-values by calling the Pr(>|t|) column from our coefficients table by using the summary() function. This eases the process by producing only the essential information for our task.

```
sort(summary(NH.lm)$coef[,"Pr(>|t|)"], decreasing=T)

rn_rate                      as.factor(ssf)Y as.factor(owner_group)2      restot
1.177988e-01                 1.125841e-04    1.508868e-06            1.079191e-08
as.factor(owner_group)3 (Intercept)         qual_rate               health_insp
3.679381e-09                 0.000000e+00    0.000000e+00            0.000000e+00
staff_rate
  0.000000e+00
```

Since the variable with the highest p-value is rn_rate, we will see if we can improve our logistic model by removing the variable from our model:

```
NH.lm2<-lm(overall ~ qual_rate + health_insp + staff_rate +
as.factor(owner_group) + restot + as.factor(ssf))

summary(NH.lm2)$adj.r.squared

      0.8622591

sort(summary(NH.lm2)$coef[,"Pr(>|t|)"], decreasing=T)
as.factor(ssf)Y as.factor(owner_group)2 restot as.factor(owner_group)3
1.120093e-04    1.598819e-06            1.592811e-08       4.295077e-09
(Intercept)     qual_rate               health_insp        staff_rate
0.000000e+00    0.000000e+00            0.000000e+00       0.000000e+00
```

Our model has only minutely decreased in adjusted R-squared value, indicating that the variable removed was not highly influential in the variability of our outcome variable. Further, our new maximal p-value appears to be quite significant, indicating that all variables are now below our critical alpha value. It may be time to cease the elimination process. Let us assess our sum of squared errors—we want to reduce this value within our model as it is an indicator of the discrepancy (error) between our estimated model and our true data.

```
sse1 <- sum(resid(NH.lm)^2)

sse2 <- sum(resid(NH.lm2)^2)
```

```
sse1

sse1
[1] 3929.764

sse2

sse2
[1] 3930.38
```

It appears that the new model only slightly increases our SSE. Let us check the correlation of our rn_rate variable against our other variables. To avoid multicolinearity, we do not want to include two variables that are highly correlated with one another—this would result in redundant information.

```
cor(rn_rate, staff_rate)

0.8072305
```

Indeed, rn_rate is highly correlated with staff_rate, so we can confidently remove this variable from our model.

Let us run a new model without the rn_rate variable and determine our highest predictors to our overall rating:

```
summary(NH.lm2)

Call:
lm(formula = overall ~ qual_rate + health_insp + staff_rate +
    as.factor(owner_group) + restot + as.factor(ssf))

Residuals:
     Min       1Q    Median       3Q      Max
 -1.19910  -0.37415  0.00949  0.33020  2.09129

Coefficients:
                           Estimate   Std. Error   t value    Pr(>|t|)
(Intercept)               -0.9896007   0.0194576   -50.859    <2e-16   ***
qual_rate                  0.3168952   0.0038990    81.275    < 2e-16  ***
health_insp                0.7802547   0.0031993   243.885    < 2e-16  ***
staff_rate                 0.2920473   0.0032790    89.067    < 2e-16  ***
as.factor(owner_group)2    0.0825192   0.0171904     4.800    1.60e-06 ***
as.factor(owner_group)3    0.0576429   0.0098103     5.876    4.30e-09 ***
restot                    -0.0004230   0.0000748    -5.654    1.59e-08 ***
as.factor(ssf)Y           -0.2092870   0.0541637    -3.864    0.000112 ***
---
Signif. codes:  0 '***' 0.001 '**' 0.01 '*' 0.05 '.' 0.1 ' ' 1

Residual standard error: 0.5016 on 15624 degrees of freedom
Multiple R-squared: 0.8623,      Adjusted R-squared: 0.8623
F-statistic: 1.398e+04 on 7 and 15624 DF, p-value: < 2.2e-16
```

The output tells us that all of our predictors are significant, as is our overall model, and that our model accounts for 86.2 percent of the total variability of our outcome variable.

The ANOVA table for our multiple regression analysis is given using the anova() function and provides a slightly different picture. This is because these tests are successive; they correspond to the stepwise removal of the terms (from the bottom up) until the only variable left becomes qual_rate.

```
                                        anova(NH.lm2)

> anova(NH.lm2)

Analysis of Variance Table

Response: overall
```

	Df	Sum Sq	Mean Sq	F value	Pr(>F)	
qual_rate	1	4347.7	4347.7	17283.052	< 2.2e-16	***
health_insp	1	18009.1	18009.1	71589.393	< 2.2e-16	***
staff_rate	1	2236.0	2236.0	8888.616	< 2.2e-16	***
as.factor(owner_group)	2	12.4	6.2	24.686	1.976e-11	***
restot	1	8.0	8.0	31.813	1.727e-08	***
as.factor(ssf)	1	3.8	3.8	14.930	0.000112	***
Residuals	15624	3930.4	0.3			

```
---
Signif. codes:  0 '***' 0.001 '**' 0.01 '*' 0.05 '.' 0.1 ' ' 1
```

We can see that all predictors are highly significant and that qual_rate and health_insp are the highest predictors of overall rating. Due to the interest in determining what predicts extremely poor overall performance (one-star on overall rating)—in short, the nursing homes that require the most improvement—the variables qual_rate and health_insp can be used to predict overall one-star ratings (the lowest possible value). We can do this via multiple logistic regression.

Multiple Logistic Regression

To begin, we will first generate a contingency table in Excel, and from the values within those cells, we will create a data frame in RStudio where we will run the multiple logistic regression.

The first step is to open the fivestar.csv file in Excel. We will generate a table to count the number of providers that have health_insp as 1, compared to the number of providers with a qual_rate of 1, compared to the number of providers with an overall score of 1. On the right side of our Excel spreadsheet, in a location where there are not data, we will generate the contingency table. See figure 12.3 for a visual of how the contingency table should be constructed in Excel.

We will include varying SUMPRODUCT functions in each of the eight cells that you generated in the spreadsheet (as shown in figure 12.3) that need to be populated in the contingency table. The purpose of the SUMPRODUCT function is to count the number of times that multiple criteria are met. To count the number of times that health_insp is 1, qual_rate is 1, and overall is 0, the following SUMPRODUCT function is used to populate a count into the contingency you created in the cell. The function populates the cell when there is a Yes for Overall 1-Star Rating, Yes for Health Inspection, and Yes for Quality (cell N5 in figure 12.3):

$$= SUMPRODUCT((B:B = 1)*(C:C = 1)*(F:F = 1))$$

Where, B:B is the column for overall and is counted when equal to 1; C:C is the column for health_insp and is counted when equal to 1; F:F is the column for qual_rate and counted when equal to 1. Only those will be counted providers when all three criteria are met. The result of the function should be 82. The other 7 SUMPRODUCT functions are shown in table 12.2.

The results from the SUMPRODUCT function are shown in table 12.3. This tells us that the majority of providers are those that do not have an overall one-star rating, did not have an overall one-star rating for quality, and did not have an overall rating of one star for the general survey. To ease the process of creating the framework for our contingency table in RStudio, we have taken advantage of Excel's SUMPRODUCT function and can now smoothly create a data frame in RStudio using the results derived from each cell. The next step is to create the data frame in RStudio to reflect the following binary variables from our contingency table. When you go back to RStudio, the contingency table that was created in Excel will be created in RStudio. The data.frame function will be used to generate four columns of data: quality, survey, overall, and count. The quality, survey, and overall columns will contain the values of 1 or 0 and defined as follows:

- Quality one-star rating where 1 = Yes and 0 = No
- Survey one-star rating where 1 = Yes and 0 = No
- Overall one-star rating where 1 = Yes and 0 = No

Following the input shown, our data frame is named NH1 and the binary variables are derived from the contingency table for logistic regression analysis, table 12.3.

Figure 12.3. Creating the contingency table in Excel

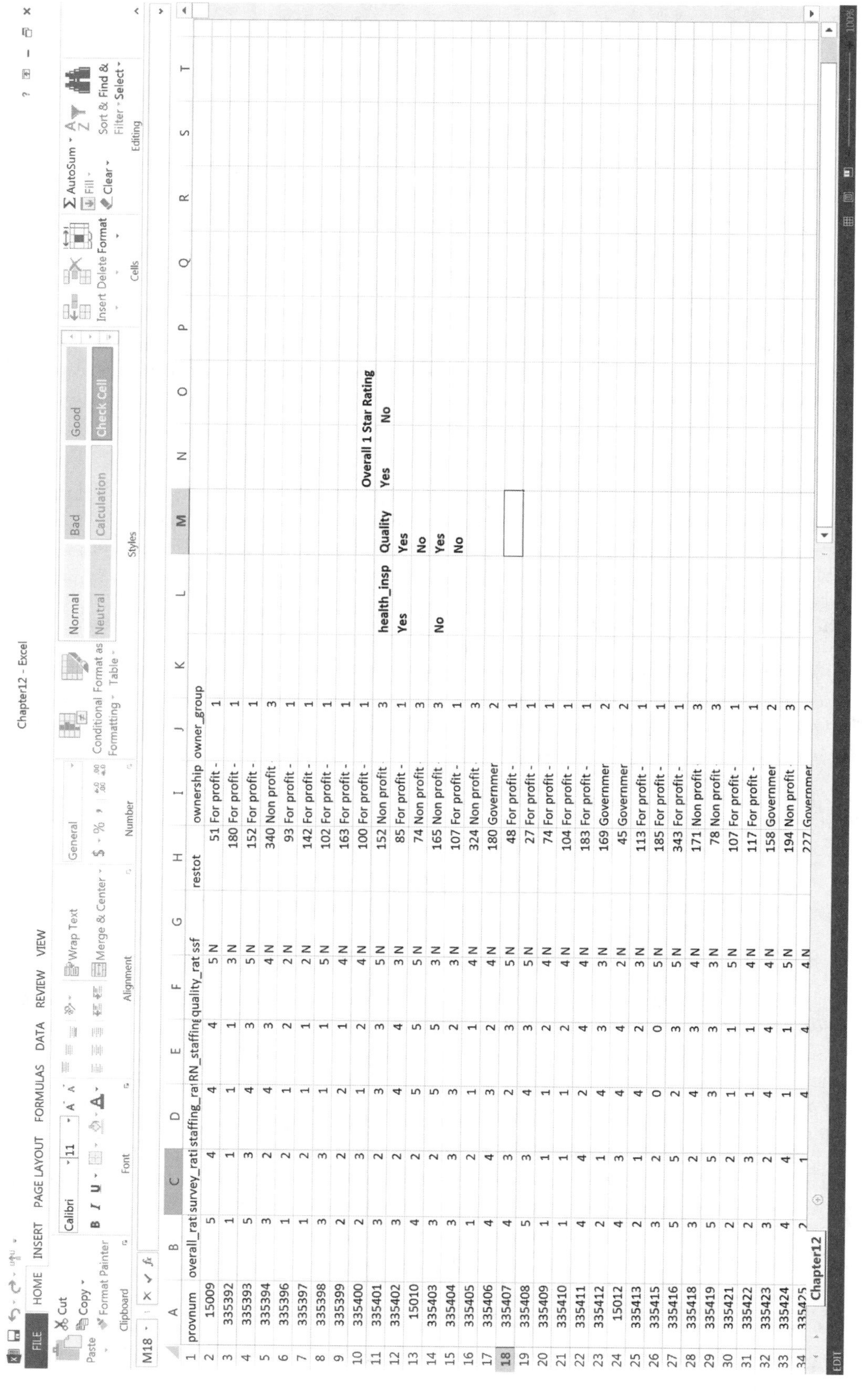

provnum	overall_rati	survey_rati	staffing_rati	RN_staffing_rat	quality_rat	ssf	restot	ownership	owner_group
15009	5	4	4	4	5	N	51	For profit	1
335392	1	1	1	1	3	N	180	For profit	1
335393	5	3	4	3	5	N	152	For profit	1
335394	3	2	2	3	4	N	340	Non profit	3
335396	1	2	1	1	2	N	93	For profit	1
335397	1	2	1	1	2	N	142	For profit	1
335398	3	3	1	1	5	N	102	For profit	1
335399	2	2	2	1	4	N	163	For profit	1
335400	2	3	2	2	4	N	100	For profit	1
335401	3	2	3	3	5	N	152	Non profit	3
335402	3	2	4	4	3	N	85	For profit	1
15010	4	2	5	5	5	N	74	Non profit	3
335403	3	2	5	5	3	N	165	Non profit	3
335404	3	3	3	2	3	N	107	For profit	1
335405	2	2	1	2	4	N	324	Non profit	3
335406	4	4	4	3	4	N	180	Governmer	2
335407	4	3	2	2	4	N	48	For profit	1
335408	5	3	4	3	5	N	27	For profit	1
335409	1	1	1	2	4	N	74	For profit	1
335410	1	1	1	1	4	N	104	For profit	1
335411	4	4	4	2	4	N	183	For profit	1
335412	2	1	3	4	3	N	169	Governmer	2
15012	4	3	4	3	2	N	45	Governmer	2
335413	4	2	2	1	3	N	113	For profit	1
335415	3	2	0	0	5	N	185	For profit	1
335416	5	5	3	3	5	N	343	For profit	1
335418	3	2	4	3	4	N	171	Non profit	3
335419	5	5	3	3	3	N	78	Non profit	3
335421	2	3	1	1	5	N	107	For profit	1
335422	2	3	1	3	4	N	117	For profit	1
335423	3	2	4	4	4	N	158	Governmer	2
335424	4	4	1	1	5	N	194	Non profit	3
335425	1	1	4	4	4	N	227	Governmer	2

Contingency table (right side):

		Overall 1 Star Rating	
health_insp	Quality	Yes	No
Yes	Yes		
	No		
No	Yes		
	No		

Chapter12

Table 12.2.   Create a contingency table in Excel using the SUMPRODUCT function

Health_ Insp	Quality	Overall 1-Star Rating Yes	No
Yes	Yes	=SUMPRODUCT((B:B=1)*(C:C=1)*(F:F=1))	=SUMPRODUCT((B:B<>1)*(C:C=1)*(F:F=1))
	No	=SUMPRODUCT((B:B=1)*(C:C=1)*(F:F<>1))	=SUMPRODUCT((B:B<>1)*(C:C=1)*(F:F<>1))
No	Yes	=SUMPRODUCT((B:B=1)*(C:C<>1)*(F:F=1))	=SUMPRODUCT((B:B<>1)*(C:C<>1)*(F:F=1))

Table 12.3.   Contingency table for logistic regression analysis

Survey	Quality	Overall 1-Star Rating Yes	No
Yes	Yes	82	0
	No	1010	1971
No	Yes	52	178
	No	228	1045054

The count variable will contain the frequency values from the contingency table where we first fill in the count values for nursing homes with an overall 1-star rating and continue by entering in the numeric count values for nursing homes without an overall 1-star rating. The R code that will be generated to create the data frame includes the following:

```
NH1<-data.frame(quality=c(1,1,0,0,1,1,0,0),
survey=c(1,0,1,0,1,0,1,0), overall=c(1,1,1,1,0,0,0,0),
count=c(82,1010,52,228,0,1971,178,1045054))
```

We want to examine the odds of having a one-star overall rating with a one-star survey rating and one-star quality rating as the predictors. We will begin by examining the main effects of one-star survey rating and one-star quality rating without interaction.

Here we use the glm() function and use the + sign to add additional terms to our model. We name our model NH1.logit. Additionally, because we are treating our variables as factors we incorporate the factor() function on our two predictor variables:

```
NH1.logit<-glm(overall~factor(quality) + factor(survey), weights=count,
data=NH1, family="binomial")

summary(NH1.logit)

> summary(NH1.logit)

Call:
glm(formula = overall ~ factor(quality) + factor(survey), family =
    "binomial", data = NH1, weights = count)

Deviance Residuals:
    1       2       3       4       5       6       7       8
0.488   46.755   12.426   62.004   0.000   -40.387   -9.564   -21.347

Coefficients:
                Estimate Std.   Error z value Pr(>|z|)
(Intercept)       -8.43076       0.06623  -127.29  <2e-16 ***
```

```
factor(quality)1   7.76234        0.07670   101.21  <2e-16  ***
factor(survey)1    7.20317        0.17058    42.23  <2e-16  ***
---
Signif. codes: 0 '***' 0.001 '**' 0.01 '*' 0.05 '.' 0.1 ' ' 1

(Dispersion parameter for binomial family taken to be 1)

Null deviance:      20959.4  on 6  degrees of freedom
Residual deviance: 8363.5   on 4  degrees of freedom
AIC: 8369.5

Number of Fisher Scoring iterations: 9
```

The logistic equation can also be stated in mathematical terms:

1. $\log(\text{odds}) = \beta_0 + \beta_1 \times \text{survey} + \beta_2 \times \text{quality}$
2. $\log(\text{odds}) = -8.43076 + 7.76234 \times \text{survey} + 7.20317 \times \text{quality}$

Notice that the survey and quality terms are both statistically significant ($p < 0.0001$).

We want to know the odds of being an overall poor performer for nursing homes that performed poorly on quality but not on survey, compared with nursing homes that performed poorly on survey but not on quality. We can use the logistic equation established and insert the values of the coefficients in order to determine the odds. This computation is performed in five steps:

1. $\log(\text{odds})\ \text{survey}(0) + \text{quality}(1) = \beta_0 + \beta_1(0) + \beta_2(1)$
2. $\log(\text{odds})\ \text{survey}(1) + \text{quality}(0) = \beta_0 + \beta_1(1) + \beta_2(0)$
3. $\log(\text{OR}) = \beta_0 + \beta_2 - [\beta_0 + \beta_1] = \beta_2 - \beta_1$
4. $\log(\text{OR}) = 7.20317 - 7.76234 = -0.55917$
5. $\text{OR} = \exp(-0.55917) = 1.75$

Nursing homes that perform poorly on quality but not on survey have 1.75 times greater odds of having a one-star rating on overall performance than nursing homes that perform poorly on survey but not on quality. Nursing homes that have lower quality are significantly more likely to have a one-star rating than do nursing homes that have higher quality but lower survey ratings. Not surprisingly, "quality" is heavily weighted in terms of the quality rankings.

Now let us compute the **odds ratio** for surveys with one star, compared to surveys with more than one star and for quality ratings with one star, compared to quality ratings with more than one star. In RStudio, we will use the exp() and coef() functions to exponentiate each coefficient in the summary output given to get these odds ratios. Or, recall from simple logistic regression (chapter 9) that we can extract each coefficient using coef() and use exp() to exponentiate to obtain the odds ratios all in one step using the following code:

```
exp(coef(NH1.logit))
> exp(coef(NH1.logit))
   (Intercept) factor(quality)1 factor(survey)1
  2.180567e-04 2.350404e+03 1.343680e+03
```

The results summary includes

1. One-star quality ratings have a 2.350 greater chance of having a one-star overall rating than do quality ratings with more than one star.
2. One-star survey ratings have a 1.344 greater chance of having a one-star overall rating than do survey ratings with more than one star.

Let us consider adding the interaction between quality and survey ratings to our model. We can use the A*B with factors to include each singular term and the interaction in the model (A:B will add only the interaction). Therefore, in RStudio, we will be creating another general linear model using the glm() function, but instead of using the plus (+) sign to add terms to a model, we will be using the asterisk (*) sign to examine interactions between terms in the model. In this case, we want to see if quality and survey ratings have an interaction on the overall star rating for nursing homes. In RStudio, use the following code to create the model:

```
NH1.logit2<-glm(overall~factor(quality) * factor(survey), weights=count,
data=NH1, family="binomial")

summary(NH1.logit2)

> summary(NH1.logit2)
Call:
glm(formula = overall ~ factor(quality) * factor(survey), family
    = "binomial",
    data = NH1, weights = count)

Deviance Residuals:
    1          2          3          4          5          6          7          8
0.007    46.757    12.435    62.002    0.000    -40.384    -9.552    -21.353

Coefficients:
                                     Estimate   Std. Error   z value   Pr(>|z|)
(Intercept)                          -8.43023      0.06623   -127.280   <2e-16 ***
factor(quality)1                      7.76164      0.07671    101.182   <2e-16 ***
factor(survey)1                       7.19969      0.17098     42.107   <2e-16 ***
factor(quality)1:factor(survey)1      8.58441    128.30314      0.067    0.947
Signif. codes: 0 '***' 0.001 '**' 0.01 '*' 0.05 '.' 0.1 ' ' 1

(Dispersion parameter for binomial family taken to be 1)

Null deviance:    20959.4 on 6 degrees of freedom
Residual deviance: 8363.2 on 3 degrees of freedom
AIC: 8371.2

Number of Fisher Scoring iterations: 10
```

The interaction is not significant (p = 0.947) and our logistic model can be written as:

log(odds) = B0 + B1(quality) + B2(survey) + B3(quality*survey)
log(odds) = –8.43023 + 7.76164(quality) + 7.19969(survey) + 8.58441(quality*survey)

The Akaike Information Criterion (AIC) is 8371.2 and is just barely larger than our model without the interaction (that is, NH1.logit AIC = 8369.5). The AIC is used to compare the performance of models on the same dataset—the closer the AIC is to zero illustrates the quality of the model. Since the AIC is only slightly larger in NH1.logti2 as compared to NH1.logit, and the interaction is not significant in NH1.logit2, we conclude that the model without the interaction (namely, model NH1.logit) is a sufficient fit.

If you have multiple predictors and interactions in your model, R can systematically select significant predictors using forward selection, backward selection, or stepwise selection. The default selection criteria are based on AIC.

In forward selection, R begins with no predictors in the model. It then selects the predictor with the smallest AIC and adds it to the model. It then selects another predictor from the remaining variables and chooses the model with the smallest AIC. It continues this process until the AIC no longer improves.

In backward selection, R begins with all of the predictors in the model and eliminates the predictors one at a time, refitting the model between each elimination step and comparing the AIC. It stops once all of the predictors remaining in the model result in the lowest AIC.

Stepwise selection combines both forward and backward selection and is the default "direction" set in R. We will employ the stepwise selection method in the next example, using the R function, step. Since we have previously fit this model and assigned to NH1.logit2, we can use this assignment as our object name:

```
step(NH1.logit2)

> step(NH1.logit2)
Start: AIC=8371.25
overall ~ factor(quality) * factor(survey)

                                       Df Deviance AIC
- factor(quality):factor(survey)        1  8363.5    8369.5
<none>                                     8363.2    8371.2

Step: AIC=8369.49
overall ~ factor(quality) + factor(survey)

                   Df Deviance        AIC
<none>                   8363.5    8369.5
- factor(survey)     1   9156.4    9160.4
- factor(quality)    1  19592.5   19596.5

Call: glm(formula = overall ~ factor(quality) + factor(survey), family
= "binomial",
          data = NH1, weights = count)

Coefficients:
   (Intercept)            factor(quality)1  factor(survey)1
       -8.431                      7.762            7.203

Degrees of Freedom: 6 Total (i.e. Null);        4 Residual
Null Deviance:          20960
Residual Deviance: 8363        AIC: 8369
```

The interaction term tested in NH1.logit2, which depicted the simultaneous influence of quality and survey, on overall rating, was not included in the final model generated by R's step() function.

Using different methods, we set out to determine the most **parsimonious** model. That is, the simplest and most robust model to define our data. This is highly important because as the model becomes complicated, it also becomes error prone. The model selected by the stepwise selection process in R contains only the survey and quality ratings as independent variables, and does not include the interaction term. This confirms our manually selected model, as the final model selected by the stepwise regression functions in R is identical to our original model, NH1.logit.

Discussion

Our research question, "What nursing home factors are most associated with the lowest ranking (one-star) on the Nursing Home Compare website?" prompted us to perform a multiple linear regression in order to identify the factors most associated with the overall rating. After identifying the top contributors, we were able to dig deeper and determine the odds of having a one-star rating for varying conditions.

We identified the top two predictors of our outcome variable overall_rating. The variables quality_rating and survey_rating were the greatest predictors of overall_rating as evidenced by their low p-value, high coefficient estimates, high t-value, and contributions to the overall model. Because these variables were the most influential in contributions to the overall rating, we selected them to determine the odds of having a one-star rating given performance on quality as compared to performance on survey. We learned from this analysis that within our data, nursing homes that perform poorly on quality but not on survey have 1.75 times greater odds of having a one-star rating on overall performance than nursing homes that perform poorly on survey but not on quality. What this may mean is that when evaluating nursing homes online one can speculate that a nursing home with a very low overall score is most likely to have low scores in QM than deficiencies in health measures. Further, the model selected by the stepwise selection process in R contained only the survey and quality ratings, as in our results, and we saw that the model without the interaction term was a sufficient fit—indicating that health measures do not necessarily contribute to quality ratings.

Conclusion

We set out to minimize the number of variables in order to increase the stability and generalizability of our logistic regression model. The most robust and parsimonious model that still fits our data is log(odds)= –8.43076 + 7.76234*Survey + 7.20317*Quality, as was computed in NH1.logit. A one-star rating on quality is 1.75 times more likely to result in an overall one-star rating than a health inspection (survey) rating.

Review Exercises

Instructions: Answer the following questions.

1. What is masking (in the context of R computing) and how can it be avoided?

2. What is the purpose of a causal analysis?

3. What is AIC and how can it be useful?

4. What is the difference between backward elimination and forward regression?

5. Which R function will produce the dimensions of a data frame?

6. For what does the adjusted r-squared value adjust?

References

Anic, G.M., E.B. Pathak, J.P. Tanner, M.L. Casper, and L.G. Branch. 2014. Transfer of residents to hospital prior to cardiac death: The influence of nursing home quality and ownership type. *Open Heart* 1(1):e000041.

Castle, N.G. 2008. Nursing home caregiver staffing levels and quality of care a literature review. *Journal of Applied Gerontology* 27(4):375–405.

Centers for Medicare and Medicaid Services. 2012. Design for Nursing Home Compare Five-Star Quality Rating System: Technical Users' Guide. http://www.cms.gov/Medicare/Provider-Enrollment-and-Certification/CertificationandComplianc/downloads/usersguide.pdf

Centers for Medicare and Medicaid Services. 2014. Medicare Provider Utilization and Payment Data: Physician and Other Supplier. http://www.cms.gov/Research-Statistics-Data-and-Systems/Statistics-Trends-and-Reports/Medicare-Provider-Charge-Data/Physician-and-Other-Supplier.html

Dall, T.M., P.D. Gallo, R. Chakrabarti, T. West, A.P. Semilla, and M.V. Storm. 2013. An aging population and growing disease burden will require a large and specialized health care workforce by 2025. *Health Affairs* 32(11):2013–2020.

Godin, J., J. Keefe, E.K. Kelloway, and J.P. Hirdes. 2015. Nursing home resident quality of life: Testing for measurement equivalence across resident, family, and staff perspectives. *Quality of Life Research* 24(10):2365–2374.

Luo, H., X. Zhang, B. Cook, B. Wu, and M.R. Wilson. 2014. Racial/ethnic disparities in preventive care practice among US nursing home residents. *Journal of Aging and Health* 26(4):519–539.

Medicare.gov. 2015. Nursing Home Compare. http://www.medicare.gov/nursinghomecompare/search.html

Mueller, C., G. Arling, R. Kane, J. Bershadsky, D. Holland, and A. Joy. 2006. Nursing home staffing standards: Their relationship to nurse staffing levels. *Gerontologist* 46(1):74–80.

The Relationship between a Quality Measure and Staffing Hours in Nursing Homes

Patricia A. Senk, PhD, RN and Sally K. Koski, PhD, RN

Learning Objectives

- Describe the process of combining multiple data sets for carrying out analytical procedures
- Demonstrate the use of t test, ANOVA, and linear regression to evaluate a quality measure in nursing homes
- Evaluate the effect of adjusted nurse staffing hours per resident per day, nursing home type, and nursing home location on percentage of high-risk long-stay residents with pressure ulcers

Key Terms

Categorical data
Descriptive statistics
Line of best fit
Pairwise comparisons
Simple linear regression
Two-sample t-test
Two-way ANOVA

Improving the quality of healthcare and quantifying health outcomes are important goals in healthcare today. Outcome quality measures are used to capture the health-related outcomes of residents in nursing homes (Bowblis 2011) and are used to quantify the healthcare processes; outcomes; perceptions of patients; and systems and structures of the organization (CMS 2014). The overall goal of quality measures are to provide effective, safe, efficient, patient-centered, equitable, and timely care to residents. CMS (2014) uses quality measures as a means to measure quality improvement, pay for reporting, and reporting to the public. Quality measures can be used by healthcare organizations to change processes of care that can lead to improved patient outcomes.

Mandatory reporting of health outcomes is required for acute-care hospitals, long-term care hospitals, skilled nursing facilities, home healthcare, and outpatient facilities. In 2002, CMS initiated Nursing Home Compare (NHC), a public reporting program about nursing homes (CMS n.d.). NHC, managed by CMS, includes data from over 15,000 Medicare and Medicaid certified nursing homes in the United States (CMS n.d.). The data from the quality measures, in the NHC database, provide information on quality measures as a means for patients, families, and clinicians to compare facilities, make informed decisions about choosing a nursing home, and evaluate the quality of care (CMS, n.d.). Data are collected from nursing homes, using the minimum data set (MDS), which is an assessment completed at regular intervals for each CMS-certified nursing home resident. The MDS focuses on health, physical functioning, mental status, and general well-being; the data are used by the nursing home to plan residents' care needs. NHC rankings provide an unbiased way to assess the services provided and comparison of quality measures between nursing homes (Lutfiyya et al. 2013).

Table 13.1.   NHC quality measures

Long-Stay Resident Quality Measures
Percentage experiencing one or more falls with major injury
Percentage with a urinary tract infection
Percentage who self-report moderate to severe pain
Percentage of high-risk residents with pressure ulcers
Percentage of low-risk residents who lose control of their bowels or bladder
Percentage who have/had a catheter inserted and left in their bladder
Percentage who were physically restrained
Percentage whose need for help with daily activities has increased
Percentage who lose too much weight
Percentage who have depressive symptoms
Percentage assessed and given, appropriately, the seasonal influenza vaccine
Percentage assessed and given, appropriately, the pneumococcal vaccine
Percentage who received an antipsychotic medication
Short-Stay Resident Quality Measures
Percentage who self-report moderate to severe pain
Percentage with pressure ulcers that are new or worsened
Percentage assessed and given, appropriately, the seasonal influenza vaccine
Percentage assessed and given, appropriately, the pneumococcal vaccine
Percentage who are newly administered antipsychotic medications

Source: CMS n.d.

There are thirteen NHC quality measures for long-stay residents (individuals whose cumulative stay is 101 days or greater) and five quality measures for short-stay residents (individuals whose cumulative stay is 100 days or less) (CMS 2014). Refer to table 13.1 for NHC quality measures. NHC data have been used in research to evaluate the effect of staffing patterns on outcome measures (Trinkoff et al. 2013), differences in outcome measures based on rurality (Lutfiyya et al. 2013), quality ratings (Unroe et al. 2012), and influenza vaccine rates (Cai and Temkin-Greener 2011). This chapter focuses on high-risk long-stay residents.

Pressure ulcers are localized skin or tissue injuries that occur due to pressure, and sometimes shear, usually over bony prominences (National Pressure Ulcer Advisory Panel et al. 2014). Preventing the development of pressure ulcers is important in all healthcare settings and guidelines have been developed that focus on prevention. Pressure ulcers have been shown to cause pain and may potentially invoke mood changes, impact self-image, and restrict activities of daily living and social participation (Gorecki et al. 2011). Long-term care settings are federally mandated to properly care for and prevent the development of pressure ulcers, which was established by the federal framework of the Omnibus Budget Reconciliation Act of 1987 (Thomas 2006). Specifically, residents admitted without a pressure ulcer should not develop one, and if a pressure ulcer is present on admission healing should be promoted and additional pressure ulcers should be prevented. NHC includes a quality measure specific to long-term residents that identifies the percentage of high-risk long-term residents with pressure ulcers; the measure includes residents at high risk of developing a pressure ulcer and actually develop a pressure ulcer while in the nursing home (CMS n.d.). This is one of the measures used in this chapter.

Currently, Federal law mandates each nursing home must have at least one registered nurse (RN) on duty for at least eight straight hours a day, seven days a week; either an RN or licensed practical nurse or licensed vocational nurse (LPN/LVN) must be on duty 24 hours per day. Certified nursing assistants (CNAs) provide care to nursing home residents 24 hours per day, 7 days a week. A number of states may have additional staffing requirements (CMS n.d.). For example, Minnesota requires that nursing homes provide the greater of 2 total nursing hours for each resident every 24 hours, or 0.95 hours per standardized resident day (Revisor of Statutes, State of Minnesota 2014). Because RNs, LPNs, and CNAs are generally the largest numbers of personnel in nursing homes, quality care is often equated with staffing levels of these individuals (Wunderlich and Kohler 2001).

CMS collects staffing data on the following: (a) registered nurses (RNs), (b) licensed practical nurses (LPNs), (c) certified nursing assistants (CNA), and (d) physical therapists (CMS n.d.). The NHC database collects nurse staffing data, which include adjusted total nurse staffing hours per resident per day and the adjusted RN total nurse staffing hours per resident per day. The adjusted total nurse staffing hours per resident per day are calculated by adding CNA, LPN, and RN hours per resident per day, and dividing by the total number of residents. The adjusted total RN hours per resident per day are calculated by dividing the total number of RN hours per day by the total number of residents (CMS n.d.). This chapter investigates the influence of adjusted nurse staffing hours per resident per day and the adjusted RN nurse staffing hours per resident per day on one outcome measure.

The relationship between nurse staffing and quality measures in nursing homes has been studied; a number of those studies have identified a link between staffing and overall quality of care in nursing homes (Wellis 2004), but results appear mixed. A recent systematic review did not find consistent results between nursing staffing and nursing home quality measures (Backhaus et al. 2014). A study from the *Journal of the American Geriatrics Society* found nursing homes with higher CNA hours had lower fall rates (Leland et al. 2012). Results from a prospective cohort study suggested that older residents in nursing homes with no RNs but more nursing assistants were more likely to develop pressure ulcers than those residents in nursing homes where there were nurses, but fewer nursing assistants (Kwong et al. 2009). A systematic review of the literature focusing on total nurse staffing and quality indicators found that while the results for pressure ulcers were mixed (some studies indicating a positive association between total nurse staffing and pressure ulcers, others indicating no association between total nurse staffing and pressure ulcer), the total nurse staffing is more likely to result in better overall outcomes (Spilsbury et al. 2011). In a longitudinal study using MDS and Online Survey Certification and Reporting data, results suggest greater levels of RN intensity, care hours per resident per day, were associated with significantly lower rates of pressure ulcers (Konetzka et al. 2008).

Research Question and Hypothesis

Do nurse staffing rates impact the percentage of high-risk long-stay residents with pressure ulcers in nursing home facilities when compared by organization type and location?

To answer a research question dependent and independent variables need to be defined. Because of the nature of this study, the dependent variable will vary depending upon the specific analysis that is being conducted. For example, we will be conducting statistical analyses where pressure ulcer rates are the dependent variable, but we will also conduct a separate analysis where nurse staffing rates are the dependent variable. Give the complexity of this project, it is important to pay close attention to the hypotheses. In the case of the proposed research question and similar to the dependent variables, the independent variables of this study will vary depending upon the specific analysis being conduct. The independent variables will include: adjusted nurse staffing hours per day, adjusted RN staffing hours per day, organization type, and the location of the nursing home.

The analysis for answering the proposed research question will have three parts:

1. Compare the percent of high-risk long-stay residents with pressure ulcers between for-profit, nonprofit, and government-owned nursing homes
2. Compare the rates of adjusted nurse staffing hours per resident per day between for-profit, nonprofit, and government-owned nursing homes
3. Determine if there is a correlation between the percent of high-risk long-stay residents with pressure ulcers and adjusted nurse staffing hours per resident per day across for-profit, nonprofit, and government-owned nursing homes

Given the research question, several hypotheses are proposed and will be tested. The hypotheses should be stated as a null (H_0) and alternative (H_A). Since our research question includes more than one independent variable the null and alternative hypotheses are developed using the dependent variable separately with each independent variable. Because the research question is measuring the percentage of high-risk nursing home residents with pressure ulcers and staffing rates for different groups of nursing homes (that is, ownership and location of nursing home), there are more than one set of hypotheses.

Hypotheses

The research question will require more than one hypothesis. The hypotheses will include the following:

$H1_0$: The percentage of high-risk long-stay nursing home residents with pressure ulcers is the same between for-profit, nonprofit, and government nursing homes.

$H1_A$: The percentage of high-risk long-stay nursing home residents with pressure ulcers is not the same between for-profit, nonprofit, and government nursing homes.

$H2_0$: The percentage of high-risk long-stay nursing home residents with pressure ulcers is the same between nursing homes located in hospitals and not in hospitals.

$H2_A$: The percentage of high-risk long-stay nursing home residents with pressure ulcers is not the same between nursing homes located in hospitals and not in hospitals.

$H3_0$: The average adjusted nurse staffing hours per resident per day in nursing homes is the same between for-profit, nonprofit, and government nursing homes.

$H3_A$: The average adjusted nurse staffing hours per resident per day in nursing homes is not the same between for-profit, nonprofit, and government nursing homes.

$H4_0$: The adjusted RN staffing hours per resident per day in nursing homes is the same between for-profit, nonprofit, and government nursing homes.

$H4_A$: The adjusted RN staffing hours per resident per day in nursing homes is not the same between for-profit, nonprofit, and government nursing homes.

$H5_0$: There is no relationship between the percentage of high-risk long-stay nursing home residents with pressure ulcers and adjusted nurse staffing hours per resident per day in for-profit, nonprofit, and government nursing homes.

$H5_A$: There is a relationship between the percentage of high-risk long-stay nursing home residents with pressure ulcers and adjusted nurse staffing hours per resident per day in for-profit, nonprofit, and government nursing homes.

Checklist

To answer the research question, a specific process of data acquisition, preparation, and discovery is required. The following steps will be explained in detail:

1. Extract data sets from MySQL
   a. Select required columns of data from database
   b. Join columns of data using MySQL queries
2. Data preparation with Microsoft Excel
   a. Review data for erroneous values
   b. Modify column headers
3. Import the data into R
4. Conduct descriptive statistics
5. Conduct statistical procedures: two-sample t-test, two-way ANOVA, and linear regression

The Analysis

Now that the research question and hypotheses are written, the data elements are identified, and the appropriate statistical procedures have been determined, the data analysis process can begin.

Step 1: Data Extraction

In order to carry out the analysis, the following data elements are needed. All data required for answering the research question are included in the database associated with this textbook.

- A list of all nursing homes in the United States
- An indicator as to whether the nursing home is for-profit, nonprofit, or government owned
- An indicator as to whether the nursing home is located in a hospital
- A measure of adjusted nurse staffing hours per day per nursing home resident
- A measure of adjusted RN staffing hours per day per nursing home resident

Two data sets need to be combined to obtain the needed data to answer the proposed research question. The first data set is named nursing_home_provider_info, and the second data set is named nursing_home_quality_measures.

The two data sets will be combined using MySQL scripts (see figure 13.1). The scripts will be constructed so that only the following data elements are extracted: nursing home NPI, quality measure code and description, detailed nursing home ownership and ownership group, whether the nursing home is located within a hospital, adjusted nurse staffing hours per resident per day, adjusted RN staffing hours per resident per day (figure 13.1).

Figure 13.1 shows the SQL script that combines the two required data sets and extracts only the relevant data elements. For the purpose of this study, two tables of data will be combined: nursing_home_quality_measures and nursing_home_provider_info. In this query, we will be selecting four columns of data. From the nursing_home_provider_info table, provnum, ownership, inhosp, adj_total, and adj_rn are selected. From the nursing_home_quality_measures table, msr_cd, msr_descr, and measure_score_3qtr_avg are selected. In our query, we can change the name of the measure_score_3qtr_avg column by including the AS after selecting the column. After the AS function, you are required to specify the new name of the column. A JOIN is also required in order to combine the two tables of data. The ON function specifies which two fields of data in our two tables match. This used to JOIN the two tables by finding matches between the matching fields. In this case, the

Figure 13.1. SQL script and returned data for combining two data sets

```
SELECT
nursing_home_provider_info.provnum,
nursing_home_quality_measures.msr_cd,
nursing_home_quality_measures.msr_descr,
nursing_home_quality_measures.measure_score_3qtr_avg
    AS avg_value,
nursing_home_provider_info.ownership,
nursing_home_provider_info.inhosp,
nursing_home_provider_info.adj_total,
nursing_home_provider_info.adj_rn
FROM
nursing_home_quality_measures
JOIN
nursing_home_provider_info
ON
nursing_home_quality_measures.nursing_home_provider_info_id= nursing_home_
provider_info.nursing_home_provider_info_id
WHERE
nursing_home_quality_measures.msr_cd=403
AND
nursing_home_quality_measures.measure_score_3qtr_avg>0
AND
nursing_home_provider_info.adj_total>0;
```

(Continued)

Figure 13.1.   SQL script and returned data for combining two data sets *(Continued)*

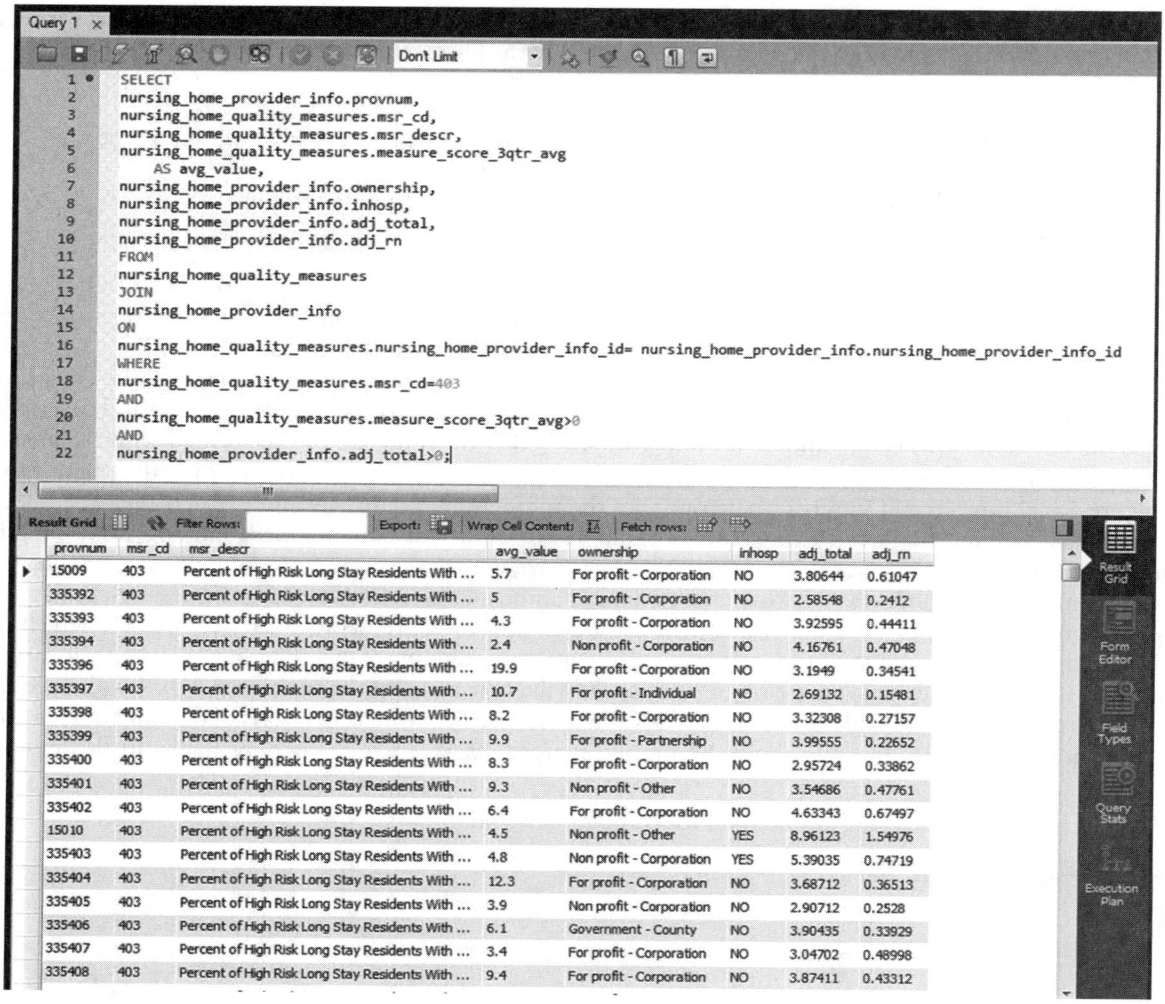

patching field is nursing_home_provider_info_id. Finally, the WHERE statement is used to specify that we only want to query data when msr_cd is equal to 403, measure_score_3qtr_avg is greater than zero, and adj_total is greater than zero. The top section of figure 13.1 depicts the MySQL script that was used to obtain the data. The bottom section of the figure depicts the first few rows of the output that was derived from the query.

Note that you must alter a setting in MySQL so that the output shows all of the results rather than just showing the first 1,000 rows (see chapter 4). After executing the query, export the data to a CSV file and save the file as nurse_staff. For detailed instructions regarding exporting data from MySQL Workbench to CSV format, see chapter 4.

Step 2: Data Preparation

Data preparation can be the most labor-intensive and, arguably, the most important step in the analytics process. The purpose of data preparation is to ensure the correct data, in the correct format, is used for the analysis. Open the nurse_staff.csv file that was exported from MySQL Workbench with Excel. You should see the following columns of data:

- provnum: The unique provider id
- msr_cd: A code for the performance measure
- msr_descr: A description of the performance measure
- avg_value: The percent of high-risk long-stay residents with pressure ulcers

- ownership: The ownership type of the provider including:
  - For-profit—corporation
  - For-profit—Individual
  - For-profit—Limited liability company
  - For-profit—Partnership
  - Government—City
  - Government—City/County
  - Government—County
  - Government—Hospital district
  - Government—State
  - Nonprofit—Church-related
  - Nonprofit—Corporation
  - Nonprofit—Other
- inhosp: Identifies whether the provider resides in a hospital; takes on a value of YES or NO
- adj_total: The adjusted total nurse staffing hours per resident per day, including certified nursing practitioner (CNA), license practicing nurse (LPN), and registered nurse (RN)
- adj_rn: The adjusted RN staffing hours per resident per day

Renaming Column Headers

Several data elements will be used in this chapter to answer the research question. The data elements that were extracted from MySQL Workbench have column names that are not particularly informative for understanding what variable we are working with for a specific analysis. To make the data easier to work with in RStudio, we will simply rename the column headers. Given the fact that RStudio is case sensitive, we will ensure that the revised names are all in lowercase. This will help to prevent errors that would otherwise occur if you tried to call a variable using the wrong case sensitivity. To rename column headers in Excel, simply click each individual cell, highlight the contents, delete the content, enter the new column name, and hit return. Repeat this process for each column header. The old and new column headers are listed in table 13.2.

Reviewing Data Sets for Erroneous Values

One of the first steps in data preparation is to carefully examine if the data include erroneous values or blanks. The CSV that was exported from MySQL does not include any erroneous values or blanks, but it is still important to review the data set for errors and issues.

Recoding a Variable in Excel

After you have reviewed the data for accuracy and completeness, you need to create a new column of data. For the purpose of this chapter one of the objectives is to compare the nursing staffing measures and percentage of high-risk long-stay residents with pressure ulcers between the different provider ownership types. However, the ownership column of data includes 10 different types. Consequently, with such a large number of groups,

Table 13.2.   Original and revised column names within Excel

Original Name	Revised Name
provnum	provnum
msr_cd	msr_cd
msr_descr	msr_descr
avg_value	ulcer
ownership	owner
inhosp	hosp
adj_total	total
adj_rn	rn

this will result in a small sample size for some of the ownership status. For example, there are only three providers in the Government—Federal group. When there are groups with very small sample sizes, this limits the quality of the analysis and also may limit the generalization of the findings. To improve the analysis, we are going to recode the owner column of data. The objective is to regroup the ownership status into three groups: for-profit, nonprofit, and government. We will group the providers based on the existing ownership status. In Excel, this task can be carried out using an IF statement.

The first step is to create a new column. The new column will be created to the right of the existing owner column. To insert a new column right click on the F column header. Next, select Insert. This will generate a blank column of data to the right of the existing owner column. Add a header to that column by typing owner_group in cell F1. In cell F2, we will enter the following formula to recode the owner column:

```
=IF(ISNUMBER(SEARCH("For profit",E2)),"For profit",IF(ISNUMBER(SEARCH
("Non profit",E2)),"Non profit",IF(ISNUMBER(SEARCH("Government",E2)),
"Government","")))
```

This formula will search for specific text in part of cell E2. When the text is found, the function will return an output. For instance, if the ownership status contains the words "for profit" the ownership status will be recoded to just "for profit." If the ownership status contains the word "nonprofit" the ownership status will be recoded to just "nonprofit." If the ownership status contains the word "government" the ownership status will be recoded to just "government." Figure 13.2 displays a screenshot of the Excel spreadsheet with this formula displayed in the formula toolbar.

After recoding the data, the data preparation phase is complete. Remember to save the file as a CSV. In Excel, click File > Save As. Under the Format drop-down window, select the Comma Separated Values option. When saving the file, name the document nurse_staff and save the file to your computer's desktop. When saving your file, you may receive a message:

Some features in your workbook might be lost if you save it as CSV (Comma defined). Do you want to keep using that format?

Figure 13.2.   A screenshot of Excel after recoding the owner column

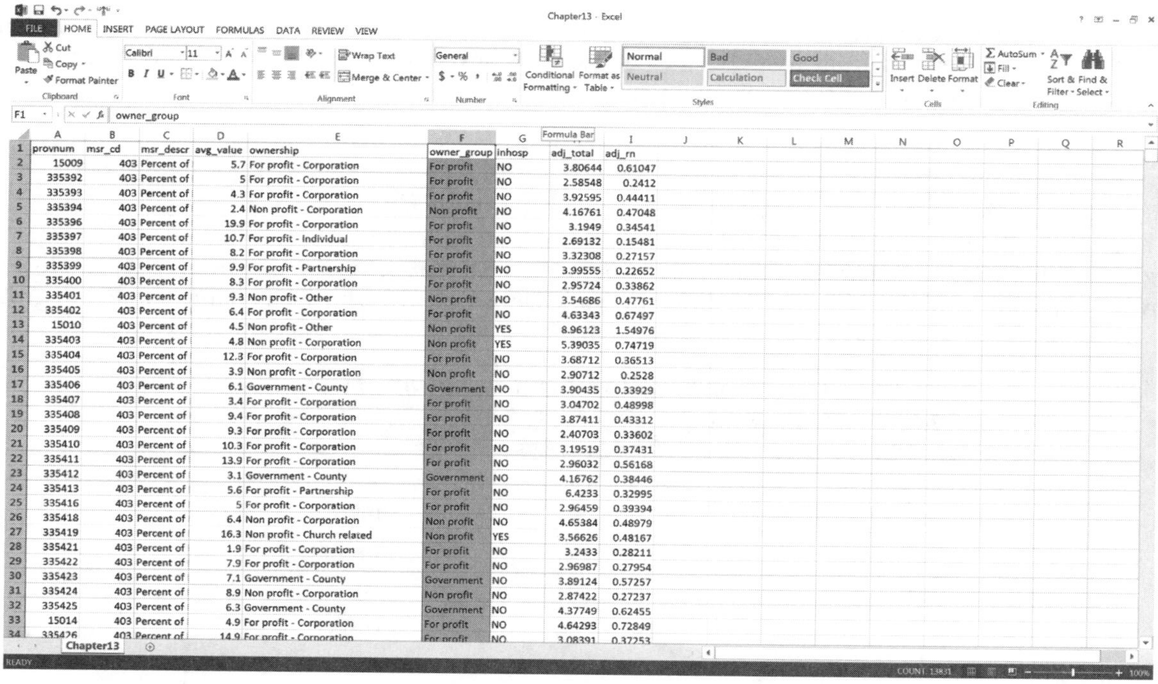

Source: Used with permission from Microsoft.

The reason Excel provides this warning is that only the active spreadsheet in your Excel workbook will be saved. If you have additional worksheets included in your file, those spreadsheets will be lost—in short, only the worksheet that is open when you save the file is retained. Click OK or Yes.

We are now ready to import the data into RStudio.

Step 3: Import the Data

Importing data into RStudio is a relatively straightforward process (see chapter 5 for detailed instructions for importing data into RStudio). To import the CSV file that was prepared for the analysis under Step 2, click Import Dataset and choose the From Text File option in the drop-down window. Navigate to the nurse_staff. csv file that was saved, highlight the file, and click Open.

After the data are imported into RStudio, open an R scripting window. The R scripting window is where you will enter the R code in order to analyze the data. To open a new R scripting window, go to File > New File > R Script. The first step is to attach the data set. The reason that the data set is attached is to make the column names accessible in RStudio. Without the use of the attach function, the only way to work with the data by the column names is to specify the name of the data frame followed by a dollar sign and the name of the column. For example, if a data set named AllData was imported into RStudio and there was a need to call out the column Age without attaching the data, a user would be required to use the following script: `AllData$Age`. If the data set is attached, a user can simply call the column by its name: Age.

To attach the data, run the following R script into the console:

```
attach(nurse_staff)
```

Step 4: Descriptive Statistics

Once the data are imported and attached into RStudio, the first type of analysis that should be conducted to familiarize yourself with the data is the **descriptive statistics**. Descriptive statistics simply refer to "a set of statistical techniques used to describe data such as means, frequency distributions, and standard deviations; statistical information that describes the characteristics of a specific group or population" (White 2013, 241).

The data we are using to answer our research question include categorical data. **Categorical data** are calculated by counting the frequency of data that occur in different categories. In this case, there are two categorical data elements: owner_group and hosp. In RStudio, the table function can be used to obtain a frequency of a data element broken down into groups.

The data element owner_group has three categories: *For profit*, *Non profit*, and *Government*. Using the table function in RStudio, the number of nursing homes that fall into each category can be obtained by running the following:

```
table(owner_group)
```

The output from this function is the following:

```
owner_group
For profit Government Non profit
9925        771        3134
```

The output tells us that there were 9,925 nursing homes that were for-profit, 3,134 that were nonprofit, and 771 that were government owned.

The same function can be used to get a frequency of each group listed under the hosp data element:

```
table(hosp)
```

The output from this function is as follows:

```
hosp
  NO     YES
13363   467
```

This output shows that the number of nursing homes located in hospitals was equal to 467. Therefore, there were many more nursing homes located outside of hospitals than within.

Cross-tabulations, also known as contingency tables, are simply a table of frequency distributions (a table that displays the number of times an observation occurs). Cross-tabulations can be beneficial for comparing the frequency of providers when defining two groups. For instance, if we wanted to know the adjusted overall nurse staffing hours per resident per day for nursing homes for each of the three different ownership types, the tapply function could be used in R:

```
tapply(total,owner_group,mean)
```

The output from this function is the following:

```
For profit Government Non profit
3.775913    4.432033   4.244119
```

The results show government-owned nursing homes have the highest adjusted nurse staffing hours per resident per day and for-profit nursing homes have the lowest. Despite these findings, we still need to conduct a statistical analysis to determine if these observed differences are statistically significant.

Another cross-tabulation that must be completed is to explore the adjusted RN staffing hours per resident per day across these same three nursing home types. The information we retrieve from the following cross-tabulation will allow us to determine if the average adjusted RN staffing hours appears to be different between for-profit, nonprofit, and government-owned nursing homes:

```
tapply(rn,owner_group,mean)
```

The output from this function is the following:

```
For profit Government Non profit
0.497240    0.656642   0.633487
```

The output shows similar results to the adjusted nurse staffing hours per resident per day. Government-owned nursing homes have the highest adjusted nurse staffing hours per resident per day (0.656642), and for-profit nursing homes have the lowest (0.497240). A statistical analysis is required in order to empirically determine if the differences in the adjusted nurse staffing hours per resident per day are statistically significantly different between nursing home types.

We also want to compare adjusted nurse staffing hours per resident per day and adjusted RN staffing hours per resident per day between nursing homes within hospitals and outside of hospitals. Again, this information will allow us to determine if total nursing staffing hours and RN staffing hours appear to be different between those nursing homes within hospitals versus those outside hospitals. Each of the following scripts should be run separately:

```
tapply(total,hosp,mean)

     NO         YES
     3.898344   4.497917

tapply(rn,hosp,mean)

     NO         YES
     0.5305379  0.7219457
```

The output shows that nursing homes located in hospitals have a higher rate of adjusted nurse staffing hours per resident per day (4.497917) and a higher adjusted RN staffing hours per resident per day (0.7219457). A statistical analysis is required in order to empirically determine if the differences in the adjusted nurse staffing hours per resident per day and adjusted RN staffing hours per resident per day are statistically significantly different for nursing homes located in hospitals.

The last three cross-tabulations we want to conduct relate to the percentage of high-risk long-stay residents with pressure ulcers across nursing homes by ownership type and by location within hospitals. Each of the following scripts should be run separately:

```
tapply(ulcer,owner_group,mean)

    For profit    Government   Non profit
    6.489441      6.067315     5.720166

tapply(ulcer,hosp,mean)

    NO            YES
    6.272828      6.828266
```

The output indicates that nonprofit nursing homes have the lowest percentage of high-risk long-stay residents with pressure ulcers (5.720166) and for-profit nursing homes have the highest percentage (6.489411). The output also indicates that nursing homes located within hospitals have higher percentages of high-risk long-stay residents with pressure ulcers (6.828266) than nursing homes not located within hospitals (6.272828). A statistical analysis is required in order to empirically determine if the differences in the percentages of high-risk long-stay residents with pressure ulcers have statistically significant differences between nursing home types.

Step 5: Statistical Analyses

As mentioned in the research question and hypotheses section, we need to conduct three statistical procedures to determine the following:

1. Is the percentage of high-risk long-stay residents with pressure ulcers different between for-profit, nonprofit, and government nursing homes?
2. Is the percentage of high-risk long-stay residents with pressure ulcers different for nursing homes located within hospitals?
3. Is the adjusted nurse staffing hours per resident per day different between for-profit, nonprofit, and government nursing homes?
4. Is the adjusted RN staffing hours per resident per day different between for-profit, nonprofit, and government nursing homes?
5. Is the adjusted nurse staffing hours per resident per day different for nursing homes located within hospitals?
6. Is the adjusted RN staffing hours per resident per day different for nursing homes located within hospitals?
7. Is there a relationship between adjusted nurse staffing hours per resident per day and percentage of high-risk long-stay residents with pressure ulcers?

To answer these questions, statistical procedures need to be conducted that can handle continuous data. A two-sample t-test, two-way ANOVA, and simple linear regression are the appropriate procedures to use in this situation. A **two-sample t-test** is used to determine if two groups are different than each other. For the purpose of this project, the two-sample t-test can be used to test whether the adjusted nurse staffing hours per resident per day, adjusted RN staffing hours per resident per day, and percentage of high-risk long-stay residents with pressure ulcers are statistically significantly different for nursing homes in hospitals compared to those not located in hospitals (that is, the two groups for the t-test are based upon location—in hospital or not in hospital). The assumptions for the two-sample t-test include that the dependent variable for each group is normally distributed and the variance should be equal between the two groups.

The **two-way ANOVA** can be used to test if more than two groups are different from each other. For the purpose of this project, the two-way ANOVA can be used to test whether the adjusted nurse staffing hours per resident per day, adjusted RN staffing hours per resident per day, and percentage of high-risk long-stay residents with pressure ulcers are statistically significantly different for nursing homes that are for-profit, nonprofit, and government owned (that is, the three groups for the ANOVA are based upon ownership type). The assumptions for the two-way ANOVA include that the dependent variable for each of the groups is normally distributed and there is equal variance between the groups (White 2013).

A **simple linear regression** is used to test if there is a relationship between two quantitative variables. The simple linear regression can be used to test if there is a relationship between adjusted nurse staffing hours per resident per day and the percentage of high-risk long-stay residents with pressure ulcers. The assumptions for the simple linear regression include that there is independence between the variables you are comparing, there are not significant outliers, and that the residuals have a mean of zero and equal variance.

To begin, we will use RStudio to conduct three two-sample t-tests to compare for significant differences between nursing homes in hospitals versus nursing homes not located in hospitals for each of the three dependent variables of percentage of high-risk long-stay residents with pressure ulcers, adjusted nurse staffing hours per resident per day, and RN staffing rates. Each of the two-sample t-tests need to be run separately. The following is the code and output for the t-test for comparing the average percentage of high-risk long-stay residents with pressure ulcers by the nursing home location:

```
t.test(ulcer~hosp,paired=F)

Welch Two Sample t-test
data: avg_value by hosp
t = -2.0759, df = 480.564, p-value = 0.03844
alternative hypothesis: true difference in means is not equal to 0
95 percent confidence interval:
 -1.08118821 -0.02968692
sample estimates:
 mean in group NO mean in group YES
   6.272828  6.828266
```

The following is the code and output for the t-test for comparing the average adjusted nursing staffing hours per resident per day by the nursing home location:

```
t.test(total~hosp,paired=F)

     Welch Two Sample t-test
data: total by hosp
t = -12.4553, df = 484.338, p-value < 2.2e-16
alternative hypothesis: true difference in means is not equal to 0
95 percent confidence interval:
 -0.6941583 -0.5049881
sample estimates:
 mean in group NO mean in group YES
   3.898344  4.497917
```

The following is the code and output for the t-test for comparing the average RN staffing rates by the nursing home location:

```
t.test(rn~hosp,paired=F)

      Welch Two Sample t-test
data: rn by hosp
t = -10.4486, df = 477.57, p-value < 2.2e-16
alternative hypothesis: true difference in means is not equal to 0
95 percent confidence interval:
 -0.2274036  -0.1554120
sample estimates:
 mean in group NO mean in group YES
   0.5305379 0.7219457
```

The RStudio output includes a variety of information. It includes the specific statistical procedure that was conducted (Welch two-sample t-test). It summarizes the data that were compared by variable name (for example, avg_value by inhosp). It also provides the test statistic (t), the degrees of freedom (df), and the p-value. The output also includes the alternative hypothesis for the test, the 95 percent confidence interval, and the sample estimates for each group. For the purposes of the text, we will be focusing primarily on the p-value, which is the value that demonstrates statistical significance based upon a predetermined significance level. R defaults to 0.05 as the significance level. If the p-value is lower than the significance level, we reject the null hypothesis and conclude that there is a significant difference.

The p-value for the first test (p < 0.05) suggests that there is enough evidence to reject the null hypothesis and conclude that nursing homes located in hospitals have significantly higher rates of high-risk long-stay nursing home residents with pressure ulcers. The p-values for following two tests (p < 0.001) suggest that there is very strong evidence to reject the null hypotheses and conclude that nursing homes in hospitals have significantly higher nurse staffing hours per resident and RN staffing hours per resident.

The next step is to use RStudio to conduct a two-way ANOVA to test for significant differences between nursing home by ownership types (for-profit, nonprofit, and government) for each of our three dependent variables of percentage of high-risk long-stay residents with pressure ulcers, adjusted nurse staffing per resident per day, and adjusted RN staffing per resident per day.

There are multiple steps associated with conducting a two-way ANOVA using RStudio. The first step is to name the ANOVA. For example, in the example that follows we named the first ANOVA "anova1a." When you use Rstudio to name this type of analysis, it is required to enter the name followed up the less than sign (<), followed by a hyphen (-). The second step is to write the function for returning the ANOVA given specific data parameters. The R function for ANOVA is aov, and the data elements we are analyzing in this analysis include ulcer, owner_group, and hosp. Thus, the first ANOVA would be developed by writing the following RStudio script:

```
anova1a<-aov(ulcer~owner_group*hosp)
```

The third step is to use RStudio to summarize the results of the ANOVA you have just conducted. The summary would be returned by simply entering the following RStudio script:

```
summary(anova1a)
```

The output from this function is the following:

```
                  Df       Sum Sq   Mean Sq  F value  Pr(>F)
owner_group       2        1451     725.3    48.15    > 2e-16  ***
hosp              1        450      449.7    29.85    4.74e-08 ***
owner_group:hosp  2        586      293.0    19.45    3.66e-09 ***
Residuals         13824    208253   15.1
---
Signif. codes:  0 '***' 0.001 '**' 0.01 '*' 0.05 '.' 0.1 ' ' 1
```

The ANOVA output includes the degrees of freedom (DF) for each variable, the sum of squares (Sum Sq), the mean of squares (Mean Sq), the test statistic (F value), and the p-value (Pr(>F)). This text will primarily focus on the p-value for determining statistical significance. Using the previous output as an example, we see significant findings in all three categories because the p-value is less than 0.05. There are significant differences by organization type, by location in hospitals, and we see an interaction between ownership type and location in hospitals. However, this output does not tell us precisely where the significant differences are, only that there are significant differences.

The fourth step is to use RStudio to conduct a post-hoc test to determine significant differences between means for each specific group (for example, it compares for-profit nursing homes in hospitals to every other nursing home type and location). The post-hoc test would be returned by simply entering the following RStudio script:

```
TukeyHSD(anova1a, ordered=T)
```

The output from this function is the following:

```
     Tukey multiple comparisons of means
     95% family-wise confidence level
     factor levels have been ordered

  Fit: aov(formula = avg_value ~ owner_group * hosp)

  $owner_group
                          diff         lwr          upr          p adj
  Government-Nonprofit    0.3471493    -0.01858118  0.7128797    0.0670824
  For profit-Non profit   0.7692749    0.58286563   0.9556841    0.0000000
  For profit-Government   0.4221256    0.08199518   0.7622561    0.0101557
```

```
$hosp

          diff         lwr          upr          p adj
YES-NO   0.9570142    0.5988641    1.315164     2e-07

$`owner_group:hosp`
                                    diff         lwr          upr          p adj
Government:NO-Non profit:NO         0.2415540    -0.2472296   0.7303376    0.7219327
Non profit:YES-Non profit:NO        0.5463174    -0.1521005   1.2447353    0.2242014
For profit:NO-Non profit:NO         0.7970736    0.5621528    1.0319943    0.0000000
Government:YES-Non profit:NO        1.0468196    0.1112674    1.9823718    0.0179334
For profit:YES-Non profit:NO        5.2388831    3.5769090    6.9008571    0.0000000
Non profit:YES-Government:NO        0.3047634    -0.4959194   1.1054462    0.8876211
For profit:NO-Government:NO         0.5555196    0.0989091    1.0121300    0.0069784
Government:YES-Government:NO        0.8052656    -0.2089155   1.8194466    0.2094500
For profit:YES-Government:NO        4.9973291    3.2898563    6.7048018    0.0000000
For profit:NO-Non profit:YES        0.2507562    -0.4255361   0.9270484    0.8983481
Government:YES-Non profit:YES       0.5005022    -0.6297374   1.6307417    0.8056629
For profit:YES-Non profit:YES       4.6925657    2.9137061    6.4714252    0.0000000
Government:YES-For profit:NO        0.2497460    -0.6694067   1.1688986    0.9718521
For profit:YES-For profit:NO        4.4418095    2.7890114    6.0946076    0.0000000
For profit:YES-Government:YES       4.1920635    2.3074384    6.0766886    0.0000000
```

The Tukey HSD post-hoc test returns a substantial amount of information. First, it provides a summary of the post hoc test and summarizes the original ANOVA. It then conducts **pairwise comparisons** of differences in means for each of the independent variables (that is, owner_group and hosp). Pairwise comparisons provide statistical differences for each group against each other group. For example, government versus non-profit or nonprofit versus for-profit. It also provides the difference in observed means for each comparison (diff), the lower end point of the interval (lwr), the upper end of the interval (upr), and the adjusted p-value after each comparison (p adj).

Based upon these results, we can conclude that there are significant differences between for-profit and government nursing, as well as between for-profit and nonprofit nursing homes, regarding rates of high-risk long-stay nursing home residents with pressure ulcers. There is not a significant difference between nonprofit and government nursing homes because the p-value is greater than 0.05. We can also conclude there are significant differences in regarding rates of high-risk long-stay nursing home residents with pressure ulcers based upon location within hospitals.

When we look at the last section of the output ($`owner_group:hosp`), we are able to see the pairwise comparisons between nursing home ownership and location within a hospital or not. Under this category, we see eight significant differences (those pairwise comparison where the p-value is less than 0.05):

```
For profit:NO-Non profit:NO, For profit:YES-Non profit:NO, For profit:
NO-Government:NO, For profit:YES-Government:NO, For profit:YES-Non
profit:YES, For profit:YES-For profit:NO, For profit:YES-Government:YES
```

Because the p-value from this test is less than 0.05, we have enough evidence to reject our null hypothesis that the average adjusted nurse staffing hours per resident per day in nursing homes is the same between for-profit, nonprofit, and government nursing homes. Therefore, we can conclude that there is a significant difference between for-profit nursing homes (both within hospitals and not) and nonprofit and government nursing homes.

Let us now conduct a two-way ANOVA to test for significant differences between nursing home ownership types (for-profit, nonprofit, and government) and overall nurse staffing rates using these same four steps. The following are the RStudio scripts and output:

```
anova2a<-aov(total~owner_group*hosp)
summary(anova2a)
```

```
                    Df      Sum Sq  Mean Sq  F value  Pr(>F)
owner_group         2       737     368.7    654.57   > 2e-16  ***
hosp                1       30      30.2     53.68    2.49e-13 ***
owner_group:hosp    2       14      6.8      12.08    5.72e-06 ***
Residuals           13824   7787    0.6
---
Signif. codes: 0 '***' 0.001 '**' 0.01 '*' 0.05 '.' 0.1 ' ' 1

TukeyHSD(anova2a, ordered=T)

Tukey multiple comparisons of means
 95% family-wise confidence level
 factor levels have been ordered

Fit: aov(formula = total ~ owner_group * hosp)

$owner_group
                             diff        lwr       upr       p adj
Non profit-For profit        0.4682057   0.4321606 0.5042509 0
Government-For profit        0.6561197   0.5903501 0.7218892 0
Government-Non profit        0.1879139   0.1171942 0.2586336 0

$hosp
             diff          lwr           upr         p adj
YES-NO       0.2481434     0.1788895     0.3173973   0

$'ownership_group:inhosp'         diff        lwr           upr         p adj
Non profit:NO-For profit:NO       0.45963942  0.414213822   0.5050650   0.0000000
Government:NO-For profit:NO       0.57579200  0.487499229   0.6640848   0.0000000
Non profit:YES-For profit:NO      0.58912113  0.458349450   0.7198928   0.0000000
For profit:YES-For profit:NO      0.61653173  0.296937397   0.9361261   0.0000006
Government:YES-For profit:NO      1.01176383  0.834031302   1.1894964   0.0000000
Government:NO-Non profit:NO       0.11615258  0.021638627   0.2106665   0.0061556
Non profit:YES-Non profit:NO      0.12948170  -0.005568304  0.2645317   0.0690270
For profit:YES-Non profit:NO      0.15689231  -0.164476344  0.4782610   0.7323069
Government:YES-Non profit:NO      0.55212441  0.371220773   0.7330280   0.0000000
Non profit:YES-Government:NO      0.01332913  -0.141495394  0.1681536   0.9998795
For profit:YES-Government:NO      0.04073973  -0.289426799  0.3709063   0.9992964
Government:YES-Government:NO      0.43597183  0.239864074   0.6320796   0.0000000
For profit:YES-Non profit:YES     0.02741061  -0.316559680  0.3713809   0.9999177
Government:YES-Non profit:YES     0.42264270  0.204093233   0.6411922   0.0000005
Government:YES-For profit:YES     0.39523210  0.030810393   0.7596538   0.0244680
```

The p-values listed in the results from this analysis indicate that there is a significant difference between adjusted nurse staffing rates per resident per day by ownership type (for-profit, nonprofit, and government), a significant difference based upon location within a hospital, and also an interaction between ownership type and location within a hospital. Again, based upon the Tukey HSD post-hoc test, we see major significant differences in adjusted nurse staffing hours per resident per day between nonprofit and for-profit nursing homes, as well as between government and for-profit nursing homes. We see less significant differences when comparing government and nonprofit nursing homes, except when comparing those nursing homes within a hospital and those not within a hospital. Nursing homes within hospitals appear to have higher adjusted nurse staffing hours per resident per day.

The final two-way ANOVA will test for significant differences between nursing home ownership types (for-profit, nonprofit, and government) and adjusted nurse staffing hours per resident per day. We will use the same process as above to conduct this two-way ANOVA. After running each of the RStudio scripts separately the following output is returned:

```
anova3a<-aov(rn~owner_group*hosp)
summary(anova3a)

                  Df     Sum Sq  Mean Sq  F value  Pr(>F)
owner_group       2      55.9    27.951   509.524  <2e-16 ***
hosp              1      4.7     4.677    85.258   <2e-16 ***
owner_group:hosp  2      0.2     0.080    1.466    0.231
Residuals         13824  758.4   0.055
---
Signif. codes:  0 '***' 0.001 '**' 0.01 '*' 0.05 '.' 0.1 ' ' 1

TukeyHSD(anova3a, ordered=T)

Tukey multiple comparisons of means
 95% family-wise confidence level
 factor levels have been ordered

Fit: aov(formula = rn ~ owner_group * hosp)

$owner_group
                            diff        lwr         upr         p adj
Non profit-For profit       0.13624698  0.124998100 0.14749586  0.0000000
Government-For profit       0.15940197  0.138876775 0.17992716  0.0000000
Government-Non profit       0.02315499  0.001084965 0.04522502  0.0371004

$hosp
          diff       lwr         upr        p adj
YES-NO    0.0975943  0.07598171  0.1192069  0

$'owner_group:hosp'
                                    diff         lwr           upr         p adj
Non profit:NO-For profit:NO         0.128910585  0.1147342773  0.14308689 0.0000000
Government:NO-For profit:NO         0.136591767  0.1090375803  0.16414595 0.0000000
For profit:YES-For profit:NO        0.145726027  0.0459878243  0.24546423 0.0004504
Non profit:YES-For profit:NO        0.220048621  0.1792377225  0.26085952 0.0000000
Government:YES-For profit:NO        0.259694367  0.2042280439  0.31516069 0.0000000
Government:NO-Non profit:NO         0.007681182  -0.0218144951 0.03717686 0.9766356
For profit:YES-Non profit:NO        0.016815442  -0.0834764860 0.11710737 0.9969228
Non profit:YES-Non profit:NO        0.091138036  0.0489919662  0.13328411 0.0000000
Government:YES-Non profit:NO        0.130783782  0.0743278279  0.18723974 0.0000000
For profit:YES-Government:NO        0.009134260  -0.0939032883 0.11217181 0.9998608
Non profit:YES-Government:NO        0.083456854  0.0351396031  0.13177410 0.0000128
Government:YES-Government:NO        0.123102600  0.0619017807  0.18430342 0.0000002
Non profit:YES-For profit:YES       0.074322594  -0.0330227948 0.18166798 0.3577659
Government:YES-For profit:YES       0.113968340  0.0002405244  0.22769616 0.0491568
Government:YES-Non profit:YES       0.039645746  -0.0285586265 0.10785012 0.5606807
```

Similar to the results from the adjusted nurse staffing hours per resident per day, the p-values of the results indicate that there are significant differences between nursing home ownership types at all levels. The results of the Tukey post-hoc analysis demonstrate that there are significant differences between for-profit nursing homes and nonprofit and government nursing homes regarding adjusted RN staffing hours per resident per day. Again, we see less significant results between government and nonprofit nursing homes, except when the nursing homes are within hospitals—nursing homes within hospitals appear to staff more nurses and more nurses who are RNs.

The final analysis for this study will be to conduct three simple linear regressions using RStudio to determine if there is a relationship between overall nurse staffing rates per resident and average pressure ulcer rates for high-risk long-stay residents in for-profit, nonprofit, and government-owned nursing homes. Similar to conducting a two-way ANOVA, there are multiple steps to conducting a simple linear regression. The first step is to determine which variables you will be including in your analysis. For the purpose of the linear regression, we will need to quantitative variables (ulcer and total). We will be plotting each of those values for each of the ownership types (for-profit, nonprofit, and government).

The second step in the process is to create and name the linear regression in RStudio. The process is very similar to conducting the linear regression. When writing the R script, you must name the linear regression (lin1) followed by the less than sign and a hyphen. You then use the lm R function to tell R to perform a linear regression. The linear regression is testing if average rate of pressure ulcers (avg_value) for for-profit nursing homes is associated with the average RN staffing rate per resident in only for-profit nursing homes. Notice that to limit only to for-profit nursing homes you must use two equal signs in brackets following the variable you are attempting to limit. The following is the RStudio script for the first linear regression

```
lin1<-lm(ulcer[owner_group=="For profit"]~rn[owner_group=="For profit"])
```

At this point, there will not be a summary of the results from the linear regression. Essentially, you have generated your linear model, but have not called for the results to be shown. The third step in the process is to use the summary function to display the results of the linear regression. To do this you use the following RStudio script:

```
summary(lin1)
```

The output from this function is the following:

```
Call:
lm(formula = ulcer[owner_group == "For profit"] ~ rn[owner_group ==
   "For profit"])

Residuals:
Min      1Q       Median   3Q      Max
-6.514   -2.838   -0.623   2.035   38.888

Coefficients:
                           Estimate   Std. Error  t value  Pr(>|t|)
(Intercept)                7.35017    0.09945     73.908   >2e-16  ***
rn[owner_group=="For profit"] -1.73101  0.18391    -9.412   <2e-16  ***
---
Signif. codes: 0 '***' 0.001 '**' 0.01 '*' 0.05 '.' 0.1 ' ' 1

Residual standard error: 3.894 on 9923 degrees of freedom
Multiple R-squared: 0.008849,   Adjusted R-squared: 0.008749
F-statistic: 88.59 on 1 and 9923 DF, p-value: < 2.2e-16
```

The output summarizes the linear regression and the data that were analyzed under Call and provides the summary of the residual statistics. The second section of the model summary (labeled Residuals) presents the regression residuals, also known as errors. As explained in chapter 8, the least squares regression line described is intended to minimize error, so the residuals should be small. The fact that we have very small numbers is a good sign for our model. The next section of the output summarizes coefficient statistics related to the variable of focus (that is, the relationship of pressure ulcers to RN staffing). The statistics include the estimate (Estimate), the standard error (Std. Error), and test statistics (t value), and the p-value (Pr (>|t|). For our purposes we will focus on the p-value for RN, which is less than 0.05 and therefore we can conclude that there is a relationship between percentage of high-risk long-stay residents with pressure ulcers and adjusted RN staffing hours per resident per day in nursing homes. However, we also need to review the statistics in the last section of the output. While the p-value is low, an important step in linear regression is to understand the strength of the association by the R-squared value. The adjusted R-squared value is about 0.009, which is very close to 0. The low R-squared value indicates that the strength of the relationship between pressure ulcers and adjusted RN staffing hours is weak. Therefore, although the relationship between the two variables is significant, the strength of the relationship is weak (see chapter 8 for more information on the linear regression).

The fourth step in the process is to plot the points on a graph using the following RStudio script:

```
plot(ulcer[owner_group=="For profit"]~rn[owner_group=="For profit"],
col="red", xlab="adj_rn", ylab="avg_value")
```

The code is telling RStudio to plot the ulcer and rn data for each nursing home on a plot. We are telling it that each point should be red (col="red"), that the RN data should be on the *x*-axis and the *x*-axis label should read adj_rn (xlab="adj_rn"), and that the pressure ulcer data should be on the *y*-axis and the *y*-axis label should read avg_value (ylab="avg_value"). The output from this script is depicted in figure 13.3.

The fifth step in the process is to add the **line of best fit** to the linear regression plot. The line of best fit is a line on a graph showing the general direction that a group of points seem to be heading. The best fit line is displayed on the graph at a location where the sum of squared residuals is the least. This means that the line is drawn through the points on the graph at a point where the total distance of all the points from the line is as small as possible. To add the line to the plot, simply use the following RStudio script:

```
abline(lin1, col="darkred")
```

Here we are telling R to add the line of best fit to the graph using the abline function using the linear regression model we have produced earlier named lin1 and to make the line dark red (col="darkred"). Figure 13.4 displays the output of the plot with the line.

Figure 13.3.   Linear regression plot of pressure ulcers and RN staffing rates in for-profit nursing homes

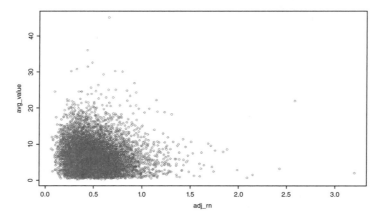

Source: Used with permission from RStudio.

Figure 13.4.   Linear regression plot of pressure ulcers and RN staffing rates in for-profit nursing homes with line of best fit

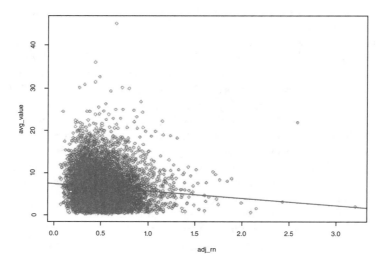

Source: Used with permission from RStudio.

The line shows that there is a weak negative correlation between the percentage of high-risk long-stay residents with pressure ulcers and adjusted RN staffing hours per resident per day in for-profit nursing homes. To complete this analysis we need to replicate these five steps for both nonprofit and government-owned nursing homes. The output of this analysis is as follows:

```
lin2<-lm(ulcer[owner_group=="Non profit"]~rn[owner_group=="Non profit"])

summary(lin2)

Call:
lm(formula = ulcer[owner_group == "Non profit"] ~ rn[owner_group ==
 "Non profit"])

Residuals:
Min      1Q       Median   3Q       Max
-5.460   -2.631   -0.749   1.777    33.638

Coefficients:
                  Estimate   Std. Error   t value   Pr(>|t|)
(Intercept)       6.1791     0.1695       36.449    < 2e-16 ***
rn[owner_group=="Non profit"         -0.7244   0.2457  -2.948 0.00322 **
---
Signif. codes: 0 '***' 0.001 '**' 0.01 '*' 0.05 '.' 0.1 ' ' 1

Residual standard error: 3.757 on 3132 degrees of freedom
Multiple R-squared: 0.002767,   Adjusted R-squared: 0.002449
F-statistic: 8.69 on 1 and 3132 DF, p-value: 0.003223
```

One difference in the process involves the following step. Rather than using the R plot function, we will use the R points function because we will be adding the points from this linear regression to the existing plot. The points function requires that you must specify where points need to be drawn on the graph. To specify where the points must be drawn, include the same arguments that were included when the corresponding linear regression was generating:

```
points(ulcer[owner_group=="Non profit"]~rn[owner_group=="Non profit"],
col="pink")

abline(lin2, col="darkgray")

lin3<-lm(ulcer[owner_group=="Government"]~rn[owner_group=="Government"])
summary(lin3)

Call:
lm(formula = ulcer[owner_group == "Government"] ~ rn[owner_group ==
 "Government"])

Residuals:
Min       1Q        Median    3Q        Max
-5.8017   -2.8584   -0.9475   1.7055    22.6394

Coefficients:
                  Estimate                      Std. Error t value   Pr(>|t|)
(Intercept)       6.6169                        0.3353     19.735    <2e-16 ***
rn[owner_group == "Government"]   -0.8370 0.4578   -1.828    0.0679.
---
Signif. codes: 0 '***' 0.001 '**' 0.01 '*' 0.05 '.' 0.1 ' ' 1

Residual standard error: 4.122 on 769 degrees of freedom
Multiple R-squared: 0.004327,   Adjusted R-squared: 0.003032
F-statistic: 3.342 on 1 and 769 DF, p-value: 0.06792
points(ulcer[owner_group=="Government"]~rn[owner_group=="Government"],
col="darkred")
abline(lin3, col="black")
```

Figure 13.5.   Linear regression output for pressure ulcer rates and RN nurse staffing rates for for-profit, nonprofit, and government nursing homes

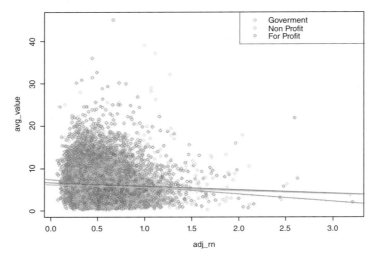

Source: Used with permission from RStudio.

The last step in the entire process is to add a legend to the linear regression graphic for each of the different colors. To add a legend we will use the R legend () function, including telling RStudio exactly where to place the legend (top right), the name of the groups for each hospital ownership status in the order that the text should appear (the first entry will be listed first), and the colors of each entry will be associated with the order they are entered. The last item in the script relates to the point type and size included in the legend (pch=c(1,1,1)). By specifying the 1 in pch, this creates an open circle for each point. The legend will be added using the following code:

```
legend("topright", c("Government","Non Profit", "For Profit"),col=c("black",
"darkgray","darkred"), pch=c(1,1,1))
```

Figure 13.5. displays the output from this script and summarizes the three disparate linear regressions in one graphic.

Discussion

The results of the analysis revealed several findings to discuss in more detail. Analysis was performed to evaluate the relationship of ownership type and nursing home location on the percentage of pressure ulcers. The location of the nursing home only made a difference with the for-profit nursing homes. In other words, when the percentage of pressure ulcers were examined comparing for-profit nursing homes in hospitals and not in hospitals there was a significant increased percentage of pressure ulcers found with for-profit nursing homes located in hospitals. There was not a significant difference in the percentage of pressure ulcers for government nursing homes, or nonprofit nursing homes located in hospitals when compared to the same ownership type not in hospitals. When examining the differences between nursing homes located in hospitals or not in hospitals based on ownership type, analysis showed that there was a statistically significant higher percentages of pressure ulcers when comparing for-profit nursing homes with both government and nonprofit nursing homes located in hospitals and also not in hospitals. Government nursing homes located both in and out of the hospital setting had mean percentages of pressure ulcers that were not significantly different than nonprofit nursing homes. The results need to be interpreted cautiously; researchers and policy makers have found the role of ownership of nursing homes a challenging issue (Stevenson et al. 2013). Simply using the proprietary status of a nursing home may not provide enough detail to evaluate the structure and operational approach of the nursing home. Using ownership data from state licensing agencies might be an option to combine with the NHC data to provide more detail (Stevenson et al. 2013).

The results related to ownership and location, with regard to adjusted nurse staffing showed that government nursing homes located in hospitals and not in hospitals had statistically significant increased adjusted nurse staffing rates when compared to both for-profit and nonprofit nursing homes located in hospitals. In addition, nonprofit nursing homes not located in hospitals had significantly higher adjusted nurse staffing rates when compared to for-profit nursing homes, but when the setting was in hospital the adjusted nurse staffing rates were not statistically different between nonprofit and for-profit nursing homes. When examining the results for ownership and location, with adjusted RN staffing hours, results showed that location (in hospitals, not in hospitals) made a difference. All nursing homes (for-profit, nonprofit, and government) located in hospitals had significantly higher adjusted RN staffing hours when compared with the same nursing home type (for-profit, nonprofit, and government respectively) not in hospitals. When nursing homes were not located in hospitals both nonprofit and government owned had significantly higher adjusted RN staffing hours than for-profit nursing homes. Further analysis of in-hospital nursing homes with regard to adjusted staffing hours and percentage of pressure ulcers is needed. One might expect that increased staffing would decrease the percentage of pressure ulcers. But residents of in-hospital nursing homes may have a higher acuity, which may have an impact on the percentage of pressure ulcers, which was not examined in this analysis.

A linear regression showed that as the number of adjusted RN staffing hours decreased the percentage of pressure ulcers increased, and was found with for-profit and nonprofit nursing homes. These results support a systematic review that found lower pressure ulcers with increased staff (Backhaus et al. 2014). The results of this analysis related to the percentage of pressure ulcers needs to be interpreted cautiously. The NHC database defines the percentage of high-risk residents with pressure ulcers to include residents who are at high risk of developing a pressure ulcer or who develop a pressure ulcer (CMS n.d.). The concepts of risk of developing a pressure ulcer and developing a pressure ulcer are different. Based on this it is difficult to know the exact percentage of residents who developed a pressure ulcer in the nursing home. In addition, a definition for "high risk" was not found in the NHC data dictionary.

There are a number of limitations to be aware of with this study. While the NHC database contains a variety of data on nursing homes, the data themselves are based on self-report. Self-report data may result in reporting bias or reporting errors due to variations in how each individual nursing home reports on the data elements. It is possible the definitions for data elements may change or evolve over time resulting in insufficient or inaccurate reporting. The staffing data may not be indicative of the overall staffing patterns for the facility. Because of a potential delay in the data entry and the ever-changing status of residents (including discharges and admissions), the data included in the NHC database may not necessarily be the most current actual data.

These results and the use of the NHC database provide some directions for future study. The role of location—in hospital and not in hospital—needs further exploration. Research was not found that examined location and the relationship with outcome measures in the nursing homes. Further exploration into factors that may impact the development of pressure ulcers in nursing home residents is warranted, including studies exploring the impact of adjusted CNA staffing hours per resident per day. Additional studies on any or all of the thirteen measures for long-stay residents and the five measures for short-stay residents would add to the knowledge base of quality care in nursing homes for both long and short-stay residents.

Conclusion

The data analysis for this chapter was conducted in order to answer the following research question: Do nurse staffing rates impact the of high-risk long-stay residents with pressure ulcers in nursing home facilities when compared by organization type and location? Additional research questions were developed, along with appropriate hypotheses. The data used to answer the research question were obtained from the Centers for Medicare and Medicaid NHC database. Results from this study suggest that as the adjusted RN staffing hours per resident per day decreased, there was an increase in the percentage of long-stay high-risk residents with pressure ulcers in for-profit, and nonprofit.

Review Exercises

Instructions: Choose the best answer.

1. When using MySQL, the function used to specify which columns of data are linked on one unique variable is called:
   a. SELECT
   b. JOIN
   c. AND
   d. ON

2. In order to create a frequency table using RStudio, what function should be used?
   a. lin1<-
   b. aov()
   c. summary()
   d. tapply()

3. When conducting an analysis of variance, what symbol should you place between two variables to determine if there are interactions between them?
   a. %
   b. $
   c. *
   d. |

4. True or False: In order to conduct pairwise comparisons between groups, the aov() function should be used.

5. True or False: When interpreting the R output from linear regression, the Pr(>|t|) element relates to the residual errors from the model.

References

Backhaus, R., H. Verbeek, E. van Rossum, E. Capezuti, and J.P.H. Hamers. 2014. Nurse staffing impact on quality of care in nursing homes: Systematic review of longitudinal studies. *Journal of the American Medical Directors Association* 15:383–393.

Bowblis, J.R. 2011. Staffing ratios and quality: An analysis of minimum direct care staffing requirements for nursing homes. *Health Services Research* 46(5):1495–1516.

Cai, S. and H. Temkin-Greener. 2011. Influenza vaccination and its impact on hospitalization events in nursing homes. *Journal of the American Medical Directors Association* 12:493–498.

Centers for Medicare and Medicaid Services. 2014. Quality Measures. http://www.cms.gov/Medicare/Quality-Initiatives-Patient-Assessment-Instruments/QualityMeasures/index.html?redirect=/qualitymeasures/03_electronicspecifications.asp

Centers for Medicare and Medicaid Services. n.d. Nursing Home Compare. http://www.medicare.gov/nursinghomecompare/search.html

Gorecki, C., S.J. Closs, J. Nixon, and M. Briggs. 2011. Patient-reported pressure ulcer pain: A mixed-methods systematic review. *Journal of Pain and Symptom Management* 42(3):443–459.

Konetzka, R.T., S.C. Stearns, and J. Park. 2008. The staffing-outcomes relationship in nursing homes. *Health Research and Educational Trust* 43(3):1025–1042.

Kwong, E.W., S.M. Pang, G.H. Aboo, and S.S. Law. 2009. Pressure ulcer development in older residents in nursing homes: Influencing factors. *Journal of Advanced Nursing* 65(12):2608–2620.

Leland, N.E., P. Gozalo, J. Teno, and V. Mor. 2012. Falls in newly admitted nursing home residents: A national study. *Journal of the American Geriatrics Society* 60:939–945.

Lutfiyya, M.N., C.E. Gessert, and M.S. Lipsky. 2013. Nursing home quality: A comparative analysis using CMS Nursing Home Compare data to examine differences between rural and nonrural facilities. *Journal of the American Medical Directors Association* 14:593–598.

National Pressure Ulcer Advisory Panel, European Pressure Ulcer Advisory Panel, and Pan Pacific Pressure Injury Alliance. 2014. *Prevention and Treatment of Pressure Ulcers: Quick Reference Guide*, 2nd ed. Osborne Park, Western Australia: Cambridge Media.

Revisor of Statutes, State of Minnesota. 2014. 2014 Minnesota Statutes. https://www.revisor.mn.gov/statutes/?id=144A.04

Spilsbury, K., C. Hewitt, L. Stirk, and C. Bowman. 2011. The relationship between nurse staffing and quality care in nursing homes: A systematic review. *International Journal of Nursing Studies* 48:732–750.

Stevenson, D.G., J.S. Bramson, and D.C. Grabowski. 2013. Nursing home ownership trends and their impacts on quality of care: A study using detailed ownership data from Texas. *Journal of Aging & Social Policy* 25(1):30–47.

Thomas, D.R. 2006. The new F-tag 314: Prevention and management of pressure ulcers. *Journal of the American Medical Directors Association* 7(8):523–531.

Trinkoff, A.M., K. Han, and C.L. Storr. 2013. Turnover, staffing, skill mix, and resident outcomes in a national sample of US nursing homes. *Journal of Nursing Administration* 43(12):630–636.

Unroe, K.T., M.A. Greiner, C. Colon-Emeric, E.D. Peterson, and L.H. Curtis. 2012. Associations between published quality ratings of skilled nursing facilities and outcomes of Medicare beneficiaries with heart failure. *Journal of the American Medical Directors Association* 13:188.e1–188.e6.

Wellis, J.C. 2004. The case for minimum nurse staffing in nursing homes: A review of the literature. *Alzheimer's Care Quarterly* 5(1):39–51.

White, S. 2013. *A Practical Approach to Analyzing Healthcare Data*, 2nd ed. Chicago, IL: AHIMA.

Wunderlich, G.S. and P.O. Kohler. 2001. Improving the Quality of Long-Term Care (Institute of Medicine Committee on Improving the Quality of Long Term Care). Division of Health Care Services, Washington, DC.

Chapter 14

Studying the Relationship between Primary Care Access and Preventive Care Utilization

Brooke Palkie, EdD, RHIA

Learning Objectives

- Combine three disparate administrative data sources to evaluate elements of hospital emergency department performance and patient satisfaction
- Determine if a relationship exists between the average time a patient waits in the emergency department after the decision to admit the patient and the patient's overall willingness to recommend the hospital to others
- Conduct a one-way ANOVA to assess the differences in emergency department efficiency based on different levels of patient satisfaction
- Utilize the linear regression model to predict the relationship between two variables
- Create graphical displays such as histograms and scatter plots to examine distribution of the data

Key Terms

Boarding
Centers for Medicare and Medicaid Services (CMS)
Crowding
Emergency department (ED) wait time
Emergency Medical Treatment and Labor Act (EMTALA)
Hospital Compare
Hospital Consumer Assessment of Healthcare Providers and Systems (HCAHPS)
National Quality Forum (NQF)
Output
Patient flow
Patient satisfaction
Quality measure
Scatter plot

The **Centers for Medicare and Medicaid Services (CMS)** post emergency department (ED) metrics via the Hospital Compare website for all Medicare participating hospitals. The intent is to hold hospitals accountable for effective and efficient ED patient care. Hospital EDs are a focus of the federal government because many EDs have reported operating at or above capacity (GAO 2009). Unfortunately this issue has not changed as validated by the Hospital-Based Emergency Departments: Background and Policy Considerations Report of 2014 (Heisler and Tyler 2014). The **Emergency Medical Treatment and Labor Act (EMTALA)** was enacted to eliminate discrimination in emergency care and has since become a national health policy with regard to the treatment of all ED patients. The provisions of EMTALA apply to all emergency care patients, not just Medicare beneficiaries. One component of the regulation focuses on timely medical screening examinations (or SME) to determine if an emergency medical condition (EMC) exists (Rosenau and Alexander 2013). Although EDs have made great strides in minimizing the initial time it takes to conduct the SME once a patient arrives to the ED, the reality is that patients are still experiencing crowding within the ED. ED crowding is one of the most common causes of excessive wait times. In 2014, the national average **ED wait time** before being seen by a doctor was 24 minutes (ProPublica 2014). The national average time spent waiting in the ED after admission but waiting to be transferred to an inpatient room is 97 minutes (ProPublica 2014). This period of time can cause overcapacity conditions that can, in turn, delay care.

Capacity problems also affect the way patients pass through the ED, which ultimately contribute to long wait times and crowding. **Crowding** is due to an influx of patients beyond the capabilities of the ED to treat them in a timely fashion (Nugus et al. 2011). One particular problem of crowding can be classified as ED **output**. Output problems are related to discharging patients to their home or to the hospital as an inpatient. Bed shortages are a common result when the issue of crowding intensifies into what the industry considers patient boarding. **Boarding** is considered the time a patient spends remaining in the ED after the decision has been made to either transfer the patient or admit the patient to the hospital.

Another important risk of boarding relates to **patient satisfaction**. EDs play an important role within a local community. According to the Agency for Healthcare Research and Quality (AHRQ), the public places trust and confidence in an organization to provide effective and efficient care (McHugh et al. 2012). Patient satisfaction surveys help to collect and identify how well hospitals provide recommended care to their patients. The **Hospital Consumer Assessment of Healthcare Providers and Systems** (**HCAHPS**) was developed to collect consumer-oriented patient satisfaction information for a hospital. HCAHPS was developed by CMS and AHRQ and has been endorsed by the **National Quality Forum** (**NQF**) as a standardized means for measuring the patient perspective of care.

Hospital Compare was developed through the efforts of Medicare and the Hospital Quality Alliance to publicly report information about quality of care (CMS 2015). Hospital Compare is considered the national standard for comparable data collection and allows for valid comparisons to be made across hospitals by looking at specific aspects of care. The Hospital Compare data are comprised of domains that include, but are not limited to, the aspects of timely and effective care as well as patients' experiences.

Research Question and Hypothesis

Is there a relationship between the average time a patient waits in the emergency department (ED) after the decision to admit the patient and the patient's overall willingness to recommend the hospital?

There are three dependent variables (the measured variables) for this research question: (1) the average percentage of patients not willing to recommend the hospital; (2) the average percentage of patients probably willing to recommend the hospital; and (3) the average percentage of patients willing to recommend the hospital. The independent variable (the comparison variable) will be the average time patients wait in the ED after a decision is made to admit them to the hospital.

Hypotheses

The research question will require more than one hypothesis. The hypotheses will include the following:

$H1_0$: There is not an association between the average time patients wait in the ED after the decision to admit and the percentage of patients not willing to recommend the hospital.

$H1_A$: There is an association between the average time patients wait in the ED after the decision to admit and the percentage of patients not willing to recommend the hospital.

$H2_0$: There is not an association between the average time patients wait in the ED after the decision to admit and the percentage of patients probably willing to recommend the hospital.

$H2_A$: There is an association between the average time patients wait in the ED after the decision to admit and the percentage of patients probably willing to recommend the hospital.

$H3_0$: There is not an association between the average time patients wait in the ED after the decision to admit and the percentage of patients willing to recommend the hospital.

$H3_A$: There is an association between the average time patients wait in the ED after the decision to admit and the percentage of patients willing to recommend the hospital.

Checklist

To answer our research question, a specific process of data acquisition, preparation, and discovery is required. The following steps will be explained in detail:

1. Extract data sets from MySQL
   a. Select the appropriate columns of data
2. Data preparation with Microsoft Excel
   a. Rename column headers to make analysis easier
3. Import the data into RStudio
4. Conduct statistical procedures in RStudio
   a. Conduct descriptive statistics
   b. Use linear regression to examine relationship between variables

The Analysis

This section will provide a step-by-step description of obtaining and analyzing the data required to answer the proposed research question.

Step 1: Data Extraction

In this chapter, we will examine three different data sets. The first data set is titled Timely and Effective Care–Hospital, and is a component of Medicare's Hospital Compare data (CMS 2015). This data set provides hospital-specific data on quality and efficiency for over 4,000 Medicare-certified US hospitals, including variables related to hospital claims, value-based purchasing, hospital readmission, and many other topics. The second data set we will be using is titled HCAPHS–Hospital and is also a component of Medicare's Hospital Compare data (CMS 2015). The data set includes patient survey results that span a wide range of topics such as cleanliness of facilities, patient provider communication, patient understanding of care upon discharge, and many other patient satisfaction-related items. The third data set is called Hospital General Information and is also a component of Medicare's Hospital Compare (CMS 2015). This data set includes geographic information about each hospital in the United States, as well as information such as hospital type and ownership.

The three data sets will be combined using MySQL scripts (as illustrated in figure 14.1). The scripts will be constructed so that only the following data elements are extracted: hospital_general_information. provider_id, timely_and_effective_care.measure_name, timely_and_effective_care.score, hcahps.hcahps_ question, hcahps.hcahps_answer_percent, hcahps.hcahps_measure_id (see figure 14.1). Note that you must alter a setting in MySQL so that the output shows all of the results rather than just showing the first 1,000 rows (see chapter 4). The final step of this process is to export the data as a CSV file. Name the file hcahps_and_efficiency and save it. See chapter 4 for detailed instruction on saving CSV files from MySQL Workbench.

Step 2: Data Preparation

In this chapter, we will do much of our work from within RStudio, but a few preliminary steps will be easier in Excel. Start by loading the files into Excel and examining them. The general structure for each is the same—a listing where each row is an individual hospital. You should see the following columns:

Figure 14.1.   SQL script and returned data for combining three data sets

```sql
SELECT
    hospital_general_information.provider_id,
    timely_and_effective_care.measure_name,
    timely_and_effective_care.score,
    hcahps.hcahps_question,
    hcahps.hcahps_answer_percent,
    hcahps.hcahps_measure_id
FROM
    timely_and_effective_care
JOIN
hospital_general_information ON timely_and_effective_care.provider_id
= hospital_general_information.provider_id
JOIN
    hcahps ON hospital_general_information.provider_id = hcahps.provider_id
WHERE
    hcahps.hcahps_measure_id LIKE '%H_RECMND_%'
        AND timely_and_effective_care.measure_id = 'ED_2b'
        AND timely_and_effective_care.score>0
        AND hcahps.hcahps_answer_percent>0;
```

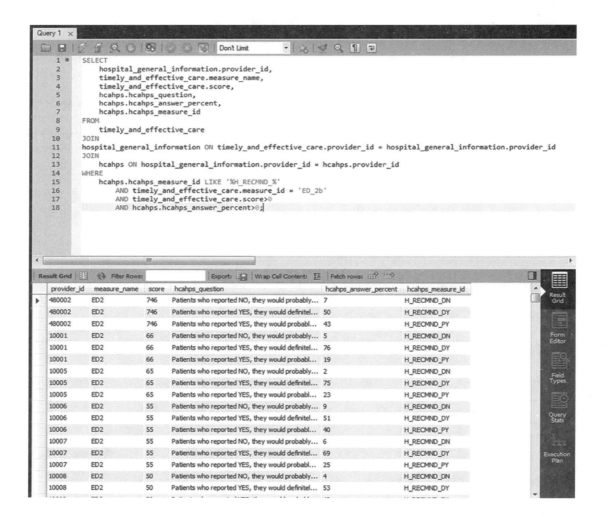

- provider_id: The unique ID for each Medicare-certified hospital in the data set.
- measure_name: The description of the measure name pulled from the timely and effective care table. For the purpose of this chapter, we are focused solely on ED2, which is defined as "admit decision time to ED departure time for admitted patient" (Medicare.gov n.d.).
- score: For the measure of ED2, the column refers to the "average time patients spent in the emergency department after the doctor decided to admit them as an inpatient before leaving the emergency department for their inpatient room" (Medicare.gov n.d.). The measure was developed by CMS and the Joint Commission as a method for the "reduction of overcrowding to reduce poor patient outcomes and compromised patient satisfaction" (Medicare.gov n.d.). The denominator is any ED patient, regardless of age, from the facility's ED and excludes patients placed into observation, patients having a length of stay greater than 120 days, and patients who are not ED patients. The measure's numerator is calculated as time (in minutes) from admit decision time to time of departure from the ED for ED patients admitted to inpatient status.
- hcahps_question: This column includes three different HCAHPS questions of interest for this study, including: Patients who reported YES, they would definitely recommend the hospital; Patients who reported YES, they would probably recommend the hospital; and Patients who reported NO, they would probably not or definitely not recommend the hospital.
- hcahps_answer_percent: Percentage of patients from the particular hospital for each of the three HCAHPS measures: Yes, definitely recommend; Yes, probably recommend; and No definitely or probably not recommend.
- hcahps_measure_id: This column represents the general HCAPHS measure related to the three specific measures of interest for this study. It is defined as "willingness to recommend the hospital (global measure)" (HCAHPS 2015).

Renaming Column Headers in Excel

When we import these data into RStudio, these column header names will become the names of different fields in a data frame. RStudio will do its best working with names that have spaces in them, but it would be better to make each of these field names shorter now while in Excel, rather than changing them in RStudio (or worse, typing long field names in RStudio each time we want to use them). Table 14.1 contains the names we will use when renaming the column headers.

Recoding a Variable in Excel

Now that we have our revised column headers, let us complete one more step to make the data set easier to work with in RStudio. Because the responses in the question column are so long, it can make the output in RStudio difficult to interpret. Create a new column by entering Q_Revised into cell G1. Under the Q_Revised column header that we added, we are going to change the questions to the following: Yes_definitely; Yes_probably; and No. Performing this change is easy using Excel. In the cell directly beneath the Q_Revised column header (cell G2), enter the following Excel function:

```
=IF(F2="H_RECMND_DN","No",IF(F2="H_RECMND_DY",
"Yes_definitely","Yes_probably"))
```

With this Excel function, we are telling Excel that if cell F2—the HCAHPS measure id—contains the text "H_RECMND_DN", then return the word "No." If that condition is found to be false, then test if cell F2 contains the text "H_RECMND_DY" and, if true, return "Yes_definitively." Otherwise, if both conditions are false, return the text "Yes_probably." Once you have input the Excel function, hit enter. Populate the entire column by clicking on cell G2 and double-clicking the auto-fill square in the bottom right hand corner of the cell. Table 14.2 shows the original and revised measure id and names. The purpose of revising the measure names is simply to make the analytics output easier to work with and interpret once we import it into RStudio. Save the file as a CSV file with the title hcahps_and_efficiency and close it.

Step 3: Import the Data

Now you are ready to import the data into RStudio. Select Import Dataset and choose the From Text File option in the drop-down window. Navigate to the hcahps_and_efficiency.csv file that was saved in the final

Table 14.1.   Original and revised column names within Excel

Original Name	Revised Name
Provider id	pid
measure_name	name
score	score
hcahps_question	question
hcahps_answer_percent	percent
hcahps_measure_id	mid

Table 14.2.   Original and revised HCAHPS question names within Excel

Original Name	HCAHPS ID	Revised Name
Patients who reported YES, they would definitely recommend the hospital	H_RECMND_DY	Yes_definitely
Patients who reported YES, they would probably recommend the hospital	H_RECMND_PY	Yes_probably
Patients who reported NO, they would probably not or definitely not recommend the hospital	H_RECMND_DN	No

action of Step 2, highlight the file, and click Open. (For more detailed instruction regarding importing data into RStudio, see chapter 5.) The R code that will populate the RStudio console will be as follows (the file location may vary depending on where you save your file on your computer):

```
hcahps_and_efficiency <- read.csv("~/hcahps_and_efficiency.csv")

View(hcahps_and_efficiency)
```

After the data are imported into RStudio, open an R scripting window. The R scripting window is where you will enter the R code in order to analyze the data. To open a new R scripting window, go to File > New File > R Script. The next step in the importing process is to use the R attach function to load the column names to make it easier to conduct the analysis. We attach the data so that we no longer need to call the name of the data set every time we call a variable or column name. This is particularly useful when we are only working with one data set and do not have the need to differentiate columns between multiple sets. To attach the data, use the following code:

```
attach(hcahps_and_efficiency)
```

Step 4: Descriptive Statistics

Before launching into the statistical modeling and analysis of our data set, we will perform some simple summary and graphical characterizations of the data. One of the first things we want to prepare is a summary of the entire data set by using R's summary function. The summary function allows us to obtain a detailed understanding of the data set we are working with, including the number of rows included in the data set (measure_name) and a breakdown of the frequency of responses to each measure (Q_revised). Here is the code for producing this summary:

```
summary(hcahps_and_efficiency)
```

Output from this function is as follows:

```
pid                          name                    score
Min. : 10001                 ED2:9958                Min.: 1.0
1st Qu.:111327                                       1st Qu.: 63.0
Median :250094                                       Median : 88.0
Mean :262022                                         Mean : 102.6
3rd Qu.:390093                                       3rd Qu.: 127.0
Max. :670082                                         Max. :1026.0
question
Patients who reported NO, they would probably not or definitely not: 3296
Patients who reported YES, they would definitely recommend: 3332
Patients who reported YES, they would probably recommend the hospital: 3330
percent                      mid                     Q_Revised
Min.: 1.00                   H_RECMND_DN:3296         No:3296
1st Qu.: 7.00                H_RECMND_DY:3332         Yes_definitely:3332
Median: 25.00                H_RECMND_PY:3330         Yes_probably :3330
Mean: 33.46
3rd Qu.: 64.00
Max.: 100.00
```

This output provides a quick and easy snapshot of the entire data set. The pid output is irrelevant for our purposes because calculating the mean of a unique hospital ID has no meaning—RStudio sees that it is a number so it is possible to calculate quantitative analysis on it. However, the name variable does provide us with useful information. We see that there are 9,998 observations of the number of minutes between decision to admit and admittance in hospital EDs in this data set. The score variable informs us that the range of values is from 1 to 1,026 (minutes), and the mean is 102 (in short, the average time a patient waits to be admitted to the hospital after the decision has been made in the ED is just over 1.5 hours). The summary also provides us the first and third quartiles, as well as the median.

The other data included in the output relate to the HCAPHS measure of percentage of patients who would recommend the hospital or not. By looking at the Q_revised variable, we can see that there is an almost even distribution of responses for the three variables. The percent variables provides us with a summary of all of the averages for each of the three measures—in other words, this variable does not provide useful information because it includes percentages for both No and Yes responses. The last two variables included in the output (Q_Revised & mid) provide us the same information in the question variable—the number of responses by hospital by question.

We will now explore the breakdown of this number by calculating some descriptive statistics for each of the specific HCAHPS measures. As mentioned previously, the summary of the percent was not meaningful because it included all of the measures in the analysis. To summarize each of the measures individually, we will use RStudio's summary function again but we will specify only to summarize the data for observation when the column for Q_Revised is equal to the specific response we are interested in examining (for example, No). The following scripts will be used to conduct this analysis:

```
summary(percent[Q_Revised=="No"])

summary(percent[Q_Revised=="Yes_probably"])

summary(percent[Q_Revised=="Yes_definitely"])
```

Output from these functions is the following:

```
summary(percent[Q_Revised=="No"])
  Min. 1st Qu.  Median   Mean 3rd Qu.   Max.
 1.000  3.000   5.000  5.356  7.000  28.000

summary(percent[Q_Revised=="Yes_probably"])
```

```
Min. 1st Qu.  Median   Mean   3rd Qu.   Max.
1.00  20.00   24.00    24.84   29.00    64.00

summary(percent[Q_Revised=="Yes_definitely"])
Min. 1st Qu.  Median   Mean   3rd Qu.   Max.
21.00  64.00   71.00    69.88   76.00    100.00
```

This analysis gives us useful information about each measure. For example, around 5.4 percent of US hospital patients would not recommend the hospital (the mean of "No") yet the maximum value in the "No" data set is 28 percent. In short, there is a hospital where 28 percent of patients would not recommend the hospital. This is an area that needs further analysis. The output also shows us that the majority of patients would definitely recommend the hospital (69.9 percent) or probably recommend the hospital (24.8 percent).

We are largely interested in examining if there is a relationship between ED process efficiency and overall patient satisfaction with hospital encounters. To explore this topic, let us create a few plots to graphically explore the data before we begin looking at the data statistically. The first graphic we will create is a histogram of the average number of minutes patients spend between the decision to admit and admission in a US hospital. Creating a histogram for this variable will allow us to determine if the data are normally distributed. Use the following R script to create the histogram:

```
hist(score)
```

The output from this script is shown in figure 14.2. The plot shows that the data are skewed to the right. This means that there are some hospitals that have a higher average time patients spent in the ED after the doctor decided to admit them as an inpatient before leaving the ED for their inpatient room.

We will examine this average time closer by looking at the distribution when broken down by the three groups showing the percentage of patients that would not, probably would, or definitely would recommend the hospital based on the HCAHPS measures.

Figure 14.2.   Histogram of average minutes between the decision to admit in ED to hospital admission

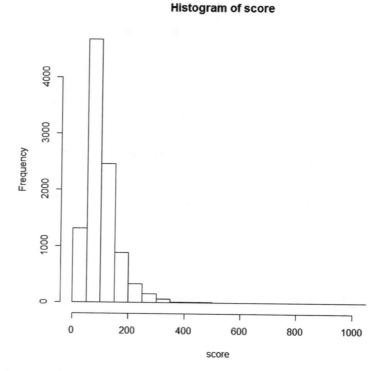

Source: Used with permission from RStudio.

The following are the scripts to create these three histograms in RStudio:

```
hist(percent[Q_Revised=="No"], main="Reported NO, they would probablyn not
or definitely not recommend the hospital", xlab="Percent")

hist(percent[Q_Revised=="Yes_probably"], main="Reported YES, they would
probablyn recommend the hospital", xlab="Percent")

hist(percent[Q_Revised=="Yes_definitely"], main="Reported YES, they would
definitelyn recommend the hospital", xlab="Percent")
```

The histograms from this code are illustrated in figures 14.3 through 14.5 (please note that the charts may look slightly different based on resolution of your screen and the size of the RStudio plot window). The histograms in figure 14.3 show that the HCAPHS measure regarding average patients reporting that they would probably or definitely not recommend the hospital is skewed to the right—the majority of hospitals have between 0 to 5 percent of patients who would probably or definitely not recommend the hospital. The histogram in figure 14.4 is normally distributed and shows that, on average, about 25 percent of patients would probably recommend the hospital. The histogram in figure 14.5 illustrates patients who would definitely recommend the hospital and is very close to a normal distribution with the majority of the hospitals having between 60 and 80 percent of patients reporting definitely recommend.

These histograms show that there is clear variation regarding the percentage of patients willing to recommend a hospital.

Step 5: Statistical Analyses

We are interested in exploring the relationship between hospital efficiency—as measured by the average time between the decision to admit in the ED and admission—and patient willingness to recommend the hospital. The outcome of interest for this study is patient recommendation and the predictor variable is ED efficiency. To examine the relationship between these two variables, we will create four different linear regression models to answer each of the research questions posed.

Figure 14.3. Histogram of average patients reporting they would not recommend the hospital

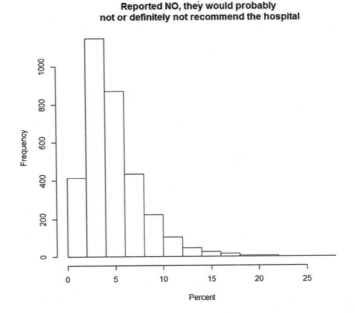

Source: Used with permission from RStudio.

Figure 14.4.   Histogram of average patients reporting they would probably recommend the hospital

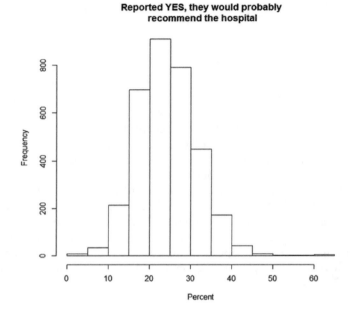

Source: Used with permission from RStudio.

Figure 14.5.   Histogram of average patients reporting they would definitely recommend the hospital

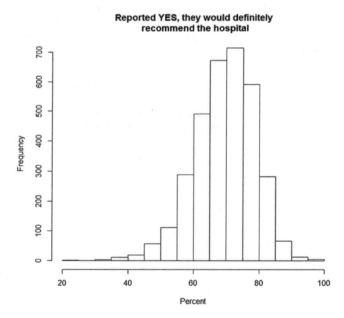

Source: Used with permission from RStudio.

Having graphically explored our data, we need to create a linear regression model predicting ED efficiency and using patient recommendations as the explanatory variable. The first step in conducting a linear regression in RStudio is to name the model and use R's lm function (lm stands for linear model) to create the linear model. Here is the R script for completing this first step:

```
lin1<-lm(score[Q_Revised=="No"] ~ percent[Q_Revised=="No"])
```

Note that we have named the linear model lin1. Following the name we have provided (lin1), we separate the name from the function by a less than sign and a hyphen. We then use the R function lm and are forcing R to predict the score variable (dependent) based upon the percent variable (independent variable) but only including those responses when the data in the Q_Revised column are equal to No.

The next step is to summarize the model by using the following code:

```
summary(lin1)
```

The output of this model is the following:

```
Call:
lm(score[Q_Revised=="No"] ~ percent[Q_Revised=="No"])

Residuals:
   Min      1Q    Median      3Q      Max
-142.39  -38.36  -13.36   24.45   932.64

Coefficients:

                          Estimate  Std. Error  t value  Pr(>|t|)
(Intercept)                81.0413    2.1390     37.89    <2e-16 ***
percent[Q_Revised == "No"]  4.1067    0.3461     11.87    <2e-16 ***
---
Signif. codes:  0 '***' 0.001 '**' 0.01 '*' 0.05 '.' 0.1 ' ' 1

Residual standard error: 61.29 on 3294 degrees of freedom
Multiple R-squared: 0.04099,    Adjusted R-squared: 0.0407
F-statistic: 140.8 on 1 and 3294 DF, p-value: < 2.2e-16
```

The regression equation is y = 81.0 + 4.1x. Based on the equation, the slope of our best-fit line is 4.1x, while the y-intercept is 81.0. Because our slope is a positive number, we know that the observed relationship will be a positive relationship. That is, our line will be sloping upward. For a detailed discussion of linear regression and interpreting RStudio output for linear regression, see chapter 13. The p-value from our linear model tests whether the slope of our best-fit line is significantly different from zero. The p-value from our linear model is <2e-16, which is scientific notation for 0.0000000000000002. If we set our alpha (namely, significant level) to 0.05 (RStudio defaults to this significance level), we observe that our p-value is much lower than 0.05. Therefore, we have enough evidence to reject the null hypothesis, and we can conclude that there is a relationship between the average wait time between the decision to admit and admission in US hospitals and the percentage of patients reporting they would not recommend the hospital. The R-squared value indicates that 4 percent of the variance is explained by the predictor variable. When conducting linear regression, the R-squared value is of critical importance. The R-squared value is a fraction that ranges from –1 to 1. The closer the R-squared value is to –1 or 1, the stronger the relationship between the predictor variable and the outcome. If the R-squared value is 0, there is no relationship between the two variables. Together, the output tells us that there is a significant relationship between the average wait time between the decision to admit and admission in US hospitals and the percentage of patients reporting they would not recommend the hospital because the p-value is less then 0.05; but because the R-squared value is 0.04 we can conclude that the observed association is weak.

The next step in conducting a linear regression is to plot the data points for the linear regression for each hospital on a **scatter plot** (the hospital's average time in minutes between decision to admit and admission by the percentage of patients reporting that they would not recommend the hospital). To create a scatter plot in RStudio, use the following R script:

```
plot(score[Q_Revised=="No"]~percent[Q_Revised=="No"], xlab="Percent who
said NO", ylab="Time")
```

The output of this code is shown in figure 14.6.

The plot's y-axis is the time in minutes between the decision to admit and admission and the x-axis represents the percentage of patients reporting that they would not recommend the hospital.

Figure 14.6.   Scatter plot showing the association between the time to admit and the percentage of patients reporting they would not recommend the hospital

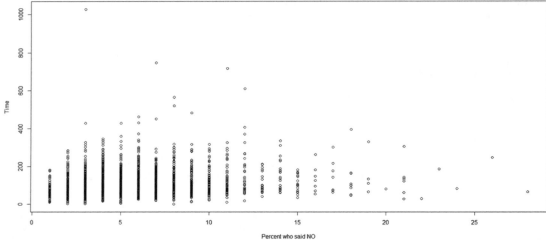

Source: Used with permission from RStudio.

The next step in the process is to add a line to the plot that represents the regression line. The regression line shows the direction of the data points by drawing a line through the center of the points. To add the regression line using RStudio, use the following code:

```
abline(lin1, col="red")
```

The output of this code is shown in figure 14.7.

Let us now replicate these steps and conduct a linear regression for the HCAPHS variables of "definitely yes" and "probably yes." The R scripts for these two linear regression are as follows, and the resulting scatter plot is shown in figure 14.8:

```
lin2<-lm(score[Q_Revised=="Yes_probably"]~percent[Q_Revised=="Yes_
probably"])

summary(lin2)

Call:
lm(score[Q_Revised=="Yes_probably"]~ percent[Q_Revised=="Yes_probably"])

Residuals:
   Min      1Q    Median     3Q      Max
-102.15  -39.37  -14.82    24.40   923.52
Coefficients:
                                    Estimate  Std. Error  t value  Pr(>|t|)
(Intercept)                         103.28767 3.92236     26.333   <2e-16 ***
percent[Q_Revised == "Yes_probably"] -0.03501 0.15173    -0.231    0.818
---
Signif. codes: 0 '***' 0.001 '**' 0.01 '*' 0.05 '.' 0.1 ' ' 1

Residual standard error: 62.64 on 3328 degrees of freedom
Multiple R-squared: 1.6e-05,    Adjusted R-squared: -0.0002845
F-statistic: 0.05324 on 1 and 3328 DF, p-value: 0.8175

plot(score[Q_Revised=="Yes_probably"]~percent[Q_Revised=="Yes_probably"],
xlab="Percent who said probably", ylab="Time")

abline(lin2, col="red")
```

Figure 14.7. Scatter plot with a trend line showing the association between the time to admit and the percentage of patients reporting they would not recommend the hospital

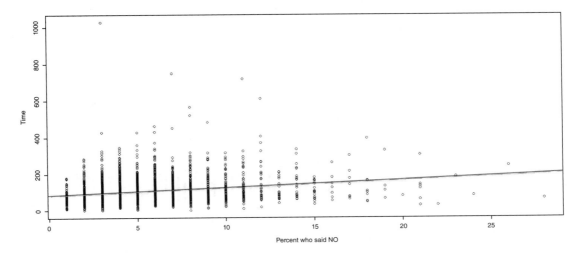

Source: Used with permission from RStudio.

Figure 14.8. Scatter plot with a trend line showing the association between the time to admit and the percentage of patients reporting they probably would recommend the hospital

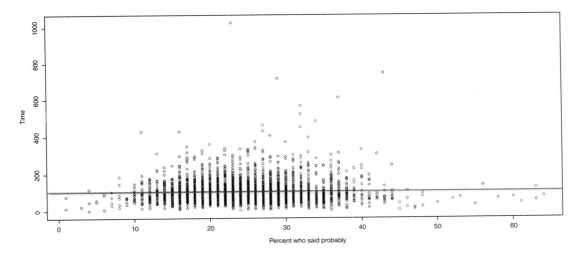

Source: Used with permission from RStudio.

The regression equation for our second linear model is y = 103.3 – 0.04x. Based on the equation, the slope of our best-fit line is – 0.04x, while the y-intercept is 103.3. Because our slope is a negative number, we know that the observed relationship will be a negative relationship. That is, our line will be sloping downward. The p-value from our linear model is 0.818. If we set our alpha (namely, significant level) to 0.05, we observe that our p-value is higher than 0.05. Therefore, there is not enough evidence to reject the null hypothesis and we must conclude that there is not a significant relationship between the average wait time between the decision to admit and admission in US hospitals and the percentage of patients reporting they would probably recommend the hospital.

The last linear regression will test if there is an association between the time to admit and the percentage of patients that reported they definitely would recommend the hospital. The following scripts are used to generate the linear regression and the graph is shown in figure 14.9:

Figure 14.9.   Scatter plot with a trend line showing the association between the time to admit and the percentage of patients reporting they would definitely recommend the hospital

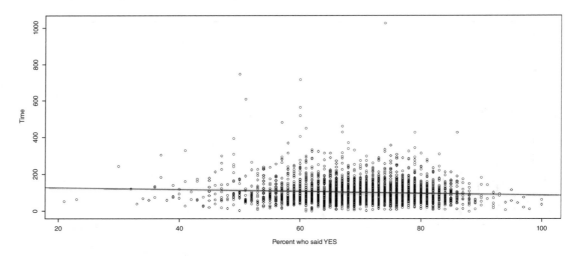

Source: Used with permission from RStudio.

```
lin3<-lm(score[Q_Revised=="Yes_definitely"] ~ percent[Q_Revised=="Yes_
definitely"])

summary(lin3)

Call:
lm(score[Q_Revised=="Yes_definitely"] ~ percent[Q_Revised=="Yes_
definitely"])

Residuals:
    Min       1Q      Median      3Q        Max
-106.91    -39.91    -14.48     24.95     925.59

Coefficients:
                            Estimate   Std. Error   t value    Pr(>|t|)
(Intercept)                 135.8550     8.2409      16.485    < 2e-16 ***
percent[Q_Revised=="Yes_     -0.4790     0.1169      -4.097    0.0000429 ***
definitely"]
---
Signif. codes:  0 '***' 0.001 '**' 0.01 '*' 0.05 '.' 0.1 ' ' 1

Residual standard error: 62.48 on 3330 degrees of freedom
Multiple R-squared:  0.005014,    Adjusted R-squared:  0.004716
F-statistic: 16.78 on 1 and 3330 DF,  p-value: 0.00004292

plot(score[Q_Revised=="Yes_definitely"]~percent[Q_Revised=="Yes_
definitely"], xlab="Percent who said YES", ylab="Time")

abline(lin3, col="red")
```

The regression equation for our last linear model is y = 135.9 – 0.48x. Based on the equation, the slope of our best-fit line is –0.48x, while the y-intercept is 135.9. Because our slope is a negative number, we know that the observed relationship will be a negative relationship. That is, our line will be sloping downward. The p-value from our linear model is 0.00004. If we set our alpha (namely, significant level) to 0.05, we observe that our p-value is much lower than 0.05. Therefore, there is enough evidence to reject the null hypothesis and we can conclude that there is a significant relationship between the average wait time between the decision to admit and admission in US hospitals and the percentage of patients reporting they definitely would recommend the hospital. The R-squared value is 0.005, which is very low. This indicates that the negative association, although significant, is weak.

Discussion

This study explored the relationship between hospital efficiency—as measured by the average time between the decision to admit in the ED and admission—and the patient's willingness to recommend the hospital based on satisfaction. The intent was to determine if the patient recommendation based on satisfaction is impacted by ED efficiency once the determination was made to admit the patient. We generated three linear models based on the answers from the HCAHPS survey to determine if there was an association between the percentage of patients that would not, probably would, and definitely would recommend the hospital and the average wait time between the decision to admit and admission in US hospitals. Based on these results we can conclude there is a significant positive relationship between average time between decision to admit in the ED and admission and percent of patients reporting they would not recommend the hospital. Organizations reporting a greater percentage of patients that would not recommend the hospital were associated with higher average minutes between the decision to admit and the admission. The R-squared value is extremely low for this linear regression and indicates that the strength of the relationship is weak. We also observed that there is a significant negative relationship between average time between decision to admit in the ED and admission and percent of patients reporting they would definitely recommend the hospital. Organizations reporting a greater percentage of patients that would recommend the hospital were associated with lower average minutes between the decision to admit and the admission. The R-squared value is extremely low for this linear regression and indicates that the strength of the relationship is weak. There is not a significant difference between the decision to admit times in the ED and patients reporting they would probably recommend the hospital. These findings are corroborated by a recent study that also identified a direct correlation between ED wait time and patient satisfaction that showed those who waited five minutes or less expressed as high as 95 percent satisfaction; and in turn, satisfaction with the experience declined with each 30-minute interval of additional wait time (Stempniak 2013).

Although this case has proven to be significant, throughput and output are not the only focus of ED wait time. An additional factor that should be researched further includes the category of input. Input is described as the cause of why people are showing up at the ED, which could include non-urgent visits (Hoot and Aronsky, 2008). Additionally, **patient flow** could also be reviewed in terms of access in addition to the element of crowding. Further research could be conducted in terms of patient satisfaction. Other criteria such as cleanliness and interactions with providers could be focused on a deeper level. It would be interesting to view the effects of boarding on different types of populations. An example of this would be to see if particular populations (such as behavioral health or elderly patients) are affected by boarding in terms of overall satisfaction versus similar patients who were not boarded.

Conclusion

The most significant finding from this analysis is that decreased patient satisfaction can be a predictor for greater ED wait times. ED flow is critical to the appropriate and timely care of patients, and ED patient flow issues have the potential to impact accreditation and reimbursement. CMS's Stage 2 of the EHR Meaningful Use Incentive Program emphasizes that eligible hospitals report on 16 of the 29 clinical **quality measures** and no less than 3 of the 6 National Quality Strategy domains (Murphy 2012). In this case, the focus was on the survey of patients' experience domain and highlights how important patient satisfaction is to overall perception of quality of care.

The link of quality measure outcomes can also be directly linked to payment, such as the hospital value-based purchasing program (HVBP), which adjusts hospitals' payments based on their performance. One such performance outcome includes the patient experience domain as used in this case. The patient experience of care domain is weighted at 30 percent of the overall total scoring (CMS 2015).

Issues with patient flow and patient boarding within the ED are not only an issue of the ED, but are also an issue with the throughput and output of patients in the healthcare facility and the patient's overall satisfaction, as well as the organizations' public reputation and financial impact.

Review Exercises

Instructions: Choose the best answer.

1. True or False: Boarding is defined as the time a patient waits between arrival and decision to admit into the hospital.

2. When recoding variables with Excel, what function can be used to rename the variable based upon the exact contents in another cell?
   a. IF
   b. SUMPRODUCT
   c. SUM
   d. RANDOM

3. When working with data in RStudio, if you want to view the data set that was imported into the RStudio platform, what function would you use?
   a. t.test()
   b. summary()
   c. lm()
   d. view()

4. After developing a linear model with RStudio, you can plot the data on a scatter plot and draw the trend line using the abline() function. The trend line is also called the:
   a. Line of fitness
   b. Best-fit line
   c. Regression fit line
   d. Trending line

5. If the slope of the regression line is negative and the R-squared value is low, we would conclude that the association is:
   a. Positive and weak
   b. Positive and strong
   c. Negative and weak
   d. Negative and strong

References

Centers for Medicare and Medicaid Services. 2015. Medicare.gov Hospital Compare. http://www.medicare.gov/hospitalcompare/search.html

Government Accountability Office. 2009. Hospital Emergency Departments. http://www.gao.gov/new.items/d09347.pdf

Heisler, E.J. and N.L. Tyler. 2014. Hospital-Based Emergency Departments: Background and Policy Considerations. *Congressional Research Service*. https://www.fas.org/sgp/crs/misc/R43812.pdf

Hospital Consumer Assessment of Healthcare Providers and Systems. 2015. HCAHPS Survey. http://www.hcahpsonline.org/files/HCAHPS V10.0 Appendix A - HCAHPS Mail Survey Materials (English) March 2015.pdf

Hoot, N.R. and D. Aronsky. 2008. Systematic review of emergency department crowding: Causes, effects, and solutions. *Annals of Emergency Medicine* 52(2):126.e1–136.e1.

McHugh, M., K. VanDyke, M. McClelland, and D. Moss. 2012. *Improving Patient Flow and Reducing Emergency Department Crowding: A Guide for Hospitals*. Rockville, MD: Agency for Healthcare Research and Quality.

Medicare.gov. n.d. Timely and Effective Care. http://www.medicare.gov/hospitalcompare/About/Timely-Effective-Care.html

Murphy, K. 2012. Stage 2 Meaningful Use Clinical Quality Measures for Eligible Hospitals. https://ehrintelligence.com/2012/09/27/stage-2-meaningful-use-clinical-quality-measures-for-eligible-hospitals/

Nugus, P., A. Holdgate, M. Fry, R. Forero, S. McCarthy, and J. Braithwaite. 2011. Work pressure and patient flow management in the emergency department: Findings from an ethnographic study. *Academic Emergency Medicine* 18(10):1045–1052.

ProPublica. 2014. ER Wait Watcher. https://projects.propublica.org/emergency/

Rosenau, D.O. and M. Alexander. 2013. Emergency Medical Treatment and Active Labor Act. Presented at: Lehigh Valley Health Network Ground Rounds, Allentown, PA.

Stempniak, M. 2013. What, no wait? *Hospitals & Health Networks/AHA* 87(11):30–35, 2.

Using Data Mining Techniques to Predict Healthcare-Associated Infections

David Marc, MBS, CHDA and Ryan Sandefer, MA, CPHIT

Learning Objectives

- Define the CRISP-DM process for conducting data mining techniques
- Illustrate the use of the data mining package Rattle for conducting data mining
- Construct a decision tree model from publicly available data
- Interpret the results of a decision tree model through the CRISP-DM process

Key Terms

Cross Industry Process for Data Mining (CRISP-DM)
Data mining
Decision trees
Knowledge discovery in databases (KDD)
Predictive Model Markup Language (PMML)
Root node
Terminal node

Healthcare-associated infections are a major patient safety concern for US healthcare organizations, and elimination of healthcare-associated infections has been deemed a priority for the Department of Health and Human Services (HHS 2012). The Centers for Disease Control and Prevention estimates that 5 to 10 percent of hospitalized patients acquire a healthcare-associated infection (Yokoe et al. 2014; Yokoe et al. 2008). According to a recent study, there were an estimated 648,000 patients in the United States with 721,800 healthcare-associated infections in 2011. Pneumonia and surgical site infections represent the most commonly reported infections (21.8 percent each), while gastrointestinal infections account for 17.1 percent of all healthcare-associated infections. *Clostridium difficile (C. diff.)* is the most commonly reported infection, accounting for 12.1 percent of all healthcare-associated infections (Magill et al. 2014; Miller et al. 2011). Figure 15.1 illustrates the significant increase in diagnoses of *Clostridium difficile* related hospital stays per capita.

Clostridium difficile infection (CDI) is "an anaerobic, spore-forming bacillus that produces two important exotoxins: toxin A, an enterotoxin, and toxin B, which is primarily a cytotoxin" (McDonald et al. 2006). CDI is defined using a two-step process. According to published clinical guidelines, CDI is defined by "the presence of symptoms (usually diarrhea) and either a stool test positive for *C. diff.* toxins or toxigenic *C. diff.*, or colonoscopic or histopathologic findings revealing pseudomembranous colitis" (Cohen et al. 2010). CDI is extremely contagious and can easily be transmitted within hospitals, and CDI is responsible for increasing levels of healthcare costs and longer hospitals stays (Cohen et al. 2010; Kyne et al. 2002).

Figure 15.1.   Trends in hospital stays associated with *Clostridium difficile* infection (CDI), 1993–2009

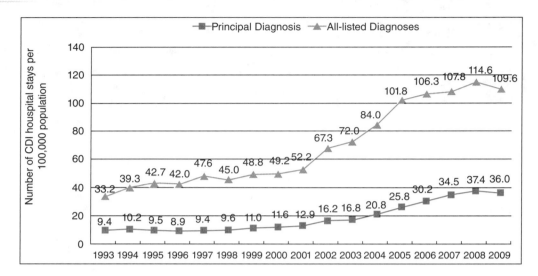

Source: AHRQ 2009, 2012.

A considerable amount of research has been conducted on CDI, including how to manage and treat the infectious disease (Magill et al. 2014; Miller et al. 2011; Cohen et al. 2010). Research has shown that CDI is more prevalent in short-stay hospitals (McDonald et al. 2006). Approximately 2 percent of all discharges from US acute-care hospitals to long-term care facilities carried CDI (Cohen et al. 2010).

Because the primary unit of analysis for most CDI-related research is the patient, much less research has been conducted on the prevalence of CDI based upon hospital characteristics. Studies have shown that CDI is significantly more prevalent in hospitals geographically located in the Northeast region of the United States and larger hospitals have significantly more discharges related to CDI (Lucado et al. 2012; McDonald et al. 2006). However, research has not been conducted on the relationship between hospital type, hospital ownership, and overall relationship between hospital quality and CDI prevalence.

The purpose of this chapter is to investigate the association between US acute-care hospital characteristics and CDI prevalence.

Research Question and Hypothesis

Do hospital characteristics predict CDI rates among US hospitals?

Data mining is "the art and science of intelligent data analysis...The aim is to discover meaningful insights and knowledge from data" (Williams 2011). Data mining involves the creation of models that can be used for gaining understanding of problems, developing insights in into processes, and using that understanding and insights for making predictions. Data mining combines skills from computer science, statistics, and machine learning.

The dependent variable for the proposed study is a hospital's measure of CDI rates within US acute-care hospitals and has three response options (Better than the US National Benchmark, No Different than the US National Benchmark, or Worse than the US National Benchmark). The independent variable is the variable we are using to compare these three groups of hospitals. In the case of the proposed research question, there are seven independent variables: hospital ownership, emergency services, overall hospital quality measure, clinical process domain score, patient experience of care domain score, readmission score, and hospital spending score. The analysis for answering the proposed research question will involve conducting the following data mining procedure(s) using Rattle (Rattle is an R package that is designed for data mining analysis): A decision tree model to predict the occurrence of CDI in US acute-care hospitals.

Hypotheses

Data mining is aimed at knowledge discovery (that is, it is focused on hypotheses generation not hypothesis testing). **Knowledge discovery in databases (KDD)** has been described as the "nontrivial process of identifying valid, novel, potentially useful, and ultimately understandable patterns in data" (Fayyad et al. 1996). Data mining research does not propose formal hypotheses. Rather, data mining projects typically follow a step-by-step process. For the purposes of this chapter we are using the **Cross Industry Process for Data Mining (CRISP-DM)** (see chapter 3 for more detail on this framework). The framework consists of the following six steps:

1. Problem understanding
2. Data understanding
3. Data preparation
4. Modeling
5. Evaluation
6. Deployment

The purpose of this chapter is to undertake a complete data mining process—from problem understanding to deployment.

Decision trees, the data mining technique employed in this chapter, are considered the "traditional building blocks of data mining and the classic machine learning algorithm" (Williams 2011). In essence, decision trees provide a simple, yet powerful, approach to gaining knowledge from data by breaking data into roots, branches, and leaves. Beginning with the root data, the data branches out based upon the characteristics of the data (for example, specific values), and ultimately terminate in a leaf node where the ultimate "decision" rests. Decision trees can be translated into rules and, therefore, be useful in deploying the knowledge to predict future events.

Of particular importance for this chapter is the deployment of data mining models using the **Predictive Model Markup Language (PMML)**. PMML is a "standards language for representing data mining models" (Williams 2011). PMML can be used to save data mining models and deploy them to commercially available analytic software or data mining tools using XML. We use PMML in this chapter.

Checklist

To answer our research question, a specific process of data acquisition, preparation, and discovery is required. The following steps will be explained in detail:

1. Extract data sets from MySQL
2. Data preparation with Microsoft Excel
   a. Review data for erroneous values and modify column headers
3. Import the data into Rattle
   a. Conduct descriptive statistics
4. Conduct data mining process

The Analysis

Now that we have our research problem identified, we can begin the data mining process.

Step 1: Data Extraction

In order to carry out the analysis, the following data elements are needed. Note: all data required for answering the research question are included in the database associated with this textbook:

- A list of all hospitals in the United States
- An indicator for the type of hospital ownership

- An indicator for the hospital's quality of patient experience
- An indicator for the hospital's clinical quality
- An indicator for whether or not the hospital provides emergency services
- An indicator for the hospital's *C. diff.* rate
- An indicator for the hospital's readmission rate

Five data sets need to be combined to obtain the needed data to answer the proposed research question. The five data sets are all part of the Centers for Medicare and Medicaid Services Hospital Compare website (CMS 2015). The data sets include the following:

- hospital_general_information
- hospital_associated_infection
- hospital_value_based_purchasing
- medicare_hospital_spending_per_patient
- readmissions_complications_deaths

Figure 15.2 provides the SQL script that combines the five required data sets and extracts only the relevant data elements from each. The scripts include the necessary joins to combine the data sets. Note that you must alter a setting in MySQL so that the output shows all of the results rather than just showing the first 1,000 rows (see chapter 4). After executing each query, export the data to a CSV file and save the file as cdiff. For detailed instructions regarding exporting data from MySQL Workbench to CSV format, see chapter 4.

Figure 15.2. SQL script and returned data for combining three data sets

```
SELECT
        hospital_general_information.provider_id,
        hospital_general_information.hospital_ownership,
        hospital_general_information.emergency_services,
hospital_value_based_purchasing.unweighted_normalized_clinical_process_of_
care_domain_score AS 'cpcd',
        hospital_value_based_purchasing.unweighed_patient_experience_of_
        care_domain_score AS 'pecd',
        medicare_hospital_spending_per_patient.score AS 'hsbp',
        readmissions_complications_deaths.score AS 'readmission',
        hospital_associated_infection.compared_to_national AS 'c_diff_
        compared'
FROM
        hospital_general_information
        JOIN
hospital_associated_infection ON hospital_general_information.provider_id =
    hospital_associated_infection.provider_id
        JOIN
hospital_value_based_purchasing ON hospital_general_information.provider_id =
    hospital_value_based_purchasing.provider_id
        JOIN
medicare_hospital_spending_per_patient ON hospital_general_information.
provider_id =
    medicare_hospital_spending_per_patient.provider_id
        JOIN
```

(Continued)

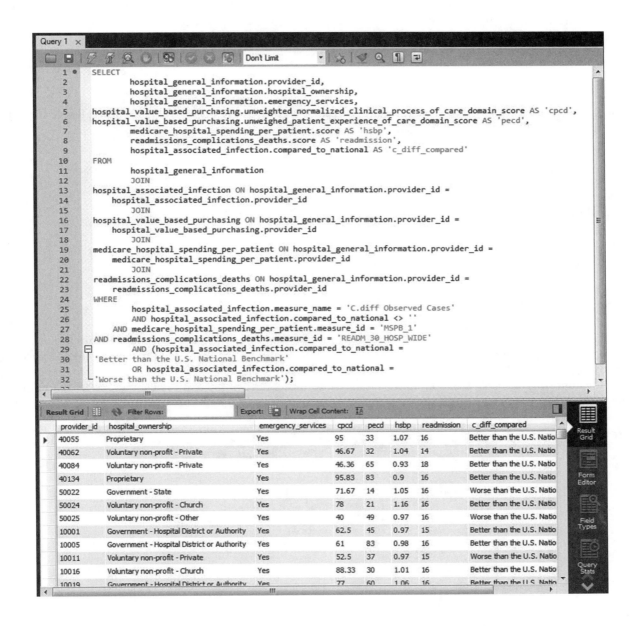

Figure 15.2.   SQL script and returned data for combining three data sets *(Continued)*

```
readmissions_complications_deaths ON hospital_general_information.provider_id =
    readmissions_complications_deaths.provider_id
WHERE
        hospital_associated_infection.measure_name = 'C.diff Observed Cases'
        AND hospital_associated_infection.compared_to_national <> ''
    AND medicare_hospital_spending_per_patient.measure_id = 'MSPB_1'
AND readmissions_complications_deaths.measure_id = 'READM_30_HOSP_WIDE'
        AND (hospital_associated_infection.compared_to_national =
'Better than the U.S. National Benchmark'
        OR hospital_associated_infection.compared_to_national =
'Worse than the U.S. National Benchmark');
```

The next step in the process is to open the Excel file with the data elements that were extracted from MySQL Workbench. You should see the following eight columns of data (each observation represents a single US hospital):

- provider_id: The code number assigned to an individual inpatient hospital.
- hospital_ownership: The category that defines the status of each hospital's ownership type.
- emergency_services: Whether or not a hospital provides emergency services.
- cpcd: Clinical process of care domain score.
- pecd: Patient experience of care domain score.
- hsbp: Spending per hospital patient with Medicare (Medicare spending per beneficiary [MSPB]). Specifically, a hospital's MSPB measure is calculated as the hospital's average MSPB amount divided by the median MSPB amount across all hospitals.
- readmission: Hospital-wide 30-day readmission rate.
- c_diff_compared: Healthcare-associated infections measures hospital-level results.

The data set includes column names that are not particularly informative for understanding what variables we are working with. The old and new column headers, as well as the definition of the data element, are listed in table 15.1.

Step 2: Starting Rattle

The first step in the analysis process is to start the Rattle software in RStudio. If you are using Rattle for the first time, you will need to install the package using the following script:

```
install.packages ("rattle")

install.packages("RGtk2", depen=T, type="source")
```

After Rattle is installed, use the following scripts to open the Rattle data mining software:

```
library (rattle)

rattle()
```

Step 3: Import the Data

By default, Rattle will load with the data tab selected. The data tab is where you manage the imported data and specify the partitions of data for the training, validation, and testing phases of the data mining protocol. Importing data into Rattle is a relatively straightforward process. Figure 15.3 displays the first step in the process for importing the CSV file. To import the data into rattle, next to the text "Filename:" select the button that reads "(None)".

Table 15.1.   Original and revised column names within Excel

Original Name	Revised Name
provider_id	id
hospital_ownership	owner
emergency_services	es
cpcd	cpcd
pecd	pecd
hsbp	hsbp
readmission	readm
c_diff_compared	c_diff

Figure 15.3.   Importing a CSV file into Rattle—step 1

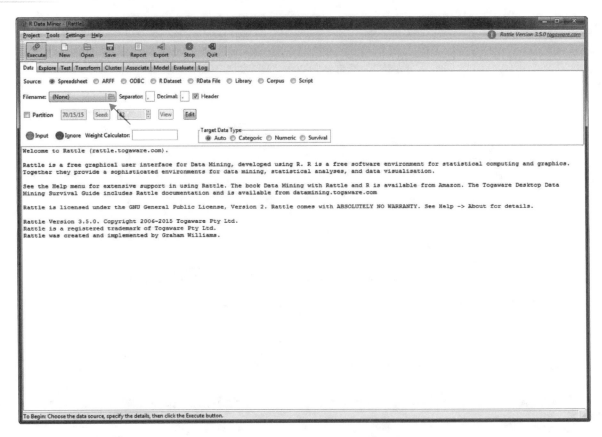

Source: Used with permission from RStudio.

A window will appear prompting you to choose a file (see figure 15.4). Find the CSV file on your computer that was exported from the MySQL query. Once found, click the file name and select Open, and then select the Execute button shown on the Rattle menu bar to load the data.

Next, you must ensure that the data are partitioned correctly for the training, validation, and testing data. In data mining, the model will be developed with the training data, validated with the validation data, and finally tested with the testing data. The training data set is typically the largest partition. Next to the word "Partition," there is an open text box with three numbers that are separated by a forward slash. The first number (70) is the percentage of our data we want to partition for the training data; the second number (15) is the percentage of the data we want to specify for our validation data; and the third number (15) is the percentage of the data we want to specify for the testing data. The sum of the three numbers must be equal to 100. The data will be randomly partitioned into each of the three data sets. You should note that because the data are randomly selected for each partition, each time you run an analysis, the results will be slightly different. Therefore, the results you derive from your analysis will be slightly different than the results shown here.

We want to make sure that the data were uploaded correctly. In the large lower windowpane, the variable names, types, and the data mining actions associated with the variables (the radio buttons) should be listed for the data that we uploaded to Rattle. You should make sure that the data type is being coded appropriately. For instance, id should be specified as an identifier variable; therefore, the Ident radio button should be selected. If id is specified as an input variable, it will be incorrectly used as a data element for the creation of our model. As an identifier, the variable is ignored as an input (see figure 15.5).

Predictive data mining requires that inputs be defined for predicting a target variable. The target variable is the data element that we would like to predict. In this case, we are predicting c_diff, which is whether a hospital has a *C. diff.* rate less than or greater than the national average (see figure 15.5). The input variables are a combination of data elements that may predict the outcome of the target variable. The data mining model uses algorithms to

Figure 15.4. Importing a CSV file into Rattle—step 2

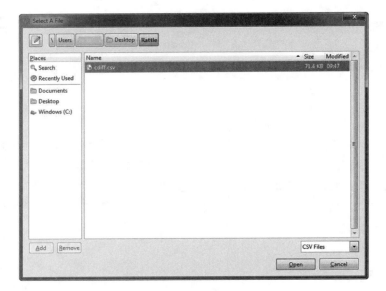

Source: Used with permission from RStudio.

Figure 15.5. Importing a CSV file into Rattle—step 3

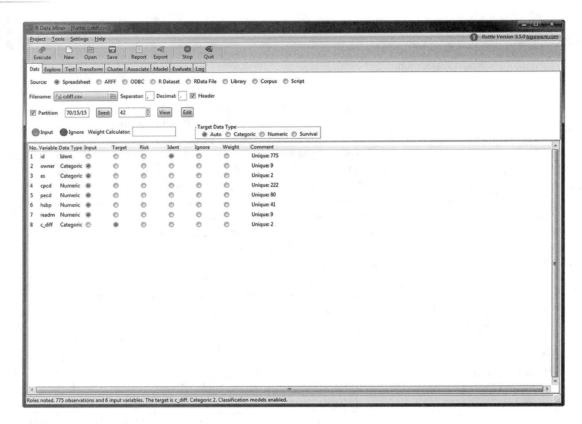

Source: Used with permission from RStudio.

detect patterns in the input variables that best predict the outcome of the target variable. When uploading the data into Rattle, an important task is to determine whether the data were categorized correctly as an input or target variable. Figure 15.5 shows that we have six input variables (owner, es, cpcd, pecd, hsbp, and readmission).

There are three categorical data variables, including owner, es, and c_diff. You can see that at the end of each row there is a comment that specifies the number of unique variables. We see that owner has nine unique variables, es has two unique variables, and c_diff has two unique variables. Note that owner and es are selected as input variables while c_diff is selected as the only target variable.

If any changes are made to the data tab, we must select the Execute button to run these changes. If we do not select Execute, all of the changes will be lost.

Step 4: Descriptive Statistics

The next phase in data mining is to explore the data. Select the Explore tab to manage this step. Under the Explore tab, there are various ways that the imported data can be analyzed. A method can be selected by choosing one of the following radio buttons: Summary, Distributions, Correlation, Principal Components, and Interactive. The Summary method offers the descriptive statistics about each variable. After selecting the Summary radio button, there are various analyses that can be carried out by selecting the appropriate check boxes. We will select the Summary and Describe check boxes (see figure 15.6). After selecting these options, choose the Execute button. As shown in figure 15.6, basic summaries of each variable are provided including the data types, levels, counts, averages, minimum, maximum values, and such. This information can be used for

Figure 15.6.   Exploring data with Rattle

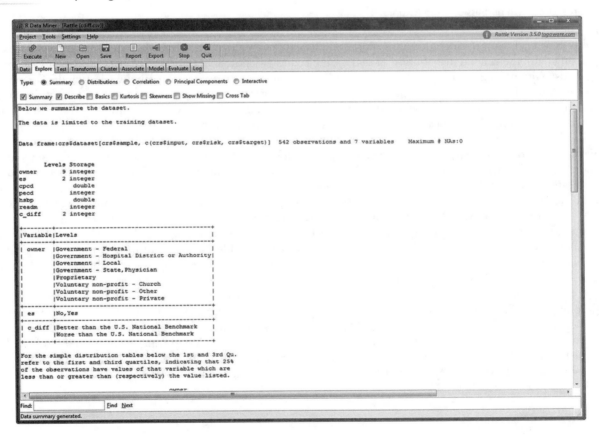

Source: Used with permission from RStudio.

Figure 15.7. Creating data visualizations with Rattle

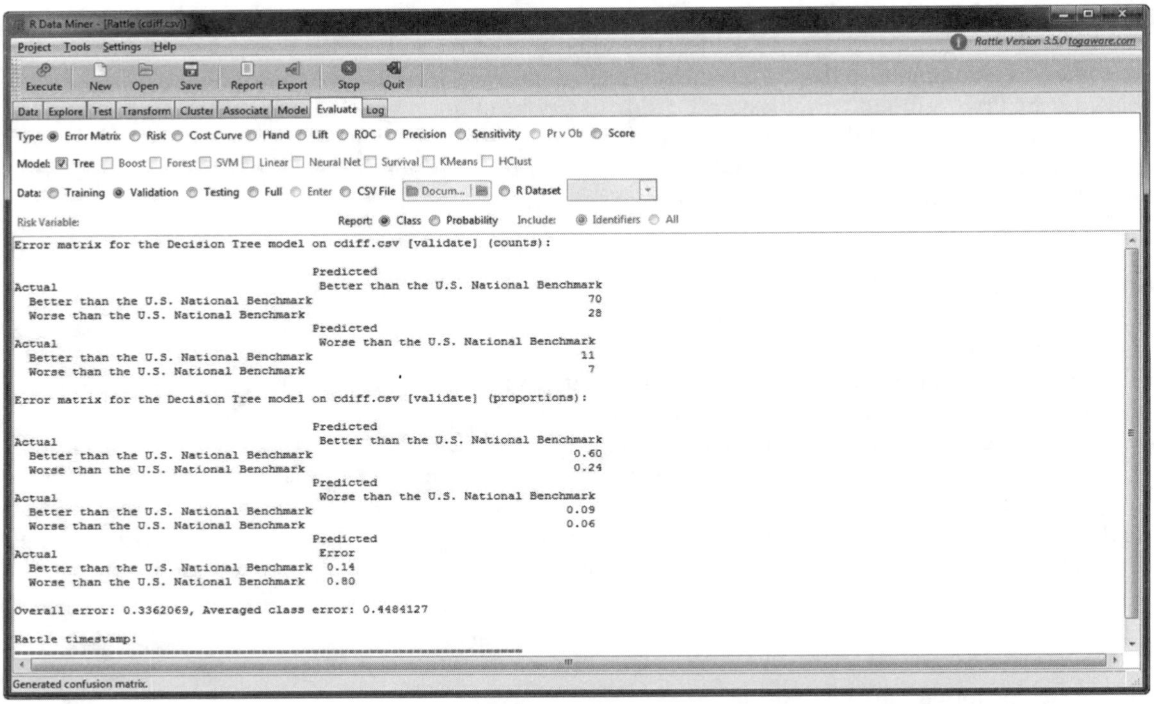

Source: Used with permission from RStudio.

describing each variable included in the data set. The data may tell you as to whether there are any variables with missing data, the general distribution of that variable, and any potential outliers that may be skewing the results.

Also within the Explore tab, you can obtain some graphical summaries of the data by selecting the Distributions radio button. The bottom windowpane will change, allowing you to select a graphical summary. Within this windowpane, numeric data are shown on the top and categorical data are shown on the bottom. It is best to choose up to three graphical summaries at one time. If you select more than three, the first three will be overwritten by any additional graphs. We can see the distribution of the numeric data by selecting the histogram textbox. Also, we can develop some barplots to see the counts of each of the categorical data variables. Visualizing the data in these ways will allow us to better understand the distribution of the data. Figure 15.7 shows how to select numeric and categorical variables in Rattle to develop visualizations. Under Histogram, check the boxes for cpcd and pecd and click Execute. Please note that all graphics produced in Rattle will appear in the RStudio Plots window.

The graphs that are created will show the overall distribution and broken down by the target. The c_diff target variable has two groups: Better than the US National Benchmark and Worse that the US National Benchmark. Figure 15.8 illustrates the frequency of c_diff variable by cpcd and pecd using a histogram. The bars of the histogram are drawn for the entire data set. The different lines show the distribution for all the data and broken down into each category.

Similarly, if we select the hsbp and readm checkboxes and click Execute, Rattle will produce two additional graphics. Figure 15.9 illustrates the frequency of hospitals by MSPB (again, the lines represent the c_diff categories of Better than or Worse than the National Benchmark). Looking at the distribution of hsbp, we find that most of the data center around 1.0. This means that on average, hospitals in the United States have an MSPB measure very close to the median MSPB amount across all hospitals. Figure 15.9 also shows the distribution of the 30-day readmission rate for hospitals. As shown, the most frequently occurring readmission rate is 16 percent.

Step 5: Statistical Analysis

We can also test for correlations between the numeric variables. Still within the Explore tab, select the Correlation radio button. Then click Execute (you may need to install an R package at this juncture). The

Figure 15.8. Sample graphic produced using Rattle

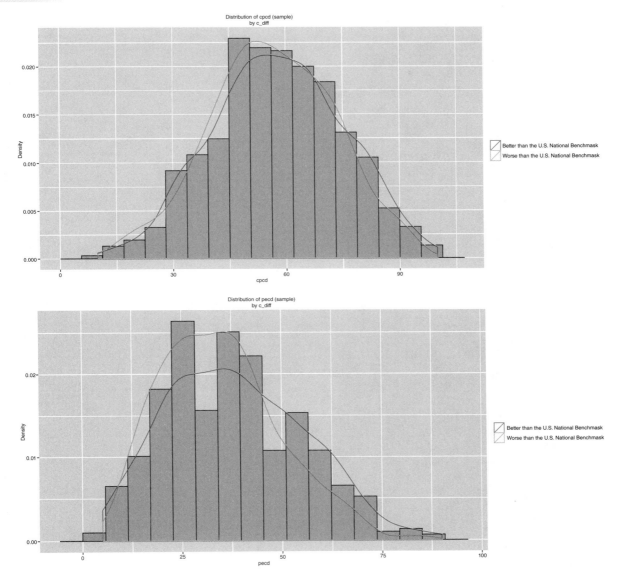

Source: Used with permission from RStudio.

result will be a table that shows the Pearson correlation coefficient for each pairwise comparison of the numeric data (see figure 15.10). A Pearson correlation coefficient refers to the measure of relationship between two numeric variables—in short, how dependent are the two variables. As you can see, the table includes each variable as a row and a column. When examining the relationship that a variable has to itself (for example, readmission versus readmission), there is a perfect correlation (1.000), which makes sense because the statistic is calculating the covariance between two variables—there is no variance when comparing one variable with itself. As you can see, the strongest negative correlation is between pecd and readmission. Also, the strongest positive correlation is between hsbp and readmission. The way to interpret the table is to look for the lowest negative number (–0.274) and the highest positive number (0.141). The closer the values are to 1 or –1, the stronger the relationship. If the values are negative, this is interpreted as a negative association. If the values are positive, this is interpreted as a positive association.

An addition to the textual output, a graph will also be generated in RStudio that shows the strength and type of the relationship between each variable (see figure 15.11). The larger the circle is in the graph, the

Figure 15.9.   Sample graphic produced using Rattle

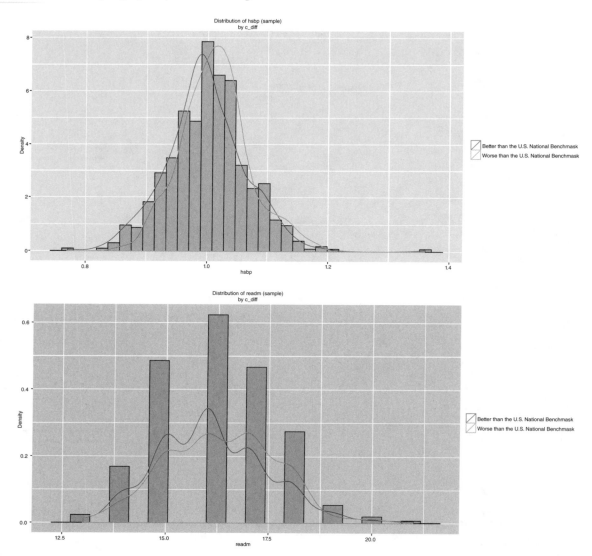

Source: Used with permission from RStudio.

stronger the association. The blue color indicates a positive relationship while the red color indicates a negative relationship. As shown, when comparing each variable to itself there is a perfect correlation. This information is redundant and really does not add to our understanding of the data. However, we also see that pecd and readmission have the largest circle closest to the color red indicating the strongest negative association. Also, hsbp and readmission have the largest circles closest to the blue color indicating the strongest positive association. As described previously, these visual representations of the data reinforce the strong negative relationships. Hospitals with higher readmission rates have lower patient experience of care scores. Moreover, the findings also show the hospitals with the highest MSPB have higher readmission rates and lower patient experience of care scores.

The next tab in Rattle is the Test tab. This is where various hypothesis-testing methods can be administered. For instance, t-tests can be run in this tab to compare the averages between two groups. For example, if you select T-test, click Sample 1 and select pecd, and then click the Execute button, a two-sample t-test will be performed comparing the average patient experience of care domain scores by hospitals with better than average and worse than average c_diff rates. Figure 15.12 shows how to conduct this test in Rattle.

Figure 15.10.   Producing correlations summaries using Rattle

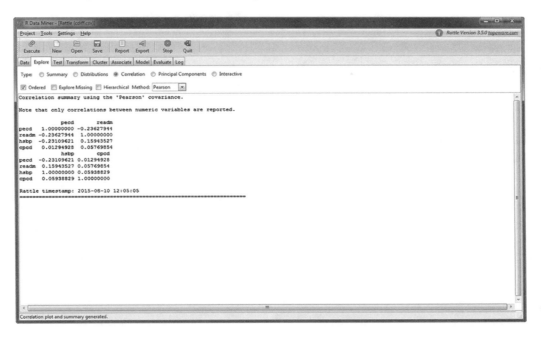

Source: Used with permission from RStudio.

Figure 15.11.   Using Rattle to visually represent correlations

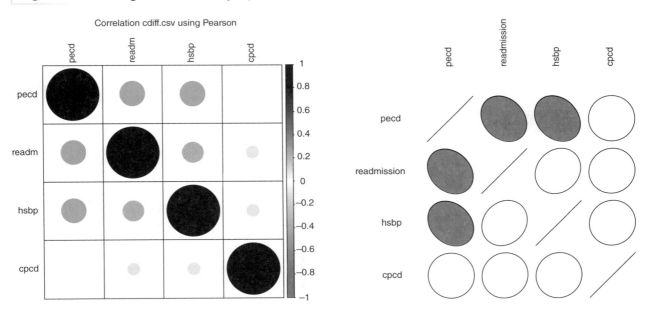

The look of the graph may vary depending on your operating system. The graph on the left was generated using a PC running Windows 7. The graph on the right was generated using a Mac running OSx Yosemite.

Source: Used with permission from RStudio.

When examining the Alternative Two-Sided p-value, we see that the output shows that the p-value is 0.01165, which is less than 0.05. Therefore, we can state that there is a significant difference in patient experience of care scores between these two hospital groups.

Figure 15.12.   Conducting a two-sample test with Rattle

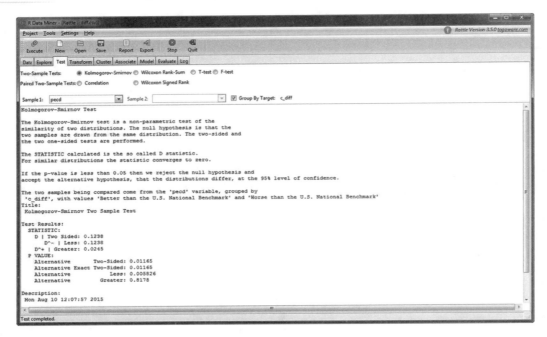

Source: Used with permission from RStudio.

The Transform tab allows you to alter the format of data. For instance, if there was a data set that we wanted to rescale by taking the natural log or wanted to rescale from numeric to binary as zeros and ones, we can select the data variable in the bottom windowpane and select the Natural Log radio or Scale [0–1] button and then click Execute (see figure 15.13). The original data variable will still exist, but will be shown as Ignore in the data tab. The new variable that is created will be coded as an input variable. We do not need to transform the data for the purposes of the study we are carrying out in this chapter.

We are now at the point where we can create our data mining model. We will be creating a decision tree with this analysis. In the Model tab, select the Tree radio button. We will be leaving the decision tree settings at their defaults. These defaults can be altered to tune your model with future iterations. After selecting the Tree radio button click Execute. Figure 15.14 shows the decision tree default settings for the decision tree model.

The result is an output that summarizes the decision tree model. As shown by n = 542, there were 542 observations of training data that were used to create the model. The model is created by rules being set automatically based on the patterns that are present in the data. The rules are shown in figure 15.15. The top of our tree is known as our **root node.** From the decision tree results shown in figure 15.15 and associated with the second rule, the rule under the root node can be interpreted as the following: "Is pecd>=54.5?" If yes, then predict that the *C. diff.* cases for that hospital are better than the national average. If no, then "Is pecd<54.5?" If yes, then "Is the hospital ownership equal to a Government—Hospital District or Authority?" If yes, then predict that the *C. diff.* cases for that hospital are better than the national average. The final decisions are known as the **terminal nodes.**

The decisions that result from the decision tree can be cumbersome to interpret. To make this interpretation easier, we can depict the rules as a graphical decision tree. To create the graphic, select the Draw button. Figure 15.16 depicts the output of a decision tree model. A graphic will be generated and appear in RStudio.

As shown in figure 15.16, the rules are much easier to interpret as a graphic. Now we can see what decision lead to the best predictions as to whether a hospital has a number of *C. diff.* cases worse than or better than the national average.

The last thing we must do is evaluate the error of the model we created. First select the Evaluate tab. Next, select the Error Matrix radio button. A checkbox should be selected for "Tree." If we were to have created other types of models, those checkboxes would also be made available. We will be testing the error rate of our model by applying our model to a new data set, the validation data set. Therefore, make sure the validation radio button is selected and then click Execute.

Figure 15.13.   Using Rattle to transform data

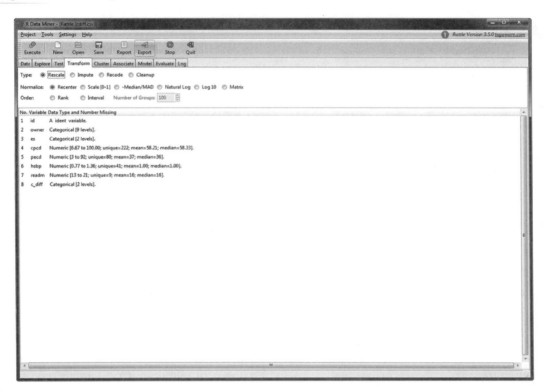

Source: Used with permission from RStudio.

Figure 15.14.   Using Rattle to create a decision tree for data mining

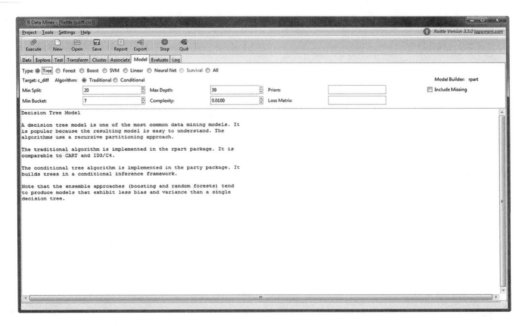

Source: Used with permission from RStudio.

Figure 15.15. Decision tree rules

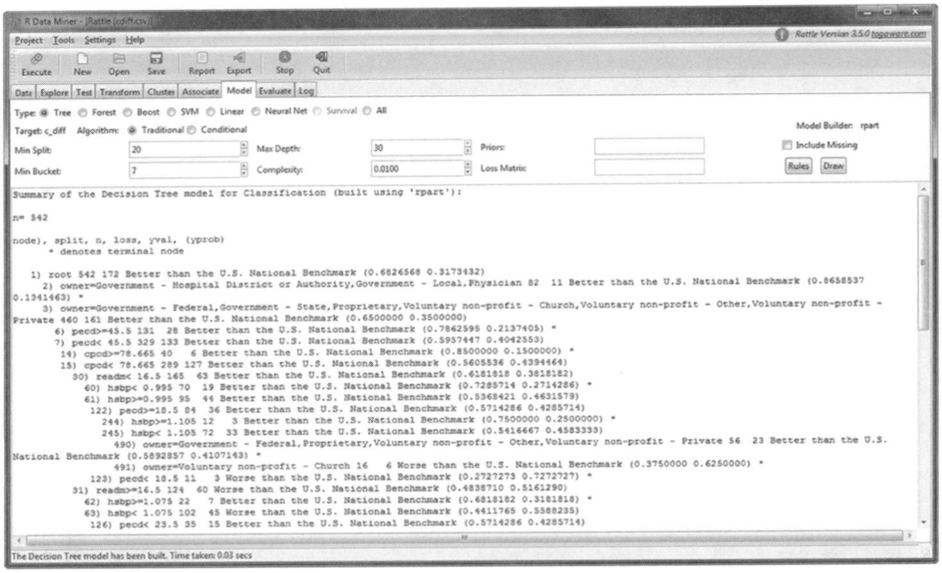

Source: Used with permission from RStudio.

The result is a table (shown in figure 15.17) that shows the predicted categorization of each observation of data as compared to the actual categorization of the data. As shown, our model correctly predicted that 70 hospitals (60 percent) would have a number of C. *diff.* cases better than the national average. However, our model also incorrectly predicted that 28 hospitals (24 percent) would have a number of C. *diff.* cases better than the national average when in fact those hospitals were worse than the national average. The total error can be summarized by the number shown after the text "Overall error." As shown, our model incorrectly categorized hospitals 34.0 percent of the time.

We should confirm this observation by examining our model a second time with another new partition of data. That is our testing data set. Select the Testing radio button under Data and then select Execute. As you can see in figure 15.18, a similar error rate was observed. With the testing partition of data, we had an error rate of 36.7 percent.

The log tab in Rattle saves all of the R code that was generated as a result of the selections made within Rattle. This code can be saved to rerun the analysis again in the future. Figure 15.19 displays the R code captured in Rattle's log tab.

The model that you generated from this exercise can be deployed into a separate existing data set. That is, the model that you created can be used to predict if the number of C. *diff.* cases will be worse or better than the national average. In order to deploy the model, we have to go back to the Model tab and select the Export button. You will be prompted to select a location to save the output file (this process is shown in figure 15.20).

The result of exporting the model is an XML file that is known as Predictive Model Markup Language (PMML). This language supports large-scale deployment and implementation of a data mining model. Figure 15.21 displays the XML format of the PMML model that was exported.

Discussion

This study utilized data mining techniques—specifically decision trees—to develop a model to predict whether US hospitals had a worse than average or better than average rate for C. *diff.* infections using multiple predictor variables. The study successfully walked through each step in the data mining process, including clearly identifying a problem with healthcare-associated infections, identifying data sources that are widely available

Figure 15.16. Decision tree rules as a data visualization

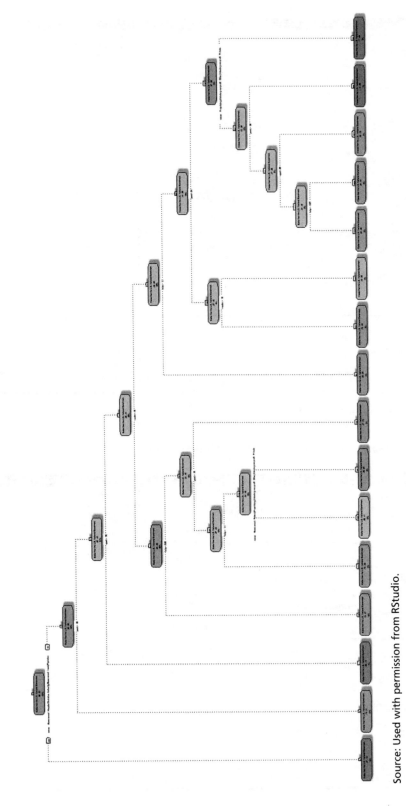

Decision Tree cdiff.csv $ c_diff

Source: Used with permission from RStudio.

Figure 15.17. Using Rattle to Predict Outcomes

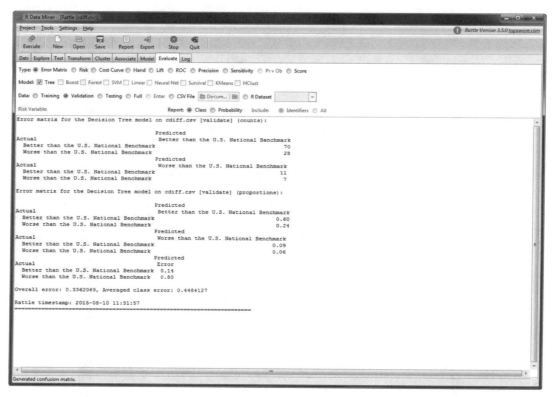

Source: Used with permission from RStudio.

Figure 15.18. Using Rattle to Evaluate Data Mining Models

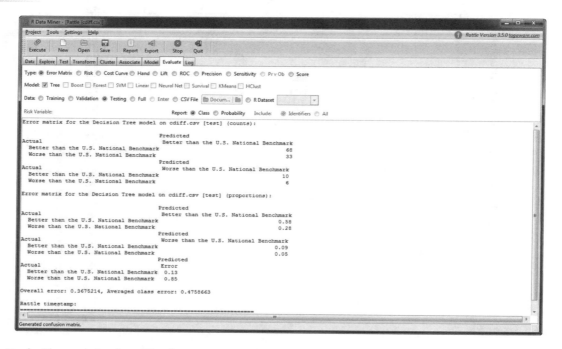

Source: Used with permission from RStudio.

Figure 15.19. Saving code for future analyses or model deployments

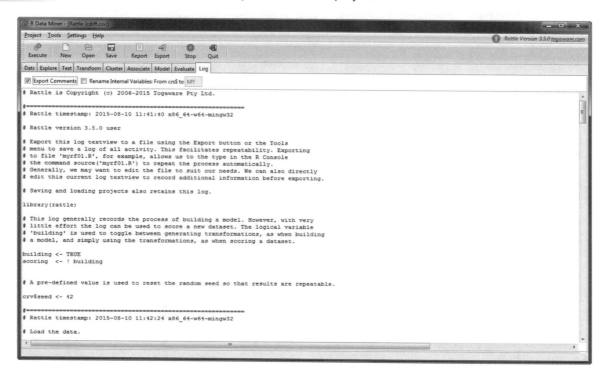

Source: Used with permission from RStudio.

Figure 15.20. Exporting decision tree model

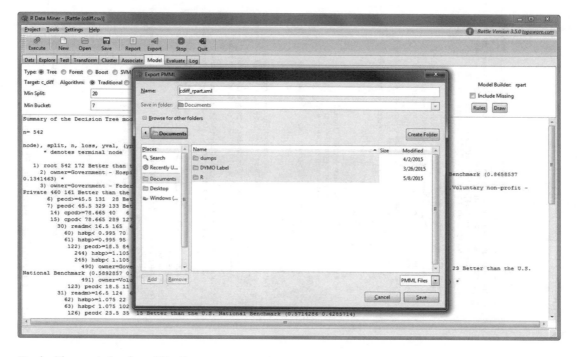

Source: Used with permission from RStudio.

Figure 15.21. Exported PMML model

```xml
<?xml version="1.0"?>
<PMML xsi:schemaLocation="http://www.dmg.org/PMML-4_2 http://www.dmg.org/v4-2/pmml-4-2.xsd" xmlns:xsi="http://www.w3.org/2001/XMLSchema-instance"
xmlns="http://www.dmg.org/PMML-4_2" version="4.2">
 <Header description="RPart Decision Tree Model" copyright="Copyright (c) 2015 ">
  <Extension extender="Rattle/PMML" value="" name="user"/>
  <Application version="1.4" name="Rattle/PMML"/>
  <Timestamp>2015-08-10 12:23:46</Timestamp>
 </Header>
 <DataDictionary numberOfFields="7">
  <DataField name="c_diff" dataType="string" optype="categorical">
   <Value value="Better than the U.S. National Benchmark"/>
   <Value value="Worse than the U.S. National Benchmark"/>
  </DataField>
  <DataField name="owner" dataType="string" optype="categorical">
   <Value value="Government - Federal"/>
   <Value value="Government - Hospital District or Authority"/>
   <Value value="Government - Local"/>
   <Value value="Government - State"/>
   <Value value="Physician"/>
   <Value value="Proprietary"/>
   <Value value="Voluntary non-profit - Church"/>
   <Value value="Voluntary non-profit - Other"/>
   <Value value="Voluntary non-profit - Private"/>
  </DataField>
  <DataField name="es" dataType="string" optype="categorical">
   <Value value="No"/>
   <Value value="Yes"/>
  </DataField>
  <DataField name="cpcd" dataType="double" optype="continuous">
   <Interval rightMargin="100" leftMargin="6.67" closure="closedClosed"/>
  </DataField>
  <DataField name="pecd" dataType="double" optype="continuous">
   <Interval rightMargin="92" leftMargin="3" closure="closedClosed"/>
  </DataField>
  <DataField name="hsbp" dataType="double" optype="continuous">
   <Interval rightMargin="1.36" leftMargin="0.77" closure="closedClosed"/>
  </DataField>
  <DataField name="readm" dataType="double" optype="continuous">
   <Interval rightMargin="21" leftMargin="13" closure="closedClosed"/>
  </DataField>
 </DataDictionary>
 <TreeModel missingValueStrategy="defaultChild" splitCharacteristic="binarySplit" algorithmName="rpart" functionName="classification" modelName="RPart_Model">
  <MiningSchema>
   <MiningField name="c_diff" usageType="predicted"/>
   <MiningField name="owner" usageType="active"/>
   <MiningField name="es" usageType="active"/>
   <MiningField name="cpcd" usageType="active"/>
   <MiningField name="pecd" usageType="active"/>
   <MiningField name="hsbp" usageType="active"/>
   <MiningField name="readm" usageType="active"/>
  </MiningSchema>
  <Output>
   <OutputField name="Predicted_c_diff" dataType="string" optype="categorical" feature="predictedValue"/>
```

Source: Used with permission from RStudio.

for analysis, transforming and preparing those data for analysis, using a decision tree to model the data and evaluate their predictive performance, and also use PMML to export the model for potential deployment in separate data sets.

Based upon the decision tree analysis, model generation, and evaluation, our model was able to successfully predict 66 percent of hospitals with lower than average or above average *C. diff.* rates. Alternatively stated, the model did not correctly categorize 34 percent of hospitals. These findings indicate that deployment of the model can be used to predict hospital-associated infections, but the model has limitations in terms of its ability to accurately predict *C. diff.* rates. Further analysis is needed, including the inclusion of additional predictor variables or the exclusion of currently included predictor variables to improve the model's performance.

Conclusion

Data mining is a powerful tool for conducting predictive analytics. This project demonstrated the power of using open source data and technology to predict clinical outcomes based upon multiple factors, but there are limitations to the study. The model that was developed had an overall poor performance—that is, the model could not correctly predict over 30 percent of hospitals based upon the current inputs. Further refinements would be necessary to improve the predictive ability of the model, such as adding key variables such as geographic location, number of discharges, number of hospitals beds, or staffing patterns.

Review Exercises

Instructions: Answer the following questions.

1. What tasks are available when exploring data for data mining?
    a. Summary, Distributions, Correlation, Principal Components, and Interactive
    b. Error Matrix, Risk, Cost Curve, Hand, Lift, ROC, Precision, Sensitivity, Pr v Ob, and Score
    c. Kolmogrov-Smimov, Wilcoxon Ranked-Sum, T-Test, F-Test, Correlation, and Wilcoxon Signed-Rank
    d. Tree, Forest, Boost, SVM, Linear, Neural Network, and Survival

2. What are the elements of a decision tree model?
    a. Fronds, trunk, and needles
    b. Bark, sap, and cones
    c. Roots, branches, and leaves
    d. Beginning, middle, and end

3. If a decision tree model has an overall error rate of 41 percent in predicting an outcome, what does this mean?

4. If we use a data mining model to predict the outcome of a malignant or benign tumor by examining patterns in a set of the following variables including age, size of tumor, sex, and tumor location, what are defined as the target and input variables?

5. The purpose of PMML is to:
    a. Prepare data for modeling
    b. Generate a data mining model
    c. Evaluate a data mining model
    d. Deploy a data mining model

References

Agency for Healthcare Research and Quality. 2009. Center for Delivery, Organization, and Markets, Healthcare Cost and Utilization Project, Nationwide Inpatient Sample, 1993–2009.

Agency for Healthcare Research and Quality. 2012. *Clostridium difficile* Infections (CDI) in Hospital Stays, 2009. http://www.hcup-us.ahrq.gov/reports/statbriefs/sb124.pdf

Centers for Medicare and Medicaid Services. 2015. Medicare.gov Hospital Compare. http://www.medicare.gov/hospitalcompare/search.html

Cohen, S.H., D.N. Gerding, S. Johnson, C.P. Kelly, V.G. Loo, L.C. McDonald, J. Pepin, and M.H. Wilcox. 2010. Clinical practice guidelines for *Clostridium difficile* infection in adults: 2010 update by the Society for Healthcare Epidemiology of America (SHEA) and the Infectious Diseases Society of America (IDSA). *Infection Control* 31(05):431–455.

Department of Health and Human Services. 2012. National Action Plan to Prevent Healthcare-Associated Infections: Roadmap to Elimination. http://www.health.gov/hcq/prevent_hai.asp

Fayyad, U., G. Piatetsky-Shapiro, and P. Smyth. 1996. The KDD process for extracting useful knowledge from volumes of data. *Communications of the ACM* 39(11):27–34.

Kyne, L., M.B. Hamel, R. Polavaram, and C.P. Kelly. 2002. Health care costs and mortality associated with nosocomial diarrhea due to *Clostridium difficile*. *Clinical Infectious Diseases* 34(3):346–353.

Lucado, J., C. Gould, and A. Elixhauser. 2012. *Clostridium difficile* Infections (CDI) in Hospital Stays, 2009. http://www.hcup-us.ahrq.gov/reports/statbriefs/sb124.pdf

Magill, S.S., J.R. Edwards, W. Bamberg, Z.G. Beldavs, G. Dumyati, M.A. Kainer, R. Lynfield, M. Maloney, L. McAllister-Hollod, and J. Nadle. 2014. Multistate point-prevalence survey of health care–associated infections. *New England Journal of Medicine* 370(13):1198–1208.

McDonald, L.C., M. Owings, and D.B. Jernigan. 2006. *Clostridium difficile* infection in patients discharged from US short-stay hospitals, 1996–2003. *Emerging Infectious Diseases* 12(3):409.

Miller, B.A., L.F. Chen, D.J. Sexton, and D.J. Anderson. 2011. Comparison of the burdens of hospital-onset, healthcare facility-associated *Clostridium difficile* infection and of healthcare-associated infection due to methicillin-resistant *Staphylococcus aureus* in community hospitals. *Infection Control* 32(04):387–390.

Williams, G. 2011. *Data Mining with Rattle and R: The Art of Excavating Data for Knowledge Discovery*. New York, NY: Springer.

Yokoe, D.S., D.J. Anderson, S.M. Berenholtz, D.P. Calfee, E.R. Dubberke, K. Ellingson, D.N. Gerding, J. Haas, K.S. Kaye, and M. Klompas. 2014. Introduction to "A compendium of strategies to prevent healthcare-associated infections in acute care hospitals: 2014 updates." *Infection Control* 35(5):455–459.

Yokoe, D.S, L.A. Mermel, D.J. Anderson, K.M. Arias, H. Burstin, D.P. Calfee, S.E. Coffin, E.R. Dubberke, V. Fraser, and D.N. Gerding. 2008. Executive summary: A compendium of strategies to prevent healthcare-associated infections in acute care hospitals. *Infection Control* 29(S1):S12–S21.

Studying the Relationship between Socioeconomic Factors and Preventive Care Utilization

Shauna M. Overgaard, MHI

Learning Objectives

- Investigate the relationship between variables graphically
- Demonstrate the use of multiple linear regression to assess the relationship between an outcome and more than one predictor variable
- Explain potential interactions between multiple variables

Key Terms

Interaction
Multiple linear regression (MLR)

Breast cancer, the most common cancer in women, is also the leading cause of cancer mortality worldwide (Shah et al. 2014). According to the American Cancer Society, one in every eight US women develops breast cancer. Indeed a major public health problem, in 2015 an estimated 40,290 US women will die of breast cancer (American Cancer Society 2015).

The sheer magnitude of breast cancer incidence reflects the urgency for preventative measures. Although not all agree that frequent mammograms are necessary, the current recommendation for breast cancer prevention is biennial screening in women between the ages of 50 and 74 (US Preventative Services Task Force 2015). The survival rate for women with breast cancer is significantly higher in those with an early diagnosis, and recent national decreases in breast cancer mortality rates are attributed to mammography and treatment developments (Berry et al. 2005). Unfortunately, women of low socioeconomic status have a statistically higher mortality rate relative to their affluent counterparts (Tao et al. 2014). To elucidate target areas for improvements, this chapter will confirm this statistic and investigate potential contributions to such disparity and to general mammography rates. The purpose of this chapter is to identify a regression model that can assist in the determination of factors affecting mammography rates in the United States.

Research Question and Hypothesis

Is there a linear relationship between rate of mammography screening and socioeconomic factors such as poverty, uninsured rate, and access to care? Are there interactions between our predictors?

A **multiple linear regression (MLR)** analysis can be used to quantify the relationship between an outcome and multiple explanatory variables. The response, or dependent variable, is a continuous measure, which we will represent by the letter y. The dependent variable for the proposed MLR model is the percentage of women of 50 years of age or older who have, within the past 2 years, undergone a mammogram. In the introduction, the current screening recommendations were noted. This is important information to consider as we set up our analysis. As the national recommendations for breast cancer screening includes an age class, we need to include this subset of women in our analysis. The independent variables may be any combination of continuous or categorical. We will symbolize the number of independent variables by the letter p. In this example, the independent variables are poverty, uninsured rate, primary care physician rate, and presence of a community health center; thus we have p = 4 independent variables. In the context of our MLR analysis, we want to test for significance of regression; therefore our null hypothesis states that no linear statistical relationship exists between our dependent variable and at least one of our independent variables. The statement for such a null hypothesis can be written in symbolic form: $H1_0$: $\beta_1 = \beta_2 = \beta_3 = \beta_4 = 0$, where β represents the coefficient estimate within the regression model, and the numbers 1 through 4 represent each of our four independent variables. Next, we determine our alternative hypothesis, the expectation that a statistically significant relationship exists between our dependent variable and at least one of our independent variables: $H1_a$: $\beta_j \neq 0$. Here we write β_j to indicate any number, and in this case we refer to the numbers 1 through 4. For the sake of a deeper understanding of our model, we may also choose to evaluate the individual effect of our independent variables on our dependent variable:

$H2_0$: $\beta_{1(Uninsured\_Rate)} = 0$; $\quad$ $H2_a$: $\beta_{1(Uninsured\_Rate)} \neq 0$

$H3_0$: $\beta_{2(Poverty)} = 0$; $\quad$ $H3_a$: $\beta_{2(Poverty)} \neq 0$

$H4_0$: $\beta_{3(Prim\_Care\_Phys\_Rate)} = 0$; $\quad$ $H4_a$: $\beta_{3(Prim\_Care\_Phys\_Rate)} \neq 0$

$H5_0$: $\beta_{4(Community\_Health\_Center\_Ind)} = 0$; $\quad$ $H5_a$: $\beta_{4(Community\_Health\_Center\_Ind)} \neq 0$

Hypotheses

The research question will require more than one hypothesis. The hypotheses will include the following:

$H1_0$: There is no relationship between the rate of mammography and poverty, uninsured rate, primary care physician rate, and presence of a community health center.

$H1_A$: There is a relationship between the rate of mammography and at least one of the following: poverty, uninsured rate, primary care physician rate, and presence of a community health center.

$H2_0$: There is no relationship between the rate of mammography and the rate of uninsurance.

$H2_A$: There is a relationship between the rate of mammography and the rate of uninsurance.

$H3_0$: There is no relationship between the rate of mammography and the rate of poverty.

$H3_A$: There is a relationship between the rate of mammography and the rate of poverty.

$H4_0$: There is no relationship between the rate of mammography and rate of primary care physicians.

$H4_A$: There is a relationship between the rate of mammography and rate of primary care physicians.

$H5_0$: There is no relationship between the rate of mammography and the presence of a community health center.

$H5_A$: There is a relationship between the rate of mammography and the presence of a community health center.

Checklist

To answer our research question, a specific process of data acquisition, preparation, and discovery is required. The following steps will be explained in detail:

1. Extract data sets from MySQL
   a. Select appropriate columns of data
2. Data preparation
   a. Review data set for erroneous values

3. Import the data into RStudio
4. Perform descriptive statistics on the variables
5. Conduct similar linear regressions to examine the relationship between lead levels and measures of infant health at the US county level

The Analysis

Which predictors and which interactions are included in a regression model should be motivated by a scientific and clinical understanding of the problem and potential solutions, and should be specified in advance. We have researched our problem, identified a gap in the literature, posed our research question, stated our hypotheses, identified our variables, and specified our methodology. The analysis can now begin.

Step 1: Data Extraction

In order to carry out the analysis, we need to extract data from the measures_of_birth_and_death table. A query will be generated to select the population size, poverty rate, mammogram rate, uninsured rate, number of primary care physicians, and whether there is a community health center for each county in the United States. All the data required for answering the proposed research question are included in the MySQL database associated with this textbook. All of the data for this analysis were made available from the Community Health Status Indicator data set that is published by CMS (CDC 2015; CMS 2015).

Figure 16.1 displays the SQL script that was used to retrieve the data and also the first few rows of the output that was derived from the query. Note that you must alter a setting in MySQL so that the output shows all of the results rather than just showing the first 1,000 rows. After executing each query, export the data to a CSV file and save the file as PreventCare. For detailed instructions regarding exporting data from MySQL Workbench to CSV format, see chapter 4.

Step 2: Data Preparation

Data preparation is critical for the analysis process. To make this data set easier to work with and meaningful for our analysis, we are going to prepare the data in Microsoft Excel prior to importing them into RStudio. Using Microsoft Excel, open the PreventCare CSV file that was exported from MySQL Workbench. Upon opening the CSV file, we should see that the data set has columns A through F, and each observation represents a single US county. The following columns of data are included:

- population_size: Count of individuals residing in the city to which the hospital is affiliated.
- poverty_rate: The percentage of individuals within each county who are living below the poverty level; therefore we expect a continuous range between 0 and 100.
- mammogram_rate: The percentage of females aged 50 years and older who have had a mammogram within the past two years.
- uninsured_rate: The percentage of uninsured individuals under the age of 65.
- prim_care_phys_rate: This is the total number of active, nonfederal physicians per 100,000 population in 2007 who practice in one of the four primary care specialties (general or family practice, general internal medicine, pediatrics, and obstetrics and gynecology).
- community_health_center_ind: A binary variable (1 = yes, 2 = no), indicates whether a community health center, considered a source of care for low-income and uninsured individuals and families, exists within the referenced county.

To make the data easier to work with in RStudio, we need to change the column names to something shorter. To rename column headers in Excel, simply click each individual cell, highlight the contents, delete the content, enter the new column name, and click return. Repeat this process for each column header. Table 16.1 contains the names we will use when renaming the column headers.

Figure 16.1.   SQL script and returned data for combining three data sets

```
SELECT
    population_size,
    poverty_rate,
    mammogram_rate,
    uninsured_rate,
    prim_care_phys_rate,
    community_health_center_ind
FROM
    measures_of_birth_and_death;
```

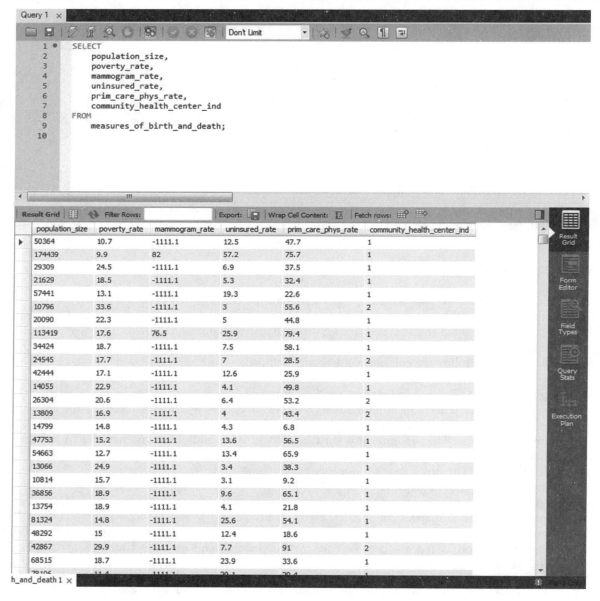

You may have noticed that our data set includes negative integers. These integers represent missing values. As we are working to simplify our data set, we will replace these negative values with a blank space so that they do not function as weighted values during our analysis. You can do this by first selecting the entire data set, then under the Home tab clicking on Find & Select icon within the top toolbar, and

Table 16.1.   Original and revised column names within Excel

Original Name	Revised Name
population_size	pop
poverty_rate	poverty
mammogram_rate	mammogram
uninsured_rate	uninsured
prim_care_phys_rate	phys_rate
community_health_center_ind	chc

Figure 16.2.   Using the Replace tool within Excel

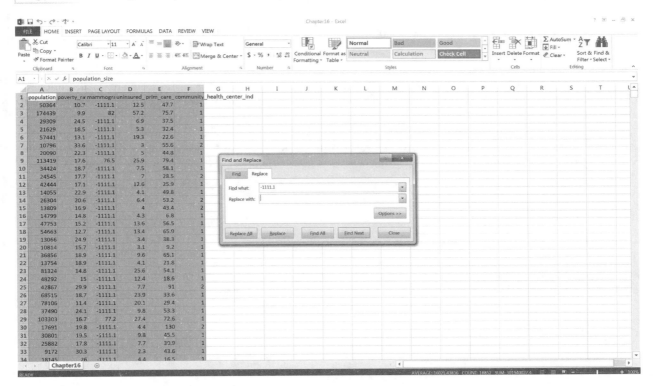

Source: Used with permission from Microsoft.

selecting Replace. When the Replace box opens, as shown in figure 16.2, enter the value −1111.1 in the "Find what:" field and leave the space below "Replace with:" empty. Select the Replace All button in order to substitute the −1111.1 values. This will replace 2,247 instances of −1111.1 within the document with a blank space.

Next, we will use the IF function to change the chc variable values from 1 and 2 to 1 and 0 (that is, 1 = yes, 0 = no). First, in column G enter chc as the name of the column in cell G1. Within cell G2 type =IF (F2=1,1,0) and press enter, to specify that if cell F2 equals 1, code as 1, otherwise code as 0. The Excel =IF() statement is shown in figure 16.3. For our purposes, logical_test = F2=1, value_if_true = 1, value_if_false = 0. To fill in the formula for the remainder of the cells in column G, click on and hover over the bottom right corner of cell G2 until the white cross turns black, then double-click to populate the rest of the column using the computation.

Now, we want to remove the formulas in column G but retain the values. The reason we want to do this is so that we can delete column F without altering the data in column G. First, copy column G by right clicking on the G, and selecting copy. Next, overwrite column G by right clicking in cell G1 and selecting the paste special as values option. The formulas are removed from column G, but the values remain. We can now delete

Figure 16.3.   Using the IF function within Excel

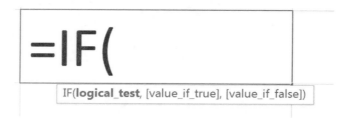

IF(**logical_test**, [value_if_true], [value_if_false])

Source: Used with permission from Microsoft.

column F from the data set. Simply right click on the F, and select Delete. Only six columns should remain: pop, poverty, mammogram, uninsured, phys_rate, and chc.

Step 3: Import the Data

Once you have made and saved these changes to the PreventCare.csv file, you can import the file to RStudio. Click Import Dataset, which can be found in the upper right quadrant of the RStudio dashboard; under the Environment tab, choose the From Text File option in the drop-down window. Navigate to the PreventCare.csv file that was saved in the final action of Step 2, highlight the file, and click Open, then click Import. For more detailed instruction regarding importing data into RStudio, see chapter 5). After the data are imported into RStudio, open an R scripting window. The R scripting window is where you will enter the R code in order to analyze the data. To open a new R scripting window, go to File > New File > R Script. The first step is to attach the file in order to call the data by the column names:

```
attach(PreventCare)
```

Step 4: Descriptive Statistics

Before moving into the statistical modeling of our data set, we need to perform some simple summary and graphical characterizations of the data. One of the first things we want to prepare is a summary of the entire data set by using R's summary function. Run following code in RStudio:

```
summary(PreventCare)
```

Output from this function is as follows:

```
      pop             poverty        mammogram        uninsured       phys_rate         chc
Min.:42         Min.:-2222.20  Min.:  58.30   Min.:  -4.40 Min.:    0.0 Min.:  0.0000
1stQu.:11014    1stQu.:10.90   1stQu.:76.50   1stQu.:  3.10 1stQu.:29.4 1stQu.:0.0000
Median:25546    Median:14.30   Median:80.60   Median:  7.00 Median:50.7 Median:0.0000
Mean:   96803   Mean:14.53     Mean:   80.03  Mean:   24.29 Mean:    56.9 Mean:  0.4912
3rdQu.:65331    3rdQu.:18.30   3rdQu.:84.10   3rdQu.:18.20 3rdQu.:74.8 3rdQu.:1.0000
Max.:9862049    Max.:54.40     Max.:   95.90  Max.:  856.00 Max.:  621.9 Max.:  1.0000
                               NA's:2247
```

In this output we see a summary of each variable within our data set that includes the minimum value of the range, 1st quartile, median, statistical mean, 3rd quartile, the maximum value of the range, and the number of missing values (NAs). To ensure an accurate representation of our data when assessing individual relationships with our response variable, we remove missing values corresponding to the mammogram variable with the following code:

```
PreventCare<-subset(PreventCare, !is.na(mammogram))
```

Now that we altered the data from the original PreventCare data set, we need to attach the data set again. If we were to run attach(PreventCare), we would receive a warning that states "The following objects are masked from PreventCare: chc, mammogram, phys_rate, pop, poverty, uninsured". This error is telling the user that there are already data attached with these column names and by attaching this data you will overwrite the data. Although our intention is to overwrite the data, we can avoid the warning by first detaching the data set and subsequently attaching the data set again. Therefore, first detach the data set with the following script:

```
detach(PreventCare)
```

Next, we can attach the data set again, but this time PreventCare will not contain NAs in the mammogram column.

```
attach(PreventCare)
```

If we run another summary of the PreventCare data set, as performed previously, it can be noted that the minimum values from variables poverty and uninsured are no longer negative, and our NA values have been removed. To run the summary again, move your cursor back to the line of code that includes summary (PreventCare). After running this script, the output will be the following:

```
pop             poverty         mammogram       uninsured       phys_rate       chc
Min.:     2060  Min.:     3.10  Min.:    58.30  Min.:     0.60  Min.:     0.00  Min.: 0.0000
1stQu.: 42526   1stQu.: 9.90    1stQu.:76.50    1stQu.:11.55    1stQu.: 54.30   1stQu.:0.0000
Median:101684   Median:13.20    Median:80.60    Median:26.15    Median: 73.45   Median:1.0000
Mean:  259924   Mean:  13.68    Mean:    80.03  Mean:    61.63  Mean:    82.49  Mean: 0.7025
3rdQu.:255645   3rdQu.:16.88    3rdQu.:84.10    3rdQu.:64.90    3rdQu.:100.78   3rdQu.:1.0000
Max.: 9862049   Max.:   35.80   Max.:    95.90  Max.:   856.00  Max.:   420.20  Max.: 1.0000
```

To ensure the data are correctly displayed within our attached variable, take a moment and look at the data set loaded into the RStudio environment to check for overall accuracy. Specifically, verify that the data set contains the five columns we preserved and that missing values have been removed from the variable mammogram. Viewing the data to ensure that our columns have been preserved can be done using R's View function (note that the V is capitalized in the View function) and the removal of missing values from the mammogram variable can be done by separately using the summary command:

```
View(PreventCare)

summary(mammogram)
```

The minimum value for the mammogram variable should now be 58.30 and the maximum value should be 95.90.

For the purpose of this study, we are largely interested in factors that may predict mammography. To explore this concept, we need to create four plots to graphically explore the data we will be working with in this chapter: mammogram versus uninsured_rate; mammogram versus poverty; mammogram versus community_health_center_ind; and mammogram versus prim_care_phys_rate. To create these plots, use the following R scripts:

```
par(mfrow=c(2,2))

plot(mammogram, uninsured,xlab="Mammography",ylab="Proportion Uninsured",
main="Mammogram vs. Uninsured")

plot(mammogram,poverty,xlab="Mammography",ylab="Rate of Poverty",
main="Mammogram vs. Poverty")

boxplot(mammogram, chc, xlab="Community Health Center",ylab="Mammography",
main="Mammogram Rates in Presence of CHC", names=c("Yes","No"))

plot(mammogram,phys_rate,xlab="Mammography",ylab="Rate of Primary Care
Physicians", main="Mammogram vs. Primary Care")
```

Graphing mammogram rates by uninsured, poverty, community health center, and primary care providers

Source: Used with permission from RStudio.

Within this code we use the command "par" to specify our graphical parameter of interest, the creation of multiple plots in one graph. The first script shown above using the function par, which is used to set graphical parameters for graphs and figures. The mfrow =c(2,2) is an argument used with the par function, which allows us to specify that this graph be filled by a matrix of two rows by two columns. That is, we will be plotting four graphs on a single display. The output of this R code is illustrated in figure 16.4.

As you can see from looking at the plots:

- A linear relationship between mammography rate and uninsured rate may be justified, as we observe a slightly negative trend between the proportion of uninsured and the rate of mammography, indicating that a low proportion of uninsured individuals per population size appears to correspond to a higher rate of mammography.
- A linear relationship between mammography rate and the rate of poverty may be justified, where a low proportion of uninsured individuals per population size appears to correspond to a higher rate of mammography.
- A difference between the rate of mammography between groups with and without a community health center is visually evident; groups with a community health center appear to have higher rates of mammography.
- Judging by the data in the plot depicting the relationship between the rate of primary care physician and mammography, it is unclear whether a linear relationship exists.

The output from the descriptive statistics and the plots provide us with very useful information about mammography rates and when considering other factors related to insurance, access to primary care providers, and poverty rates, a statistical analysis is required in order to empirically determine if there is a relationship between mammography rates and these other factors.

Having graphically explored our data, let's create an MLR model predicting mammography using our selected variables.

Step 5: Statistical Analyses

More often than not, as investigators we are interested in the relationship between an outcome and more than one predictor variable. In such cases, our model contains more than one independent variable, and it is often important to investigate an **interaction** between those variables. MLR in RStudio is quite similar to linear regression with the major differences being that more variables are added to the model statement and interaction terms ought to be considered.

We will be using MLR in RStudio to determine the following:

1. Is there a linear relationship between rate of mammography screening and socioeconomic factors such as poverty, uninsured rate, and access to care?
2. Are there interactions between the predictors?

The first step in conducting MLR in RStudio is to name the model and use R's lm function to create the linear model. Here is the R script for completing this first step:

```
US_Mammogram_lm <- lm(mammogram ~ poverty + uninsured + as.factor(chc) +
phys_rate)
```

Note that we have named the linear model US_Mammogram_lm. The model we have created regresses the rate of mammography on the rate of poverty, followed by the proportion of uninsured, the presence of a county community health center, and the rate of primary care physician. Because chc is a nonweighted binary variable we need to treat it as a factor as we have done by specifying as.factor(chc) within the lm() function.

The next step is to summarize the model by using the following code:

```
summary(US_Mammogram_lm)
```

The output of this model is the following:

```
Call:
lm(formula = mammogram ~ poverty + uninsured + as.factor(chc) +
phys_rate)

Residuals:
Min        1Q        Median    3Q       Max
-19.3015   -3.6105   0.1623    3.6838   16.7369

Coefficients:
                  Estimate    Std. Error   t value   Pr(>|t|)
(Intercept)       81.094997   0.683504     118.646   < 2e-16   ***
poverty           -0.250300   0.036263     -6.902    9.72e-12  ***
uninsured         0.003643    0.001996     1.826     0.0682    .
as.factor(chc)1   0.724069    0.435238     1.664     0.0965    .
phys_rate         0.019747    0.004505     4.383     1.31e-05  ***
---
Signif. codes: 0 '***' 0.001 '**' 0.01 '*' 0.05 '.' 0.1 ' ' 1

Residual standard error: 5.643 on 889 degrees of freedom
Multiple R-squared: 0.09335,    Adjusted R-squared: 0.08927
F-statistic: 22.88 on 4 and 889 DF, p-value: < 2.2e-16
```

Specification of our model is accomplished by setting up our formula with a "+" to separate our explanatory variables. This can be read as mammogram is described using a model that is additive in poverty, uninsured, chc, and phys_rate. We use our coefficient estimates to write our multiple regression equation, which is good form in regression modeling and also provides a platform from which to compute predictions (rounding to the nearest decimal): y = 81.1 − 0.25*poverty + 0.004*uninsured + 0.72*chc(1) + 0.02* phys_rate.

Notice that there is not only one t-value; rather there is a t-value awarded to each of our variables, and there is one overall F statistic. The magnitude of the t statistics can be used as a means to judge the relative importance of an independent variable in the multiple linear model. The F statistic allows us to assess whether there is at least one effect within our model. The R-squared value indicates the proportion of the variance that can be explained by our predictors; we can see that about 9 percent of the variance in mammography is explained by our independent variables in the model. Because the model contains more than one independent variable, however, we abide by the adjusted R-square value instead of the R-squared value in our interpretation of variance explained by the independent variables (8.9 percent) for a conservative estimation, comparable to a statistical adjustment for multiple comparisons. To test whether all of the variables taken together significantly predict the outcome variable, mammogram, we use the overall F-test.

The test statistic (F* = 22.88) and associated p-value (<0.001) are found in the last line of output. Because the p-value is less than 0.05, we reject the null hypothesis and conclude that taken together, poverty, uninsured rate, CHC, and primary care physician are significantly related to rate of mammography.

To test the significance of an individual variable in predicting rate of mammography, we use the test statistic (t value) and associated p-value for that particular variable (Pr>|t|) taken from within our summary columns.

For example, the test of whether poverty is significantly related to rate of mammography, we evaluate using the t statistic: $t* = -6.902$, $p < 0.0001$. Therefore we reject the null hypothesis and conclude that the rate of poverty is significantly related to rate of mammography. Note that the "−" sign in our t value indicates a negative value; thus we describe a negative association between the rate of mammography and poverty. That is, with a high rate of poverty, we expect a low rate of mammography.

Because we have more than one predictor variable, it is important to consider whether those variables interact. The letter A will represent any one variable within our model (for example, poverty). The letter B will represent any other variable within our model (for example, uninsured). We will use the following formulas to review the R syntax for interaction:

Y ~A+B+A:B	The inclusion of each individual term, A and B, as well as the interaction between both, A:B.
Y ~A*B	Equivalent to Y ~A+B+A:B.
Y ~A:B	The inclusion of only the interaction between A and B.

We include the interaction terms between each predictor in our model and call a summary of the model using the following R script:

```
US_Mammogram_interact_lm <- lm(mammogram ~ poverty * uninsured *
as.factor(chc)* phys_rate)

summary(US_Mammogram_interact_lm)
```

The output of this model is the following:

```
Call:
lm(formula = mammogram ~ poverty * uninsured * as.factor(chc) *
phys_rate)

Residuals:
Min        1Q        Median    3Q        Max
-18.6958   -3.5446   0.1447    3.6116    17.3867

Coefficients:
```

	Estimate	Std. Error	t value	Pr(>|t|)	
(Intercept)	7.564e+01	2.245e+00	33.701	< 2e-16	***
poverty	2.317e-01	1.764e-01	1.314	0.189299	
uninsured	1.558e-01	6.684e-02	2.330	0.020007	*
as.factor(chc)1	5.025e+00	2.773e+00	1.812	0.070258	
phys_rate	8.671e-02	2.491e-02	3.480	0.000526	***
poverty:uninsured	-1.397e-02	7.243e-03	-1.929	0.054080	.
poverty:as.factor(chc)1	-4.093e-01	2.061e-01	-1.986	0.047339	*

```
uninsured:as.factor(chc)1        -1.407e-01 6.929e-02  -2.031      0.042592 *
poverty:phys_rate                -6.967e-03 2.138e-03  -3.258      0.001163 **
uninsured:phys_rate              -1.460e-03 4.885e-04  -2.990      0.002871 **
as.factor(chc)1:phys_rate        -5.192e-02 3.064e-02  -1.694      0.090546 .
poverty:uninsured:
as.factor(chc)1                   1.329e-02 7.349e-03   1.809      0.070813
poverty:uninsured:phys_rate       1.830e-04 7.053e-05   2.594      0.009638 **
poverty:as.factor(chc)1:          6.028e-03 2.461e-03   2.449      0.014520 *
phys_rate
uninsured:                        1.316e-03 5.169e-04   2.547      0.011043 *
as.factor(chc)1:phys_rate
poverty:uninsured:               -1.744e-04 7.144e-05  -2.442      0.014819 *
as.factor(chc)1:phys_rate
---
Signif. codes:  0 '***' 0.001 '**' 0.01 '*' 0.05 '.' 0.1 ' ' 1

Residual standard error: 5.617 on 878 degrees of freedom
Multiple R-squared: 0.1127,     Adjusted R-squared: 0.09756
F-statistic: 7.436 on 15 and 878 DF, p-value: 1.04e-15
```

The tests of interactions are shown when there is a colon between two variable names. For instance, the interaction of poverty and uninsured (povertry:uninsured) has a p-value of 0.054, which is nearing significance but still greater than the 0.05 significance level. As we can see from the t-values and corresponding p-values, there are several interactions existing with poverty and other independent variables including chc ($p = 0.047$), phys_rate ($p = 0.001$), chc and phy_rate together ($p = 0.0145$), uninsured and phys_rate together ($p = 0.0096$), and uninsured, chc, and phys_rate together (0.0148) on the rate mammography. In addition, there are interactions with uninsured and phys_rate ($p = 0.0029$), and chc and phys_rate together ($p = 0.011$) on the rate of mammography. Notably, the lowest p-value indicates that the strongest interaction exists between poverty and phys_rate. Based on the negative t-value, this indicates the relationship between the rate of mammography is negative. Therefore, in counties that have a combination of high poverty rates and a high proportion of physicians, there is a lower rate of mammography.

You may notice that some of the p-values for the interaction terms are greater than 0.05; these interactions are not significant. Additionally, we notice that the adjusted R-square value is 0.098, indicating that 9.8 percent of the variability in mammogram is explained by our independent variables and their interactions. This number is slightly larger than the R-squared value derived from our original model, and this lends support for including the interaction terms in the model. Therefore, the final model should include the interactions between our four independent variables: poverty, uninsured, phys_rate, and chc. Formally, we reject the null hypothesis, $H1_0: \beta_1 = \beta_2 = \beta_3 = \beta_4 = 0$, and conclude that a statistically significant relationship exists between our response variable and at least one of our predictor variables: $H1_a: \beta_j \neq 0$.

Discussion

The purpose of this chapter is to identify a regression model that can assist in the determination of factors affecting mammography rates in the United States. We have determined that poverty, proportion of uninsured individuals, primary care physician rate, and the presence of a community health center are all significantly associated with the rate of mammography. Also, there are significant interactions between these variables.

Particularly evident given the inverse relationship between rates of mammography and rates of poverty and proportion of uninsured ($p < 0.0001$), our findings confirm the need to address socioeconomic status so that all women have equal access to preventative medical care such as mammography is of high importance. In addition, in counties where there are high rates of poverty and high proportions of physicians, there is a lower rate of mammography. In this case, the higher proportion of physicians may be related to urban settings. That is, urban areas may have a higher proportion of physicians than rural areas. If this is the case, then urban counties with high poverty rates are predicted to have lower mammography rates.

As breast cancer is the leading cause of cancer mortality for women worldwide (Shah et al. 2014), and that a better outcome is linked with an early diagnosis, an organizational structure that targets early intervention areas of low socioeconomic status has the potential to bring about important change.

Conclusion

Poverty, insurance, the presence of a primary care physician, and a community health center significantly affect the rate of mammography in the United States. In other words, we can confirm the notion that women of lower socioeconomic status receive less preventative care, by way of mammography, than do individuals of higher socioeconomic status. This is concerning, specifically when we have prior evidence to believe that mammography directly affects likelihood of survival. It is important to note that we are not evaluating the rate of breast cancer; rather, for this analysis we are interested in contributing factors to the rate of use for a known prevention method. In light of reports naming breast cancer comorbidities such as obesity and race as chief predictors of disease, the access to or use of preventative measures should be thoughtfully considered in the planning of national efforts to reduce the rate of this disease.

Review Exercises

Instructions: Answer the following questions.

1. In a new data set, the multiple regression analysis of the continuous outcome variable obesity rate involves the binary variable sex. How do you interpret the results for this variable?

2. Write a command to prepare the graphical interface for the showcasing of four tables displayed in the order of columns × rows.

3. Why did we first compute our standardized variable before eliminating negatives? Please provide an example to support this logic.

4. Why did the negative minimum values in the poverty and prop_uninsured disappear after we removed the NA values from our mammogram variable?

5. What code can be used to specify that a variable be considered nonweighted categories?

References

American Cancer Society. 2015. What Are the Key Statistics about Breast Cancer? http://www.cancer.org/cancer/breastcancer/detailedguide/breast-cancer-key-statistics

Berry, D.A., K.A. Cronin, S.K. Plevritis, D.G. Fryback, L. Clarke, M. Zelen, and E.J. Feuer. 2005. Effect of screening and adjuvant therapy on mortality from breast cancer. *New England Journal of Medicine* 353(17):1784–1792.

Centers for Disease Control and Prevention. 2015. Community Health Status Indicators. http://wwwn.cdc.gov/CommunityHealth/homepage.aspx

Centers for Medicare and Medicaid Services. 2015. Medicare.gov Hospital Compare. http://www.medicare.gov/hospitalcompare/search.html

Shah, R., K. Rosso, and S.D. Nathanson. 2014. Pathogenesis, prevention, diagnosis and treatment of breast cancer. *World Journal of Clinical Oncology* 5(3):283.

Tao, Z., A. Shi, C. Lu, T. Song, Z. Zhang, and J. Zhao. 2014. Breast cancer: Epidemiology and etiology. *Cell Biochemistry and Biophysics* 72(2):333–338.

US Preventative Services Task Force. 2015. Breast Cancer: Screening. http://www.uspreventiveservicestaskforce.org/uspstf/uspsbrca.htm

Answer Key

Chapter 1

1. b
2. c
3. a
4. d
5. **Design and capture:** Analytics can be an impetus for improving data dictionaries across systems and collecting data with closer attention to their eventual use.

   Content and record management: Analytics creates new data set, database, and report library management needs, all which need policies and procedures grounded in sound practice with governance oversight.

   Access and use: Analytics will drive key organizational priorities regarding how trusted data and information are used both centrally and locally at multifacility organizations.

   Integrity and quality: As data are cleansed for analytics, data quality problems will be identified and can be used to identify improvements in data capture moving forward.

   Privacy, confidentiality, and security: Rules are required regarding who is authorized to access what levels of analytic data. These may be role-based authorizations and may require some level of analytic training.

Chapter 2

1. True
2. b
3. a
4. b
5. False
6. a
7. True
8. d
9. d
10. b

Chapter 3

1. a
2. b
3. b
4. False
5. True

Chapter 4

1. c
2. b
3. d
4. False
5. False

Chapter 5

1. b
2. Concatenate refers to the function of combining individual items into a list or series, also known as a vector.
3. True
4. a
5. The reason that the data set needs to be attached is to create the column names into R objects in order to make them easier to work with in RStudio.

Chapter 6

1. d
2. d
3. c
4. a
5. c

Chapter 7

1. A contingency table is a table of frequency distributions (a table that displays the number of times an observation occurs).
2. b
3. The smokers have a higher than expected number of people with heart disease compared to the nonsmokers. The nonsmokers have a lower than expected number of people without heart disease.
4. False
5. True

Chapter 8

1. a
2. b
3. b
4. d
5. d

Chapter 9

1. The odds of being better than the national average for hospitals without emergency services versus with emergency services is

    OR = (13/2) / (164/134) = 5.31

    The odds of being worse than the national average for hospitals without emergency services versus with emergency services is

    OR = (2/13) / (134/164) = 0.19

    Hospitals without emergency services have an 81 percent (1–0.19) lower odds of being worse than the national rate than do hospitals with emergency services.

```
>mortality.logit <-glm(mortality ~ eservices, weights=count,
data=mortalityid, family="binomial") # we use family="binomial" to
specify logistic regression (binomial = binary outcome)

mortalityid <- data.frame(mortality=factor(c("1","1","0","0")),
    eservices=factor(c("1","0","1","0")), count=c(13,164,2,134))

str(mortalityid) # verify that mortality and eservices are factors

> summary(mortality.logit)

Call:

glm(formula = mortality ~ eservices, family = "binomial", data =
mortalityid, weights = count)

Deviance Residuals:

1  2  3  4

1.929  13.996  -2.839  -14.636

Coefficients:

              Estimate     Std. Error          z value Pr(>|z|)

(Intercept)   0.2020   0.1164   1.735    0.0828.

eservices1    1.6698   0.7684   2.173    0.0298 *

- - -

Signif. codes: 0 '***' 0.001 '**' 0.01 '*' 0.05 '.' 0.1 ' ' 1

(Dispersion parameter for binomial family taken to be 1)

Null deviance: 428.52 on 3 degrees of freedom

Residual deviance: 421.87 on 2 degrees of freedom

AIC: 425.87

Number of Fisher Scoring iterations: 4

> exp(coef(mortality.logit))

(Intercept) eservices1

1.223881 5.310976
```

The value below eservices1 is our odds ratio.

2. An odds ratio is a descriptive statistic that can be derived from a contingency table or the coefficients of a logistic regression, for example. It is a measure of effect size and provides an index for the strength of association (or nonindependence) between two values.

    Oddsgroup1/Oddsgroup2

Chapter 10

1. False
2. Because the r-squared value measures the strength of the association between two variables on a scale of 0 to 1, a value of 0.99 would indicate a strong association between two variables.
3. c
4. a
5. True

Chapter 11

1. c
2. False
3. a
4. True
5. Reimbursement data can be found in the CMS and other third party payment files. Data found in reimbursement data sets include demographic data such as patient age, gender, and race. All of these factors have been shown to impact patient readmission.

    Data describing the hospital can be found in CMS hospital information file or the American Hospital Association file describing all hospitals across the United States. The data found in these files would include information regarding the size of the hospital, its location, and ownership type, among other data.

    Information to categorize the hospitals by geographic location can be found the US Census files. This file would provide the data needed to classify the hospital as urban or rural or to designate the particular geographic location in which the hospital is located.

    The electronic health record system or clinical data warehouse could be utilized to identify additional clinical details regarding each patient who was readmitted.

Chapter 12

1. Masking covers objects that have already been attached with objects with the same name. To avoid masking, use attach(), but remember to use the detach() function to clear the object from memory. Alternatively, do not use attach() and instead call the data set along with the variable name.
2. The purpose of causal analysis is to determine which independent variables affect the dependent variable and, if in existence, to understand the magnitude of the effect.
3. AIC stands for Akaike information criterion and estimates the amount of information lost in approximating a model on a data set. The measure can be used to compare the quality of different models of the same data; where the AIC index is closer to 0 it indicates a better model fit.
4. Forward regression adds predictors; backward elimination removes predictors from its model to find the best fit.
5. dim()
6. It adjusts for the number of explanatory terms (independent variables) in a model relative to the number of data.

Chapter 13

1. b
2. d
3. c
4. False
5. False

Chapter 14

1. False
2. a
3. d
4. b
5. c

Chapter 15

1. a
2. c
3. The model incorrectly categorized the outcome 41.0 percent of the time.
4. Target = Tumor (malignant or benign)
   Input variables = Age, size of tumor, sex, and tumor location
5. d

Chapter 16

1. The regression coefficient describes the value to add to our reference category to describe the obesity rate of female relative to male.
2. par(mfcol=c(2,2))
3. We chose to first compute our standardized variable before eliminating negative numbers because the proportions computed with a blank value in either the numerator or the denominator could result a misleading number. An example of this could appear as = D2/0 would equal #DIV/0!, Or 0/D2 would equal 0.
4. The negative minimum values in the poverty and prop_uninsured variables corresponded to the mammogram NA values and were removed when rows associated with those missing mammogram values were removed.
5. as.factor()

Glossary

Accounting of disclosure. 1. Under HIPAA, a standard that states (1) An individual has a right to receive an accounting of disclosures of protected health information made by a covered entity in the six years prior to the date on which the accounting is requested, except for disclosures: (i) To carry out treatment, payment, and health care operations as provided in 164.506; (ii) To individuals of protected health information about them as provided in 164.502; (iii) Incident to a use or disclosure otherwise permitted or required by this subpart, as provided in 164.502; (iv) Pursuant to an authorization as provided in 164.508; (v) For the facility's directory or to persons involved in the individual's care or other notification purposes as provided in 164.510; (vi) For national security or intelligence purposes as provided in 164.512(k)(2); (vii) To correctional institutions or law enforcement officials as provided in 164.512(k)(5); (viii) As part of a limited data set in accordance with 164.514(e); or (ix) That occurred prior to the compliance date for the covered entity (45 CFR 164.528 2002) 2. On May 31, 2011 a notice of proposed rule-making (NPRM) was issued that would modify the AOD standard. The purpose of these modifications is, in part, to implement the statutory requirement under the Health Information Technology for Economic and Clinical Health Act ("the HITECH Act" or "the Act") to require covered entities and business associates to account for disclosures of protected health information to carry out treatment, payment, and health care operations if such disclosures are through an electronic health record. Pursuant to both the HITECH Act and its more general authority under HIPAA, the department proposes to expand the accounting provision to provide individuals with the right to receive an access report indicating who has accessed electronic protected health information in a designated record set. Under its more general authority under HIPAA, the department also proposes changes to the existing accounting requirements to improve their workability and effectiveness (HHS 2011)

Adjusted R-squared. A modified version of R-squared that has been adjusted based on the number of independent variables included in the regression model. The value will always be lower than the R-squared value. In cases where there is more than one independent variable, the adjusted R-squared should be used. If there is only one independent variable, the R-squared or adjusted R-squared can be used interchangeably

Administrative safeguards. Under HIPAA, are administrative actions and policies and procedures, to manage the selection, development, implementation, and maintenance of security measures to protect electronic protected health information and to manage the conduct of the covered entity's or business associate's workforce in relation to the protection of that information (45 CFR 164.304 2013)

Alternative hypothesis. A hypothesis that states that there is an association between independent and dependent variables

Analysis of variance. Comparing means between groups when the data are normally distributed, also known as ANOVA

Association. A relationship between two measured variables

Attribute. (1) Data elements within an entity that become the column or field names when the entity relationship diagram is implemented as a relational database. (2) Properties or characteristics of concepts; used in SNOMED CT to characterize and define concepts

Argument. Object that is modifiable by the user in order to alter the way a function works

Authorization. (1) As amended by HITECH, except as otherwise specified, a covered entity may not use or disclose protected health information without an authorization that is valid under section 164.508. (2) When a covered entity obtains or receives a valid authorization for its use or disclosure of protected health information, such use or disclosure must be consistent with the authorization (45 CFR 164.508 2013)

Backward elimination. A variable selection procedure that begins with all predictors in the model, removes the predictor with the highest p-value that is greater than the prespecified critical alpha value, and refits the model

Bar chart. A graphic technique used to display frequency distributions of nominal or ordinal data that fall into categories

Best-fit line. Provides the best approximation of the trend based upon all data points included in a scatterplot

Boarding. The time a patient spends remaining in the emergency department after the decision has been made to either transfer the patient or admit the patient to the hospital

Boxplot. A way to graphically summarize the range and center of data

Breach notification. As amended by HITECH, a covered entity shall, following the discovery of a breach of unsecured protected health information, notify each individual whose unsecured protected health information has been, or is reasonably believed by the covered entity to have been, accessed, acquired, used, or disclosed as a result of such breach (45 CFR 164.404 2013)

Business associates. (1) A person or organization other than a member of a covered entity's workforce that performs functions or activities on behalf of or affecting a covered entity that involve the use or disclosure of individually identifiable health information. (2) As amended by HITECH, with respect to a covered entity, a person who creates, receives, maintains, or transmits PHI for a function or activity regulated by HIPAA, including claims processing or administration, data analysis, processing or administration, utilization review, quality assurance, patient safety activities, billing, benefit management, practice management, and repricing or provides legal, actuarial, accounting, consulting, data aggregation, management, administrative, accreditation, or financial services (45 CFR 160.103 2013)

Cardinality. Explains which number of records in one table can be associated with which number of records in another

Categorical data. Four types of data (nominal, ordinal, interval, and ratio) that represent values or observations that can be sorted into a category

Centers for Medicaid and Medicare Services. The Department of Health and Human Services agency responsible for Medicare and parts of Medicaid. Historically, CMS has maintained the UB-92 institutional EMC format specifications, the professional EMC NSF specifications, and specifications for various certifications and authorizations used by the Medicare and Medicaid programs. CMS is responsible for the oversight of HIPAA administrative simplification transaction and code sets, health identifiers, and security standards. CMS also maintains the HCPCS medical code set and the Medicare Remittance Advice Remark Codes administrative code set (CMS 2013)

Chi-squared goodness of fit test. Used to test for relationships between categorical variables. The assumptions for the test include that the data are categorical, the observations are independent (for example, the same individual is not observed multiple times), the groups are mutually exclusive (that is, for each categorical variable each individual observation can only be in one group), and there must be at leave five expected frequencies in each categorical variable (Laerd n.d.)

Clinical trial. (1) The final stages of a long and careful research process that tests new types of medical care to see if they are safe (CMS 2013). (2) Experimental study in which an intervention or treatment is given to one group in a clinical setting and the outcomes compared with a control group that did not have the intervention or treatment or that had a different intervention or treatment

Common Rule. A rule of medical ethics concerning human research and testing governed by the Institutional Review Boards

Continuous variables. Discrete variables measured with sufficient precision

Correlation. The existence and degree of relationships among factors

Core-based statistical areas (CBSA). Statistical geographic entity consisting of the county or counties associated with at least one core (urbanized area or urban cluster) of at least 10,000 in population, plus adjacent counties having a high degree of social and economic integration with the core as measured through commuting ties with the counties containing the core. Metropolitan and micropolitan statistical areas are two components of CBSAs (US Census Bureau 2010)

Covered entity. As amended by HITECH, (1) a health plan, (2) a health care clearinghouse, (3) a health care provider who transmits any health information in electronic form in connection with a transaction covered by this subchapter (45 CFR 160.103 2013)

Cross Industry Process for Data Mining (CRISP-DM). A step-by-step process that follows the framework consisting of the following six steps: problem understanding, data understanding, data preparation, modeling, evaluation, and deployment

Cross-tabulations (contingency table). A table of frequency distributions (a table that displays the number of times an observation occurs)

Crowding. An influx of patients beyond the capabilities of the ED to treat them in a timely fashion (Nugus et al. 2011)

Data analytics. The science of examining raw data with the purpose of drawing conclusions about that information. It includes data mining, machine language, development of models, and statistical measurements. Analytics can be descriptive, predictive, or prescriptive

Data analytics life cycle. Identifies the phases of a data mining project in which data are obtained and analyzed to determine trends or patterns (LaTour et al. 2013)

Data dictionary. A descriptive list of the names, definitions, and attributes of data elements to be collected in an information system or database whose purpose is to standardize definitions and ensure consistent use

Data governance. The overall management of the availability, usability, integrity, and security of the data employed in an organization or enterprise (Data Governance Institute 2012)

Data mining. The process of extracting and analyzing large volumes of data from a database for the purpose of identifying hidden and sometimes subtle relationships or patterns and using those relationships to predict behaviors

Data normalization. In a relational database, it is the process of organizing data to minimize redundancy

Data use agreement. An agreement into which the covered entity enters with the intended recipient of a limited data set that establishes the ways in which the information in the limited data set may be used and how it will be protected (HHS-NIH 2014)

Data visualization. The presentation of data in a graphical format

Database. An organized collection of data, text, references, or pictures in a standardized format, typically stored in a computer system for multiple applications

Database management system. Software that allows the user to create and manage databases

Decision tree. A structured data-mining technique based on a set of rules useful for predicting and classifying information and making decisions

Deidentification. Health information that does not identify an individual and with respect to which there is no reasonable basis to believe that the information can be used to identify an individual is not individually identifiable health information (HHS 2012)

Dependent variable. A measurable variable in a research study that depends on an independent variable

Descriptive statistics. A set of statistical techniques used to describe data such as means, frequency distributions, and standard deviations; statistical information that describes the characteristics of a specific group or a population

Dichotomous. The outcome will always be one of two factors

Emergency department (ED) wait time. The amount of time a patient waits in the emergency department before being seen by a doctor

Emergency Medical Treatment and Labor Act (EMTALA). Enacted to eliminate discrimination in emergency care and has become a national health policy with regard to the treatment of all ED patients

Enterprise information management (EIM). (1) Ensuring the value of information assets, requiring an organization-wide perspective of information management functions; it calls for explicit structures, policies, processes, technology, and controls. (2) The infrastructure and processes to ensure the information is trustworthy and actionable

Entity. Groups of data that represent things that exist in the real world

Entity-relationship diagram. A specific type of data modeling used in conceptual data modeling and the logical-level modeling of relational databases

Expert determination method. Done by applying a statistical and scientific method to determine the risk of protected health information being identified based on the specific identifiers that are within the protected health information (Warner 2013; HHS 2012)

Exploratory data analysis (EDA). Aims to depict data graphically to help identify outliers, detect trends and patterns, and suggest hypotheses for formal testing

Flat file database. A specific type of database, such as a spreadsheet

Filler. A default value to indicate a blank field

Function. A command that executes specific processes on either a vector or an object of data

Health Insurance Portability and Accountability Act of 1996 (HIPAA). The federal legislation enacted to provide continuity of health coverage, control fraud and abuse in healthcare, reduce healthcare costs, and guarantee the security and privacy of health information; limits exclusion for pre-existing medical conditions, prohibits discrimination against employees and dependents based on health status, guarantees availability of health insurance to small employers, and guarantees renewability of insurance to all employees regardless of size; requires covered entities (most healthcare providers and organizations) to transmit healthcare claims in a specific format and to develop, implement, and comply with the standards of the Privacy Rule and the Security Rule; and mandates that covered entities apply for and utilize national identifiers in HIPAA transactions (Public Law 104-191 1996)

Histogram. A graphic technique used to display the frequency distribution of continuous data (interval or ratio data) as either numbers or percentages in a series of bars

HITECH-HIPAA Omnibus Privacy Act. strengthens the privacy and security of patient health information, modifies the breach notification rule, strengthens privacy protections for genetic information by prohibiting health plans from using or disclosing such information for underwriting, makes business associates of HIPAA covered entities liable for compliance, strengthens limitations on the use and disclosure of PHI for marketing and fundraising, and allows patients increased restriction rights (Key Health Alliance n.d.)

Hospital Compare. Developed through the efforts of Medicare and the Hospital Quality Alliance to publicly report information about quality of care (CMS 2015)

Hospital Consumer Assessment of Healthcare Providers and Systems (HCAHPS). Developed to collect consumer-oriented patient satisfaction information for a hospital

Hospital Readmissions Reduction Program. Requires payment penalties for hospitals with excess readmissions for specified conditions beginning with discharges on or after October 1, 2012 (US Congress 2010)

Hospital Value-Based Purchasing Program. A component of CMS that rewards acute-care hospitals with incentive payments for providing quality care

Independent variable. The factors in experimental research that researchers manipulate directly

Information governance. The accountability framework and decision rights to achieve enterprise information management (EIM). IG is the responsibility of executive leadership for developing and driving the IG strategy throughout the organization. IG encompasses both data governance (DG) and information technology governance (ITG)

Information management (IM) life cycle. Illustrates how information moves from origination to archival and/or deletion. The steps are comprised of design, acquire, process, use, and dispose

Informed consent. (1) A legal term referring to a patient's right to make his or her own treatment decisions based on the knowledge of the treatment to be administered or the procedure to be performed. (2) An individual's voluntary agreement to participate in research or to undergo a diagnostic, therapeutic, or preventive medical procedure

Institutional Review Board (IRB). An administrative body that provides review, oversight, guidance, and approval for research projects carried out by employees serving as researchers, regardless of the location of the research (such as a university or private research agency); responsible for protecting the rights and welfare of the human subjects involved in the research. IRB oversight is mandatory for federally funded research projects

Interaction. A communication between more than one independent variable

Knowledge discovery in databases (KDD). The "nontrivial process of identifying valid, novel, potentially useful, and ultimately understandable patterns in data" (Fayyad et al. 1996)

Least squares regression line. A straight line through all of the data points in the analysis in a simple linear regression

Logistic regression. Compares multiple independent variables simultaneously against one dependent variable

Limited data set. Protected health information that excludes direct identifiers of the individual and the individual's relatives, employers, or household members but still does not deidentify the information

Model. The representation of a theory in a visual format, on a smaller scale, or with objects

Multiple linear regression. Can be used to quantify the relationship between an outcome and multiple explanatory variables

MySQL Workbench. A software that allows the user to talk to a MySQL database

National Quality Forum. A private, not-for-profit membership organization created to develop and implement a nationwide strategy to improve the measurement and reporting of healthcare quality (NQF 2013)

Normal distribution. A theoretical family of continuous frequency distributions characterized by a symmetric bell-shaped curve, with an equal mean, median, and mode; any standard deviation; and with half of the observations above the mean and half below it

Null hypothesis. A hypothesis that states there is no association between the independent and dependent variables in a research study

Object. The basic component in an object-oriented database that includes both data and their relationships within a single structure

Odds ratio. A descriptive statistic that can be derived from a contingency table or the coefficients of a logistic regression. It is a measure of effect size and provides an index for the strength of association (or nonindependence) between two values

One-way ANOVA. Used to compare a mean across more than two groups

Open Government Initiative. Aims to "increase accountability, promote informed participation by the public, and create economic opportunity; each agency shall take prompt steps to expand access to information by making it available online in open formats" (Orszag 2009)

Open source software. Software that can be freely used, changed, and shared (in modified or unmodified form) by anyone. There are a variety of benefits of using open source technology, including customization, lower cost, and the community of users that support the product. Open source software is made by many people, and distributed under licenses that comply with the open source definition (OSI 2015).

Operator. Symbol that expresses specific actions or criteria

Organizational safeguards. Arrangements that are made to protect e-PHI between organizations (Key Health Alliance n.d.)

Output. Discharging patients to their home or to the hospital as an inpatient

Pairwise comparison. Provides statistical differences for each group against each other group. For example, government versus nonprofit

Parsimonious. The simplest and most robust model to define data

Patient flow. The stream of patients throughout a healthcare setting

Patient satisfaction. An "individual's evaluation of his or her healthcare experience" (Shirley and Sanders 2013) and "the degree to which the individual regards the healthcare service or product or the manner in which it is delivered by the provider as useful, effective, or beneficial" (NLM 2015)

Physical safeguards. As amended by HITECH, security rule measures such as locking doors to safeguard data and various media from unauthorized access and exposures, including facility access controls, workstation use, workstation security, and device and media controls (45 CFR 164.310 2013)

Population health. The capture and reporting of healthcare data that are used for public health purposes. It allows the healthcare provider to report infectious diseases, immunizations, cancer, and other reportable conditions to public health officials

Predictive Model Markup Language (PMML). A "standards language for representing data mining models" (Williams 2011)

Primary data analysis. Data analyzed for the primary reason that they are collected (for example, a lab test)

Privacy Rule. The federal regulations created to implement the privacy requirements of the simplification subtitle of the Health Insurance Portability and Accountability Act of 1996; effective in 2002; afforded patients certain rights to and about their protected health information

Protected health information (PHI). As amended by HITECH, individually identifiable health information: (1) Except as provided in paragraph (2) of this definition, that is: (i) transmitted by electronic media;

(ii) maintained in electronic media; or (iii) transmitted or maintained in any other form or medium. (3) Protected health information excludes individually identifiable health information: (i) in education records covered by the Family Educational Rights and Privacy Act, as amended, 20 U.S.C. 1232g; (ii) in records described at 20 U.S.C. 1232g(a)(4)(B)(iv); (iii) in employment records held by a covered entity in its role as employer; and (iv) regarding a person who has been deceased for more than 50 years (45 CFR 160.103 2013)

Quality measure. A gauge used to assess the performance of a process or function of any organization (CMS 2013)

Reidentification. Assigning specific codes to the data or other means of record identification (HHS 2012)

Relation. The verb that describes how the entities are related

Relational database. A type of database that stores data in predefined tables made up of rows and columns

Research. 1. An inquiry process aimed at discovering new information about a subject or revising old information. Investigation or experimentation aimed at the discovery and interpretation of facts, revision of accepted theories or laws in the light of new facts, or practical application of such new or revised theories or laws; the collecting of information about a particular subject 2. As amended by HITECH, a systemic investigation, including research development, testing, and evaluation, designed to develop or contribute to generalized knowledge (45 CFR 164.501 2013)

Residual. The distance a data point is from the least squares regression line

Root node. The top of the decision tree

R-squared value. The proportion of the observed values of y explained by the linear regression of y on x. The R-squared value explains the strength of the relationship between the two quantitative variables

Safe harbor method. Requires the removal of 18 specific identifiers from the protected health information (HHS 2012)

Scatterplot. A visual representation of data points on an interval or ratio level used to depict relationships between two variables

Secondary data analysis. Data analyzed for a reason other than the primary reason (for example, clinical quality measures)

Security Rule. The federal regulations created to implement the security requirements of HIPAA

Simple linear regression. Used to examine the correlation between two variables and "to characterize the linear relationship between a dependent variable and one independent variable" (White 2013)

Simple logistic regression. A statistical procedure that is used when you have one categorical variable with two values and one quantitative variable to know whether variation in the quantitative variable causes variation in the categorical variable

Structured Query Language (SQL). A fourth-generation computer language that includes both DDL and DML components and is used to create and manipulate relational databases

Technical safeguards. As amended by HITECH, the Security Rule means the technology and the policy and procedures for its use that protect electronic protected health information and control access to it (45 CFR 164.304 2013)

Terminal node. The final decisions in a decision tree

Tukey HSD. Performs a significance test using single pairwise comparisons of the dependent variable across pairs of the independent variable

Tuple. A single record that is an ordered set of elements

Two-sample t-test. Used to determine if two groups are different than each other

Two-way ANOVA. Used to test if more than two groups are different from each other

Unified Modeling Language (UML) model. A standard notation that can be used for depicting entities, attributes, and relations, and are used for many diagrams including an entity-relationship diagram

Vector. A list of items, which may include numbers, characters, words, sentences, or a combination

Zip code tabulation area (ZCTA). The general assigned zip codes for the United States Postal Services

References

45 CFR 160.103. 65 FR 82798, Dec. 28, 2000, as amended at 78 FR 5687, Jan. 25, 2013. www.ecfr.gov

45 CFR 164.304. 68 FR 8376, Feb. 20, 2003, as amended at 78 FR 5693, Jan. 25, 2013. www.ecfr.gov

45 CFR 164.310. 68 FR 8376, Feb. 20, 2003, as amended at 78 FR 5694, Jan. 25, 2013. www.ecfr.gov

45 CFR 164.404. 74 FR 42767, Aug. 24, 2009, as amended at 78 FR 5695, Jan. 25, 2013. www.ecfr.gov

45 CFR 164.501. 65 FR 82802, Dec. 28, 2000, as amended at 78 FR 5695, Jan. 25, 2013. www.ecfr.gov

45 CFR 164.508. 67 FR 53268, Aug. 14, 2002, as amended at 78 FR 5699, Jan. 25, 2013. www.ecfr.gov

Centers for Medicare and Medicaid Services (CMS). 2013. www.cms.gov

Centers for Medicare and Medicaid Services. 2015. Medicare.gov Hospital Compare. http://www.medicare.gov/hospitalcompare/search.html

Data Governance Institute. 2012. Defining Data Governance. http://www.datagovernance.com/gbg_defining_governance.html

Department of Health and Human Services (HHS). 2011. HIPAA Privacy Rule Accounting of -Disclosures Under the Health Information Technology for Economic and Clinical Health Act. Federal Register. https://www.federalregister.gov/articles/2011/05/31/2011-13297/hipaa-privacy-rule-accounting-of-disclosures-under-the-health-information-technology-for-economic

Department of Health and Human Services. 2012. Guidance Regarding Methods for Deidentification of Protected Health Information in Accordance with the Health Insurance Portability and Accountability Act (HIPAA) Privacy Rule. http://www.hhs.gov/ocr/privacy/hipaa/understanding/coveredentities/De-identification/hhs_deid_guidance.pdf

Department of Health and Human Services-National Institutes of Health. 2014. How Can Covered Entities Use and Disclosure Protected Health Information for Research and Comply with the Privacy Rule? http://privacyruleandresearch.nih.gov/pr_08.asp

Key Health Alliance. n.d. Healthcare Data Analytics Portal. http://www.khareach.org/portal/data-analytics

Laerd. n.d. Chi-Square Goodness-of-Fit Test in SPSS. Laerd Statistics. https://statistics.laerd.com/spss-tutorials/chi-square-goodness-of-fit-test-in-spss-statistics.php

LaTour, K.M., S. Eichenwald Maki, and P.K. Oachs. 2013. Health Information Management: Concepts, Principles and Practice. Chicago, IL: AHIMA

National Quality Forum (NQF). 2013. Who We Are. http://www.qualityforum.org/Home_New/Who_we_are.aspx

National Library of Medicine. 2015. Patient Satisfaction. http://www.ncbi.nlm.nih.gov/mesh/68017060

Nugus, P., A. Holdgate, M. Fry, R. Forero, S. McCarthy, and J. Braithwaite. 2011. Work pressure and patient flow management in the emergency department: Findings from an ethnographic study. *Academic Emergency Medicine* 18(10):1045–1052

Open Source Initiative. 2015. Open Source Initiative. http://opensource.org

Orszag, P.R. 2009. Memorandum for the Heads of Executive Departments and Agencies. Washington DC: Executive Office of the President Office of Management and Budget. https://www.whitehouse.gov/sites/default/files/omb/assets/memoranda_2010/m10-06.pdf

Public Law 104-191. 1996. 110 Stat. 1936. Short title see 42 U.S.C. 201 note. www.uscode.house.gov/

Shirley, E.D., and J.O. Sanders. 2013. Patient satisfaction: Implications and predictors of success. *Journal of Bone & Joint Surgery* 95(10):e69, 1–4

US Census Bureau. 2010. Geographic Terms and Concepts. http://www.census.gov/geo/-reference/gtc/gtc_cbsa.html

US Congress. 2010. The Patient Protection and Affordable Care Act. http://www.gpo.gov/fdsys/pkg/BILLS-111hr3590enr/pdf/BILLS-111hr3590enr.pdf

Warner, D. 2013. Regulations Governing Research (2013 update). American Health Information Management Association. http://bok.ahima.org/doc?oid=300270#.VL1fOkfF-So

White, S. 2013. *A Practical Approach to Analyzing Healthcare Data*, 2nd ed. Chicago, IL: AHIMA

Williams, G. 2011. *Data Mining with Rattle and R: The Art of Excavating Data for Knowledge Discovery*. New York: Springer

Index